WORK WITH DISPLAY UNITS 94

WORK WITH DISPLAY UNITS 94

Selected Papers of the
Fourth International Scientific Conference on
Work with Display Units
Milan, Italy, 2–5 October, 1994

edited by

ANTONIO GRIECO
GIOVANNI MOLTENI

Institute of Occupational Health
University of Milan
Milan, Italy

ENRICO OCCHIPINTI

Center for Preventive Occupational Medicine
National Health Service
Milan, Italy

BRUNO PICCOLI

Institute of Occupational Health
University of Milan
Milan, Italy

1995

ELSEVIER
Amsterdam – Lausanne – New York – Oxford – Shannon – Tokyo

NORTH-HOLLAND
ELSEVIER SCIENCE B.V.
Sara Burgerhartstraat 25
P.O. Box 211, 1000 AE Amsterdam, The Netherlands

ISBN: 0 444 82145 7

© 1995 Elsevier Science B.V. All rights reserved.

No part of this publication may be reproduced, stored in a retrieval system, or transmitted, in any form or by any means, electronic, mechanical, photocopying, recording or otherwise, without the prior written permission of the publisher, Elsevier Science B.V., Copyright & Permissions Department, P.O. Box 521, 1000 AM Amsterdam, The Netherlands.

Special regulations for readers in the U.S.A. - This publication has been registered with the Copyright Clearance Center Inc. (CCC), 222 Rosewood Drive, Danvers, MA 01923. Information can be obtained from the CCC about conditions under which photocopies of parts of this publication may be made in the U.S.A. All other copyright questions, including photocopying outside of the U.S.A., should be referred to the copyright owner, Elsevier Science B.V., unless otherwise specified.

No responsibility is assumed by the publisher for any injury and/or damage to persons or property as a matter of products liability, negligence or otherwise, or from any use or operation of any methods, products, instructions or ideas contained in the material herein.

This book is printed on acid-free paper.

Printed in The Netherlands

Preface

This Book collects approximately one third of all the papers presented and discussed at the WWDU' 94 International Conference, organized by the Institute of Occupational Health "Clinica del Lavoro Luigi Devoto" of the University of Milan.

The criteria adopted by the Editors were aimed at reaching two basic goals: on one hand, accepting major scientific contributions and, on the other hand, providing an as much as possible organized and complete survey of outstanding topical subjects from the body of knowledge on VDU use.

The support by the International Scientific Advisory Committee has been extremely valuable in the preliminary stages of the Conference by suggesting the experts to be invited.

The Session Chairs, beside organizing their own sessions, provided scientific referees on request by Editors for each paper presented in their own sessions.

A special acknowledgement is also due to the International Social Advisory Commitee which, in addition to financial support, provided suggestions and information to better investigate actual problems affecting manufactures and users of information technologies and office furniture.

Special thanks are also due to Daniela Fano for her kind effectiveness in starting and maintaining contacts between Editors and Authors, and to all the staff of the Institute of Occupational Health, in particular Marco D'Orso, Maria Grazia Semenzato, Antonio Sesia.

President WWDU'94
Prof. Antonio Grieco

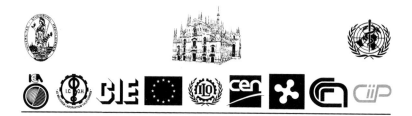

Patronage

European Union (E.U.)
World Health Organization (W.H.O.)
International Labour Office (I.L.O.)
Italian Ministry of Labour
Italian Ministry of Health
Italian Ministry of Industry
Italian Ministry of the University and Scientific and Technological Research
National Research Council (C.N.R.)
University of Milan
Region of Lombardia
Municipality of Milan
International Commission on Occupational Health (I.C.O.H.)
International Ergonomics Association (I.E.A)
Aspects in Computing (I.C.H.A.C.)
Italian Council of Scientific Societies for Prevention (C.I.I:P.)
Italian Ergonomics Society (S.I.E.)

Main Sponsoring Organizations

International Social Advisory Committee (I.S.A.C.)

The task of the Committee has been to contribute to the choice of the topics of Conference and to the implementation and management of the different Conference themes with the aim of improving the dialogue between the world of research and the world of work.

-ASSILS (Voluntary Mutual Assistance of Telecommunication Workers)

-ENEL (National Electric Power Company)

-IBM

-ITALTEL

-OLIVETTI

-INPS (International Institute of Social Security)

-DAUPHIN (Office Furniture Manufacturers)

A major support for the Conference organization has been provided by the above Companies and Institutions.

Cosponsoring Organizations

-Banca Commerciale Italiana

-Essilor Italia S.p.A.

-Mitsubishi Electric Europe Coordination Centre

International Scientific Advisory Committee

Aresini G., European Union - Luxembourg (L)
Berthelette D., Universite' du Quebec - Montreal (C)
Cakir A., Ergonomic Institut - Berlin (D)
Corlett E.N., Institute of Occupational Health - Notthingham (UK)
Fine L.J., National Institute for Occupational Safety and Health - Cincinnati (USA)
Gamberale F., National Institute of Occupational Health - Solna (S)
Hernberg S., Institute of Occupational Health - Helsinki (SF)
Knave B., National Institute of Occupational Health - Solna (S)
Kroemer K.H.E., Virginia Polytechnic Institute and State University -Blacksburg (USA)
Krueger H., Eidgenossische Technische Hochschule - Zurich (CH)
Le Leu L.A., Woden Valley Hospital - Garran (Aus)
Luczak H., Forschungsinstitut fur Rationalisierung Lehrstuhl fur Arbeits - Aachen (D)
Mayer H., Medizinische Klinik der Universitat - Heidelberg (D)
Munipov V.M., Russian Research Institute of Industrial Design - Moskow (Rus)
Noro K., Waseda University - Tokorozawa (J)
Ong C.N., National University of Singapore - Republic of Singapore
Queinnec Y., Universite' Paul Sabatier - Toulouse (F)
Sheedy J.E., California University - Berkeley (USA)
Sherwood R.J., Harward School of Public Health - Boston (USA)
Stewart T., System Concept Ltd. - London (UK)
Wideback P.G., Swedish Agency for Administrative Development - Stockholm (S)

National Scientific Advisory Committee

Abbritti G., Istituto di Medicina del Lavoro - Universita' di Perugia
Arbosti G., Ospedale S. Carlo - Milano
Bandini Butti L., Societa' di Ergonomia Applicata - Milano
Bergamaschi A., Istituto di Medicina del Lavoro Universita' " Tor Vergata "- Roma
Cortili G., Dip. di Scienze e Tecnologie Biomediche Universita' degli Studi - Milano
Di Giulio A., Politecnico - Milano
Fanelli C., Istituto Superiore Prevenzione e Sicurezza sul Lavoro - Roma
Farulla A., Istituto di Medicina del Lavoro Universita' "La Sapienza" - Roma
Ferrario M., Istituto di Medicina del Lavoro Universita' degli Studi - Milano
Grandolfo M., Istituto Superiore di Sanita' - Roma
Miglior M., Istituto di Clinica Oculistica 1a Universita' degli Studi - Milano
Novara F., Olivetti S.p.A. - Ivrea
Pedotti A., Centro di Bioingegneria "Fondazione Don Gnocchi" - Milano
Peruzzo G.F., Istituto di Medicina del Lavoro Universita' degli Studi - Milano
Rubino G., Istituto di Medicina del Lavoro Universita' degli Studi - Torino
Troiano P., Istituto di Clinica Oculistica 1a Universita' degli Studi - Milano

CONTENTS

PREFACE v

Work with display units: present situation and prospects - Introductory lecture
A. Grieco 1

Work with display units in perspective - to the better or worse?
B. Knave, G. Widebäck 9

VDU WORK AND HEALTH

An overview in different countries

An alternative perspective on the VDT health hazards debate: folk hazards and health panics
B. Pearce 15

Comparison of VDU workplaces in Australia and Sweden
A. Johansson, H. Shahnavaz 21

Skin symptoms and VDT work - Reports from three continents
B. Stenberg 27

Epidemiological aspects

The relationship between video display terminal use and pregnancy outcome
F. Parazzini, L. Luchini, P. G. Crosignani 33

A longitudinal study of quality of working life among computer users: preliminary results
P. Carayon 39

Follow-up of job stress and its relation to characteristics of VDT use among insurance employees
K. Lindström, T. Leino, M. Puhakainen, I. Torstila 45

Gender and computing: is change occurring?
A. Durndell, P. Lightbody 51

Musculoskeletal disorders

Psychosocial work factors and upper extremity musculoskeletal discomfort among office workers
S. Y. Lim, P. Carayon 57

Psychosocial and physiological effects of reorganizing data-entry work - a longitudinal study
C.Åborg, E. Fernström, M. O. Ericson...63

Musculoskeletal disorders, working posture, psychosocial environment in female VDU operators and conventional office workers
D. Camerino, P. Lavano, M. Ferrario, G. Ferretti, G. Molteni...67

VDU workplace: experimentation in an electronics firm of a methodology of clinical functional evaluation of the spine
A. Malcangi, M. Fregoso, G. Galletta, G. Ferretti, F. De Marco, D. Colombini, E. Occhipinti 73

Asthenopia

Symptoms and reading performance with peripheral glare sources
J.E. Sheedy, I.L. Bailey...77

Eye discomforts during work with visual display terminals
U. Bergqvist, B. Knave, R. Wibom..83

Asthenopia, anxiety and neuropsychological functions in VDU workers
P. Apostoli, R. Lucchini, C. Frontali, L. Alessio..89

Relationship between vertical gaze direction and tear volume
S. Abe, M. Sotoyama, S. Taptagaporn, S. Saito, M. B. G. Villanueva, S. Saito.....................95

Vision screening for display screen users
T.J. Horberry, A.G. Gale, S. P. Taylor..101

Vision physiopathology

Using visual acuity to measure display legibility
J.E. Sheedy, I.L. Bailey...107

Eye strain syndrome, contrast sensivity and critical flicker fusion frequency: a comparative study
C. Manganelli, C. M. Locarno, G. Fasolino, A. Capobianco, F. Focosi..............................113

Which is more comfortable for VDT workers: spectacles or contact lenses ?
T. Suzuki, N. Hirose, K. Ibi, T. Iwasaki, S. Saito, S. Akiya..119

Dark vergence of the eyes in relation to fixation disparity at different luminances and amounts of blur on a visual display
W.Jaschins Kruza..125

The vertical horopter and the angle of view
D. R. Ankrum, E. E. Hansen, K. J. Nemeth...131

VDT work with different gaze inclinations
I. Lie, K. I. Fostervold *137*

Stress and health problems due to alteration of binocular vision at visual display units
K. Faßbender, M. Georgi, J. Wahl, H. Mayer, E. Kraus-Mackiw, D.B. Braun, C. Danckwardt, J. Dürr *143*

Ergophthalmological surveillance

Results of an ergophthalmologic and oculistic survey on a sample of video display unit workers and non-exposed subjects
F. De Marco, D. Colombini, M. Meroni, E. Occhipinti, A. Petri, A. Soccio, E. Tosatto, C. Vimercati *149*

Testing a proposed ergophthalmic protocol for monitoring the health of video display unit workers
A. Petri, D. Colombini, F. De Marco, M. Meroni, E. Occhipinti, A. Soccio, E. Tosatto, C. Vimercati *155*

Eye disorders in employees working at VDU: longitudinal study
B. Bagolini, R.. Bellucci, B. Boles Carenini, S. Borra, C. Ceccarelli, G. Coccia, A. Di Bari, F.M. Grignolo, D. Lepore, G. Maina, M. Miglior, F. Molle, E. Monaco, R.. Morbio, C. Rechichi, B. Ricci, G. F. Rubino, L. Scullica, G. Sibour, P. Troiano, M. Turbati *161*

Risk assessment

Assessment of mechanical exposures in ergonomic epidemiology: A research program and some preliminary data
J. Winkel, I. Balogh, G.-Å. Hansson, P. Asterland, M. Kellermann, J. Byström, K. Ohlsson *167*

ELF magnetic field exposures in an office environment
P. Breysse *173*

The definition assessment of quality of images on VDUs
Part 1: **Relationships with asthenopia**
B. Piccoli *179*
Part 2: **Physical aspects**
S. Orsini, L. Milanesi *183*
Part 3: **Visual-cognitive factors**
N. Bruno, A De Angeli, W Gerbino *187*

Psycophysiological aspects

VDTs : problems arising when the physical ergonomics are perfect
L. A. Le Leu *191*

Behavioral Cybernetics, quality of working life and work organization in computer automated offices
M. J. Smith *197*

of the cell nuclei have also been found—for example, in the neurosecretory system of the hypothalamus. NIEBROJ considers this as a possible cause for other diurnal body functions.

For further examples, see HOFER u. BIEBL, BIEBL u. HOFER, SCHÖLM (plant cells), MÖDLINGER-ODORFER (animal cells with neurosecretory functions), and QUAY and RENZONI (in the pineal). In most cases, not only changes in the volume but also accompanying changes in the structure of the nucleus were observed, as well as remarkable changes in nucleolar volume (FISCHER; WEBER; SCHÖLM).

Other indications of diurnal variations in the nucleus are circadian differences in ^{14}C-leucine incorporation into protein of liver nuclei in rats (SESTAN).

KLUG reports a diurnal periodicity of the nuclear volume in the corpora allata of *Carabus nemoralis*. Evidently it is related to the circadian rhythm of this animal's activity (see Figs. 40 and 41).

Mitotic cycles. These facts are also interesting in another respect: mitosis may be one of the processes controlled by the circadian rhythm. The small temperature dependence shown in Fig. 102 demonstrates how closely mitosis can be tied to the endodiurnal system. A diurnal rhythm of cell division is known to occur in many other plants and animals, at least under normal LD cycles. Decades ago the continuation of the rhythm in cell division under constant conditions was described. Subsequent observations in animals also showed continuation of the mitotic rhythm under constant conditions (see *HALBERG et al.; UTKIN

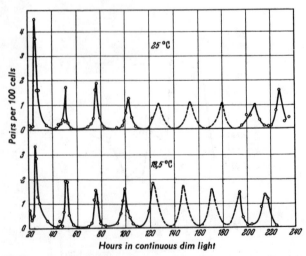

Fig. 102. *Gonyaulax polyedra*. Diurnal rhythm of cell division at 18.5 and at 25°C, as measured by the percentage of paired cells present in a cell suspension. Constant dim light. After HASTINGS and SWEENEY

Design of usability laboratories for computer networking products
C. Bracci, M. Taylor 203

Customer information system
R. Garetti 209

WWDU '94 and impact on job content, human interaction and cooperation, work organization
F. Novara 215

Human information processing in man-machine interaction
M. Rauterberg 221

A study on VDT work and psycho - physiological load
T. Okubo, K.. Sang Park 227

Psychophysiological investigation of system response time and of different break schedules in highly demanding work with display units
W. Boucsein, M. Thum 233

The effect of anticipatory mismatch in work flow on task performance and event related brain potentials
F. Schaefer, O. Kohlisch 241

Design aid tools for user interface design
H. Reiterer, S. Schäfer 247

Problem solving strategies in shop-floor control systems
G. Zülch, K. Grießer 253

Additional sound feedback in man-computer interaction: two empirical investigations
M. Rauterberg, E. Styger, A. Baumgartner, A. Jenny, M. de Lange 259

Designing multi media user interfaces with eye recording data
M. Rauterberg, P. Berny, G. Lordong, A. Schmidt, M. Zemp, T. Zürcher 265

Ergonomic aspects in designing automative displays with route guidance information
R. Den Buurman 271

WORKPLACE

"Alternative keyboards" and "alternatives to keyboards"
K. H. E. Kroemer 277

Do split keyboards help to reduce strain?
A.E. Çakir 283

Evaluation of seated posture in VDT works
H. Miyamoto, C.-S. Wu, K. Noro 289

Seated work posture: a comparative study of two chair types
M. Graf, H. Krueger 293

Check-list for studying VDU workplaces in order to observe where minimum levels, laid down by EEC Directive 270/90, are not being respected.
D. Colombini, E. Occhipinti, G. Bernazzani, G. Bocchi, A. Petri, A. Soccio, E. Tosatto, F. DeMarco 299

ENVIRONMENT

New methods to evaluate VDU screen glare
I.C. Pasini, D. K. Tiller, G. R. Newsham 305

Brightness: highest luminance or background luminance?
G. P. J. Spenkelink, J. Besuijen 311

Daylighting potentials in display office workplaces: Japan, the U.S., and Sweden
G. Sweitzer 317

Thermal environments in workplaces with video display terminals (VDTs): a draft standard
G. Alfano, F. R. d'Ambrosio 323

An application of "Adaptation level theory" to experimental data concerning temperature judgement. -quantification of the KANSEI (Human Sensitivity) attribute.
E. Masuyama 329

Biological and subjective responses to EMF exposure. A double-blind provocation study
B. Andersson, B. Arnetz, M. Berg, L. Melin, I. Langlet, S. Lidén 335

Whatever happened to MPR3 ?
D. Sawdon 339

EMERGING ASPECTS

Environmental issues

Hypersensitivity to electricity:- A round table discussion
U. Bergqvist 345

Hypersensitivity to electricity and preferred remedial measures
A.C. Blomkvist, S. Almgren 351

Facial skin symptoms in office workers. A five year follow-up study.
N. Eriksson, J. Höög, B. Stenberg, M. Sandström 357

Measurements of some physical factors in the office environment of employees who consider themselves hypersensitive to electricity
Ö. Medhage, C. Wadman, G. Linder, U. Bergqvist, B. Knave 363

Overview of the special session on melatonin and VDU work and personal results
B. Piccoli, R. Assini, F. Fraschini 369

Mouse-arm syndrome

Mouse input devices and work-related upper limb disorders
T. J. Armstrong, B. J. Martin, A. Franzblau, D. M. Rempel, P. W. Johnson 375

The "mouse-arm syndrome" - concurrence of musculoskeletal symptoms and possible pathogenesis among VDU operators
M. Hagberg 381

Special work-places and new techniques

Application of a Fuzzy Model to a Control-Room Ergonomic Design
L. Compagno 387

VDU workplace : ergonomic evaluation between a VDU worplace and a CAE-CAD-CAM workstation
L. Masseroni, M. Fregoso, G. Galletta 393

Computers for social integration of the disabled people
A. Pedotti 397

Displays for visually impaired: studies of cognitive and perceptual characteristics of speech synthesis
E. Hjelmquist, B. Jansson 403

Haptic devices in Human-Computer Interaction
H. Luczak, M. Göbel, J. Springer 409

STRATEGIES AND POLICIES

Management

The popularisation of ergonomics
T.F.M.Stewart 415

Ergonomics on video display units - lessons at the federal high school for officials of non technical administration in Germany
H. Schmidt 421

Country-specific aspects of computer/VDU safety information
A. Donagi, M. Chereisky 427

A systems analysis for integrating macroergonomic research into office and organizational planning
M.M. Robertson, M. J. O'Neill 433

Findings of the office ergonomics research committe
R. F. Bettendorf 439

Legislation and standards

Round table: an unholy alliance - experience of the development and implementation of standards and legislation on display screen equipment in Europe - The CEN/ISO experience
T.F.M. Stewart 445

A new Japanese Industrial Standard (JIS) corresponding to Part 3 of ISO 9241 (Visual display requirements) - JIZ Z 8513 - 1994
N. Koizumi 449

Implementation of the EC Directive 90/270 in the Netherlands
P. Voskamp, R.. H. Hagen, P. Biemans 455

PC-FIT User-Saver - VDU Ergonomics for Users
S. Bachinger, W. Hackl-Gruber, M. Molnar, A. Pribil 459

Testing conformance to software standards: a usability evaluation of ISO 9241 DIS Part 14 - Menu dialogues
R. E. Granda, S. L. Stanners 465

Future trends

A general modeling framework for the human-computer interaction based on the principles of ergonomic compatibility requirements and human entropy
W. Karwowski 473

Humanizing WWDU'S: a macroergonomic TQM strategy for work system and job design
H. W. Hendrick 479

Fusion of eastern and western civilisations in WWDU
H. Miyamoto 485

Statement on the European Directive on work with display screen equipment (90/270/EEC) by the International Commission in Human Aspects in Computing (ICHAC).
T.F.M. Stewart, U. Bergqvist, B. Piccoli, P.G. Wideback 491

Annex: Council Directive of 29 May 1990 on the minimum safety and health requirements for work with display screen equipment (fifth individual Directive within the meaning of Article 16 (1) of Directive 87/391/EEC)..................................505

Work With Display Units: present situation and prospects.
Introductory lecture.

A. Grieco[a]

[a] Institute of Occupational Health "Clinica del Lavoro L. Devoto"
- University of Milan (Italy)

1. INTRODUCTION

As the President of the 4th International Scientific Conference on Work With Display Units (WWDU'94), I would first of all like to give a heartfelt welcome to all the Participants for having accepted our invitation to Milan. Their valuable contribution of research, knowhow and ideas in a friendly atmosphere guaranteed the success of this scientific initiative, which is the result of a decision taken by the International WWDU Group in early February 1992, and then unanimously accepted by all the Participants to the Berlin Scientific Conference.
I would also like to pay tribute to two unforgettable masters, Etienne Grandjean and Enrico Carlo Vigliani, who both died in the early nineties, by just reminding you of their history.
They organized the First International Workshop on "Ergonomics Aspects of Visual Displays Terminals", March 17 - 19, 1980 here in Milan, under the auspices of the Permanent Commission and International Association on Occupational Health (now International Commission on Occupational Health - ICOH) and the Carlo Erba Foundation Occupational and Environmental Health Section (1).
These two scientists who honour the glorious tradition of Occupational Health, were also close family friends for over thirty years: the former, Etienne Grandjean, in Zurich, the founder of Ergonomics at an international level, the latter, Enrico Carlo Vigliani, the President of ICOH from 1975 to 1981 and Director from 1945 to 1977 of the Institute of Occupational Health of the Milan University, the oldest Clinic in the world for the study, diagnosis treatment and prevention of occupational diseases (2).
Since that International Workshop in 1980, attended by over a hundred researchers and several groups of delegates from large companies and Trade Unions, all the other initiatives have been held without interruption every three years. Even better, thanks to the commitment and organising ability of Bengt Knave, helpfully supported by Per-Gunnar Wideback, they became from 1986 in Stockholm "International Scientific Conferences" with the fourth now being held in Milan. Ever since then, the number of participants has multiplied by five, giving the feeling of being a new protagonist within the international scientific community (3).
Therefore I leave to my Colleague, Bengt Knave, the task of relating, with the deserved authority, the milestones of this original scientific path, whose origins date back to events preceding the foundation of other scientific associations in the same field (HCI, ICHAC).

2. WHY WWDU?

I am pretty sure that all of you, when speaking about WWDU, within the scientific Community or more generally, have been asked the following question at least once: why do we hold international conferences on workplaces with video displays units?
In other words why have hundreds of experts from over thirty countries who often work in quite different areas, decided to meet periodically for over 15 years to present and discuss the results of thousands of researches, from the laboratory and on the field, on VDU workplaces and more generally on the interaction between human operators and VDU computerised systems? Did they not have more important problems to tackle, more serious diseases to investigate, major health hazards to prevent, nowadays, on a planet that must face problems such as chemical pollution, infections and infestations, cancer, AIDS,and many other diseases?
I would like to try to give a reply to this question, also with hindsight, to give a sense to the work we have all done and to the major human and financial resources involved and the many expectations it has stirred up in the society.
There is no doubt that at the beginning of this particular history, with the introduction and progressive spreading of the new techniques starting from the middle of the seventies in all manufacturing sectors and services, the phenomenon has been perceived and lived, with a certain emphasis especially by operators. In fact, though the first generation VDU were rather lacking in ergonomics (symbol flicker, no luminance control, VDU-assisted keyboard with VDT, poor software usability), this roughness, subsequently amended by the third generation machines, is not sufficient in itself to justify the multiplicity and intensity of symptoms suffered by operators in a great variety of organs and apparatus, in so many different countries.
In some cases, quite a few actually, there was the sincere fear that VDU were the source of severe ionising radiations: a fear that subsequent technical investigations proved to be totally groundless.
The conspicuous amount of original knowhow produced by our WWDU International Conferences allowed us to understand that there was much more behind those symptoms and those complaints.
First of all, such transformations have taken place too quickly with unprecedented acceleration in the history of human activities. Just to make an example, think how many years of preparation were devoted to implementing a change, certainly a minor one, such as the adoption of the metric system in some countries: in Great Britain it took no less than 15 years, and during that period all the media were skillfully used to launch effective information messages.
Second, and above all, the introduction and rapid spread of the so-called new technologies in all manufacturing sectors and services have been decided and implemented by entrepreneurs with two main goals: labour cost reduction, and product and service quality improvement.
The poor attention paid during the first ten years to the operators' physiological, psychological and sociological requirements as well as the increasing reduction in employment levels devastatingly contributed to giving a negative perception of the role and perspectives of new technologies. The workers' Trade Unions on the other hand, concentrated most of their efforts on safeguarding employment levels, sometimes in a stubborn and economically unprofitable way, as prisoners of such a sectorial concept of transformations and development.
So, what happened was that both *social partners as a whole could not manage and skillfully govern the great opportunity of an anthropocentric transformation of work organisation and systems offered by the new machines.*
Ergonomically speaking, we cannot define as innovative all technical changes which fulfil some aspects of enterprise and market economy and productivity. An innovative change must also meet the need for work and the vocation of protagonist inherent in the

human operator within complex systems.
In this international scenario, comprehensive of manifold political, economic and social variables, alien to ergonomics and also to macroergonomics which therefore cannot be examined here in more detail, Video Display Units and more generally information technology have become in the operators' eyes the physical symbol of several social, sometimes dramatic, incongruencies. In WWDU International Conferences we have tried to understand such effects on health, well-being and efficiency, with priority on prevention.

3. MAGNITUDE OF THE PROBLEM

Nowadays, there are millions and millions of information technology users, and their number is progressively increasing in all manufacturing sectors and services. To this number we have to add all those who use it individually at home or for leisure purposes: but this category should be considered separately.
It is not easy to obtain official data on the growth of the phenomenon at an international level and, under certain aspects, it does not even seem to be useful in the frame of ergonomic researches since working conditions and procedures may record major differences often hampering the opportunity of an overall study.
The definition itself "VDU users" or "VDU operators" should be abandoned at present, when the investigation is aimed at studying work-well-being-efficiency relationship, the biological variables at stake being so many and so different when shifting from one homogeneous series of conditions to the others.
However given a certain degree of approximation, I think that the number of information technology machines and systems that have been sold and the yearly turnover may give an idea of the magnitude and dynamics of the phenomenon and of the associated problems (4).
1993 was not any worse for the Information Technology market than the previous year despite the current situation. In fact, whilst 1992 was the lowest point of a negative cycle that began toward the end of the eighties' characterised by a considerable fall in all major work areas, last year did not proceed along this line, showing on the contrary, positive signs and factors in certain major areas (Fig. 1).
These signs can already be seen in the aggregate market dynamics that increased by 4% in 1993, with constant exchanges and rates generally in line with those of the previous year, therefore a variation similar to that of 1991 (4.8 %) reaching a value of 478 billion dollars.
Once again the demand for information technology solutions was closely correlated with the investments made in machines and equipment and the general economic trend in the various areas.
World market growth in 1993 is the result of three different and contrasting trends, recognisable even in geographic terms:
a) a considerable recovery in those countries in which markets recorded considerably recessive trends in recent years (e.g: USA and UK);
b) very high growth rates in certain developing countries (South East Asian Countries, India, Israel, certain Latin American Countries) where the information technology market is still in an expansive phase or just taking off: China has established itself in this group being a new market with a great deal of potential;
c) a considerable reduction in growth rates and, in certain cases, a recessive situation in those countries that lead the market in the eighties such as Europe or Japan.
North America, which had already experienced an above average growth rate in 1992, recorded a very positive trend in 1993 (+ 7.6%) thanks, in particular, to the performance of the United States market, consolidating its leadership and increasing its share of the world market from 37% to 39%.

The new North American Common Market (NAFTA), including not only the United States and Canada but also a developing country with a great deal of potential such as Mexico, will help this area develop even further.
Asia, and South East Asia in particular, however, presented a situation polarised between the considerable downward trend in Japan, signs of problems of a structural nature and not simply of the economic situation, and the considerable development of the markets of the developing countries (Singapore, Hong Kong, Taiwan, South Korea) that, having taken off, entered a more up-to-date development phase.
The European Information Technology market recorded in 1993 one of the lowest growth rates in the world, that is 1.4% as compared to the 3.1% of the previous year, with a slight increase in absolute value from 154 billion dollars to 156 billion dollars. Therefore it can be said that 1993 was the worst ever year for the European Information Technology market.
Moreover the differences in the dynamics of the various European Market segments further increased in 1993. Whilst hardware and technical assistance fell by more than 2%, software and information technology services rose by 5.8%. This is a sign of a shift towards new ways of adopting and using information technology that emerged in 1993.
The satisfactory performance of the European software and information technology service segments is a sign that the role of information technology systems in companies is being reconsidered.

4. THE PROBLEM

I think that before concluding this Introductory Lecture it is worth making some general considerations concerning the relationship between information technology and operators'well-being and efficiency in the work setting.
First of all, there is no doubt that under certain aspects, that will be more evident later on, *the scientific knowledge already available is broader than that applied by manufacturers and, to a lesser extent, by user companies.*
This is not so surprising since the same occurs when evaluating the biological knowledge application coefficient also in other fields. In other words, the gap between the availability of knowhow and its applications is always wider when shifting from the other disciplines to the biological area.
One example is enough: at present we know everything about malaria, provoking parasite, pathogenetic mechanisms, diagnostic procedures, drugs for prophylaxis and treatment. Well, even today, about 50 million people die every year in the world from malaria!
This gap between available knowledge and its practical applications is however more significant in the use of information technology machines and systems in the various workplaces rather than for the design and implementation of the machines and the systems and within them, it is more significant for software than for hardware.
I mean that while in these past twenty years information technology machines and systems have exhibited a positive ergonomic evolution, with regard to hardware rather than to software, the greatest drawback now is the way they are used in work organisation of user companies.
However, science, considered in the light of what we know, is not without sin! It is divided into thousands of trickles often flowing under ground, without seeing the light. An excess of fascinating specialisms, of hermetic languages getting to an ever increasing number of scientific journals which are read with sharing interest by an ever lower number of prestigious experts.
Tens of microdisciplines crowd the field and this is no doubt a positive fact since we are facing a complex demand: such is our arduous attempt to match not only the machines but work as a whole with its contents and significant points and the world around

us, to the requirements, the limits and the aspirations of human beings.
However the increasing complexity to be faced must be respected as such and cannot be fulfilled by a scientific offer which suffers from such a high level of fragmentation, somehow hindering the outcoming issue (5).
Maybe this was what meant Hamlet when speaking to Horatio "there are more things in heaven and earth, Horatio, than are dreamt of in our philosophy".
On the other hand the solution of this problem is one of the highest challenges that society offers science.
In other words, how can we fulfil the complexity without impoverishing or, even more, offering enrichments to each one of the valuable specializations we have been able to create and develop? It is not by chance and not only today, that the crucial point of the ergonomic approach is "interdisciplinarity", as its unique original peculiarity. If this is so, and I think it is not so far from the truth, that is, if we are aware that the lack of some synthesis hinders the transfer of scientific knowhow from research to application, then it may be time to ask ourselves if that synthesis could be found by just summing up the available data.
I do not think this is the right way, on the contrary, it would be another simplification, an inadequate way of facing the complexity which we have already admitted and recognised.
On the other hand, such a complexity, even though some peculiarities associated with the application of new technologies are not to be excluded, is not only present in innovative working conditions but enters the picture everytime biological interactions of human operators within organised work are to be exhaustively investigated, to prevent health hazards and performance decrease. Nor is it possible to imagine the use of scientific data regardless of the deep knowledge of real life conditions.
Here is the core of the problem: I think that ergonomics should make a step forward to build a new conceptual picture in order to describe and interpret organized work correctly, be it traditional or innovative.
An interesting contribution in this sense was provided by Kurt Landau and Walter Rohmert in Germany using the AET method (6). These same Authors, by the end of an International Seminar organized in 1987 in Hohenheim, had proved that none of about thirty job analysis methods previously reported in the literature could be considered adequate ergonomically speaking (7).
More recently, in Italy, Bruno Maggi, with the help of organisational knowledge and occupational health knowledge, again dealt with problem emphasising epistemological considerations which orientate such job analysis methods (8,9,10). The outcoming issue was an explicit tendency to the Theory of Organisational Action, elaborated by the Nobel Prize winner, H.A. Simon, supported by J. D. Thompson, as this ensures a sound interdisciplinary base, and fits ergonomics and occupational health goals, as well. From this theory Maggi himself derived the Method of Organisational Congruencies, whose manifold applications in the field for the study of organized work and health relationships have been since 1988 the object of an interdisciplinary research Group "Organisation and Well-Being" at the Institute of Occupational Health of the Milan University.
Finally the Method of Organisational Congruencies provides ergonomics with an adequate tool for biologically oriented analysis of all working situations, considered as process systems, as ordered paths of organisational actions and decisions, overcoming not only the tayloristic (mechanistic) ways of seeing work organisation but also the organismic conception.
Thus, through biologically oriented analytical indicators, possible "organisational incongruencies" arise producing "organisational constraint elements" finally allowing the clarification of "organisational etiopathogenesis" of some risk conditions in traditional and innovative work.
I do not think it is possible to concretely achieve an interdisciplinary approach if each one of the activated disciplinary areas refers to its own epistemological choices, to dif-

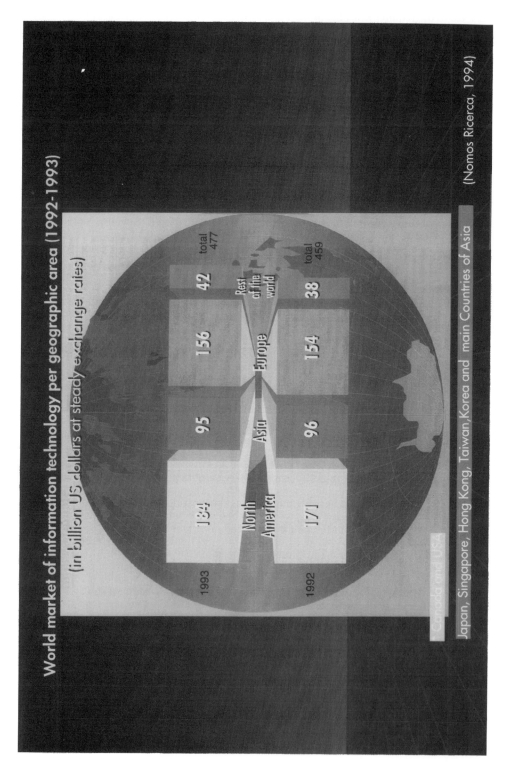

ferent conceptual frameworks producing different methods to analyse and evaluate the presence of the human operator within systems, however simple or complex they may be.

Therefore, either ergonomics definitely gives up interdisciplinarity, thus missing the last opportunity offered by applied science to design and implement anthropocentric machines and systems, or the decision must be taken to formulate consistent epistemological choices to reach such an ambitious goal.

Much depends on the reply to this question, and the stake is higher than it seems.

For example, education and training cannot be considered as alien to this problem. Each educational choice has an epistemological foundation concerning the way the social system is seen. Education is useful if it effectively helps the process, without distinctions between training in the classroom and that regarding activity performance (11).

But also the fate of our future WWDU Conferences is not independent of those choices: there is the risk that they become the opportunity to hear many interesting by unrelated seminars, and this risk increases if we do not try to identify a unique conceptual picture assuring a sound interdisciplinary basis.

On the other hand, if I am not wrong, Holgar Luczak, the President of the previous WWDU Conference in Berlin, aimed to go right in this direction when he prepared and illustrated his extremely interesting conceptual model (12).

Then, at the end of this Introductory Lecture, I think it may be useful to make a working proposal: it is addressed to all the participants and in particular to the WWDU Group, who may like to devote some attention to this problem, also in view of choosing the most convenient procedures and time schedules for the next WWDU International Conference in Tokyo.

As the starting point of this epistemological reflection, I would like to suggest the conceptual model proposed by Holgar Luczak in Berlin, which offers the advantage of collecting the first class scientific contributions of the previous WWDU International Conference in an organic manner.

REFERENCES

1. E. Grandjean and E.C. Vigliani: "Ergonomics Aspects of Visual Display Terminals". Proceedings of the International Workshop, Milan, March 17-19, 1980. Taylor and Francis (eds) 1981.
2. Institute of Occupational Health of the University of Milan: "The Clinica del Lavoro Luigi Devoto: ninety years after its foundation". Grafica Comense, Tavernerio (Como) 1993.
3. B. Knave and P.G. Wideback: "Work With Dispaly Units '86" North-Holland, Amsterdam, 1987.
4. Assinform: "Rapporto sull'informatica e le telecomunicazioni". Promobit srl (eds), Cronografica Europea, Rho (MI), 1994.
5. A. Grieco: " Il contributo della scienza per la promozione della salute nei luoghi di lavoro". La Medicina del Lavoro 84, 1:3-17, 1993.
6. W. Rohmert and K. Landau: "Das Arbeitswissenschaftliche Erhebungsverfahren zur Taetigkeitsanalyse (AET)". Haus uber verlag, Bern - Stuttgard - Wien, 1979.
7. K. Landau and W. Rohmert: " Recent developments in job analysis". Taylor and Francis (eds), 1989.
8. B. Maggi: "Questioni di organizzazione e sociologia del lavoro". Tirrenia Stampatori (ed), Torino, 1984.
9. B. Maggi: "Razionalità e Benessere. Studio interdisciplinare dell'organizzazione". Etas Libri (ed), Milano 1990.

10. B. Maggi: A. Grieco: "Il Metodo delle Congruenze Organizzative per lo studio dei rapporti tra lavoro organizzato e salute. Un esempio di applicazione nel settore metallurgico". G. Battista e P. Catalono (eds.). "Aspetti emergenti dei rischi e della patologia nel settore della metallurgica leggera e delle fonderie di seconda fusione". Atti del Convegno della Regione Toscana- USL n.19, Poggibonsi, Colle Val d'Elsa, S. Gimigniano, 1986.

11. B. Maggi: "Epistemological foundations of education choices". Paper presented at the Round Table during 11th Congress of the International Ergonomics Association (IEA), July 15-20, 1991- Paris (not published).

12. H. Luczak and A. Cakir: "Welcome address". "Work With Display Units '92", 3-12, North-Holland, Amsterdam, 1993.

Work with display units in perspective - to the better or worse?

B. Knave and P.G. Widebäck

National Institute of Occupational Health
S-171 84 Solna, Sweden

In a broader development perspective, with all our efforts during more than twenty years, we now bring forward the question: Does the VDT working environment show any real progress? We can realize some improvements, for sure, but at the same time changes for the worse do appear. These are the questions on which the paper will focus:
 - Does society take its responsibility in desired action programmes?
 - Does education in school reflect the work requirements and the society we want to live in?
 - Have only the machines improved and not the working routines and environments?
 - What are the major research areas, of yesterday, today and tomorrow?

1. BACK TO THE SEVENTIES

Twenty years ago VDTs became the symbol for the interactive work with computers. The new technology was scarcely spread over the workplaces. Applications were studied within military projects. In offices we could find clusters of programmers and operators with tasks as data entry, word processing, and data base interactions.

The VDT operator became a specialist worker. How was the new tool to be used efficiently? The curiosity of what the new technique could do for you engaged developers. Experience was exchanged and gathered to manuals and other guidance. Already in the mid-seventies standardization efforts, specially within Germany, were substantial.

The implementation of the VDTs to the offices, however, caused complaints from the operators, often brought forward to the company health officers. Therefore, VDTs began early to be a problem area within occupational health services. The hardware problem dominated: keyboard design, image quality, lighting and vision aids for the operator; and also radiation. Breakdowns and respond times of the system were discussed. Ergonomic measures were taken but not enough to ensure god working conditions.

2. PREVIOUS CONFERENCES

2.1. Conferences in Milan 1980 and Turin 1983

Around 1980 the interest was more directed toward work posture, work organization, stress and monotony. Postural discomfort from the neck, shoulders and upper parts of the back, neck-back disorders related to viewing axis, head position and furniture height, were in focus. In Turin different solutions of work postures were items that caused vivid discussions. The discomforts among men and women and the accommodation of the eye during and after longer VDT work attracted attention in large field studies.

2.2. WWDU'86

The planning for the conference in Stockholm started in summer 1983. The long marketing period of three years was evaluated as necessary for running a new large conference. The scope was to concentrate efforts to gather knowledge to state and solve problems; to inspire research within special fields as well as interdisciplinary attacks. We also found that one conference is not enough because you need subsequent conferences to reach scientific results. The conference in Stockholm and the following 1989 in Montreal and 1992 in Berlin gathered attendees with a professional interest in occupational health, occupational hygiene, image quality and vision, work physiology, work place design, work organization, or human computer interaction. The scientific heritage of the WWDU conferences is kept in the Selected Papers published a year after each conference.

Typical for the event - above all the rest - was the amount of large-scale and important field studies that were presented and discussed. The political interest was bound to electromagnetic fields emitted by the VDTs. Image polarity was treated in both image quality and lighting sessions. Alternative display technologies to CRTs and functional disabilities were sessions that were brought in at late stage. Sedentary work and physical inactivity imply the importance of work organization when designing the work and work place. Reported postural discomfort, eye discomfort and stress manifestations were often found to be related to work organization problems. Also in the relay to Montreal there was a demand on continued research: pregnancy outcome, skin disorder, alternative VDT technologies and human computer interaction.

2.3. WWDU'89

Work with VDTs as causing a higher risk of adverse reproductive outcomes could not be confirmed after the discussion of several epidemiological studies and some research hypotheses. The research on electromagnetic fields continue. However, we now know that we have to go for more complicated relationships between variables! Reviews in different areas featured the conference. Still the central issues concerning health are on visual and other ergonomics factors, job design and work organization. Ageing as well as VDTs in developing countries became important areas. VDT in schools became a new topic. Quality of life was addressed.

2.4. WWDU'92

In Berlin topics connected with the new technique appeared as video and hypermedia for communication within group, Kansei engineering and multimodal interfaces. This meant that analysis of relations of variables in complex situations now were standard. The reviewing sessions were frequent. Strategies for prevention and some other sessions indicated recommendations which could ensure better guidance. And in the year "Europe 1992" the interest in regulations and standards was not less than before.

2.5. WWDU'93 Tokyo Seminar

Last year WWDU had two technical meetings in Tokyo: "Human sciences on virtual environment" and "Hypermedia". A round table of Japanese scientists ended up with recommendations of agenda topics for WWDU conferences, as for instance forecast and evaluation of influences of new technologies, evaluation of handwritten input, ethics standards, ethnical and cultural differences in research and evaluation of electronic publication and virtual environment.

3. WWDU'94

Now in Milan we expect new items and statements. It is obvious that we look at characteristics connected with the VDT worker, his task, equipment and environment, and their interactions. The complex situation of the worker is now mapped. So, the health and well-being effects may be calculated.
There are still clusters of operators with an intensive VDT work load. Some of the monotonous jobs have diminished in frequency, however, or are distributed as a natural part of the job. Nowadays, it is a real problem to get a suitable control group of non-VDT users for field studies because of the widespread use of VDTs.

3.1. More elderly people, fewer young people, more women and more migrants in the work force

Age changes in the general population obviously affect the supply of labour. Population trends in Sweden, with corresponding changes also taking place in other parts of Europe, have been unambiguous. There will be a major increase in the number of older people in the work force by the end of the 1990s and a corresponding decline in the number of young people in working life (Figure 1). There have been speculations about whether this means that the work force will acquire more people with handicaps and chronic diseases and that employers will be forced into fierce competition with one another for the dwindling supply of young employees. This is valid under the presumption that the unemployment rate is low, but unfortunately this is not the case for the time being.

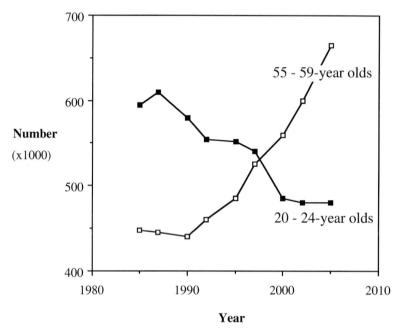

Figure 1. Supply of labour for 1990-2005

We know that young people in the future will be even better educated than was previously the case. Recent attitude studies have shown that young people have heightened expectations about work and are more critical in their perception of work hazards. The studies have also shown that the work environment, and not just the work itself, is an important factor in the choice of employment.

Another change which has become apparent in recent decades is the relative increase in the number of women in the work force. In the Nordic countries, the increase has been considerable, to some extent because men are now taking on an increasing share of household responsibilities. In Sweden, men have a legal right to leaves-of-absence to care for their children, thereby making it easier for their female partners to pursue their own careers.

A third change concerns migrants. As a result of improved communications between countries and various other parts of the world, people now have greater opportunities to leave their countries and settle elsewhere. As a result of political upheavals in eastern Europe, we can expect a major increase in migrants from that part of the world. Immigration has created problems in a number of countries, e g language problems, lower levels of education etc. Increased opportunities for a better balance between the supply and demand of labour is one of the advantages conferred by immigration. In the long run, the advantages are likely to outweigh the disadvantages.

So, to state that computer systems should be adapted to users' level of knowledge is not enough. A challenge for the society is that it should be able to educate its members up to levels qualifying them to participate fully in worklife and in the society life. Education in school for children is as important as for adults.

3.2 "Winners and losers"

As to the psycho-social effects of computerization the concept of "winners and losers of computerization" was introduced. Some people will benefit from the "new" technique (new stimulating work tasks, better paid than before) and others won´t. The "losers" will in stead will get the monotonous, dull, low-paid jobs.

In Sweden data processing know-how has been traditionally regarded as a "technical" subject for math teachers and students primarily interested in learning how computers work. The courses still cover operative systems and programming. An effect of the Swedish system is that an "A-team" of compulsory school students with computer and program experience acquired at home or else developed. But many other students, girls in particular, may enter working life or higher education with virtually no knowledge of computers as working tools. This could relegate such students to the labour market´s "B-team". Of course, we have to be on the alert to avoid the segregation of winners and losers to start already in school.

3.3. Criteria for acceptable work load

The development of equipment and systems is important. We have to develop better standards and also anticipate a continuous competition between producers. However, criteria for acceptable work load for different human functions are a challenge under development.

Mental stress has been shown to be associated with what is called high and low mental workload, where "workload" is defined in terms of the demands made by the work task and the capacity with which workers are able to accommodate these demands. Mental stress can arise as the result of "overloading" (demands > capacity) or "underloading" (demands < capacity). Cognitive aspects of software and the user interface and the organizational design of systems and networks are capable of affecting the mental health and well-being of operators and represent factors to which attention must be devoted.

Work postures, tasks and design are closely related to work organization and work tasks. A recent study of VDT work and sickness absenteeism showed that groups with a low degree of control over their work and few opportunities for obtaining new skills have higher rates of absenteeism than people with greater skills, greater control and more varied tasks. Analyses have also demonstrated the existence of a relationship between the time spent on VDT's and rates of absenteeism.

The risk presented by excessive sedentary work should also be noted. We now know that musculoskeletal disorders develop both when the physical workload is too great and when the physical workload is too little. Computerized work must be modified to reduce sedentary components.

4. CONCLUSIONS

It is clear from what have been stated above that there are more to be done as to information and action programmes where the society takes responsibility. A good example of this is student education at school, where the risk of segregation into winners and losers is imminent. It should be said, however, that machines and working routines have improved during the years, but still we face problem areas, e g eye discomfort, electromagnetic fields and health outcomes, and mental work load and work organization. Here we have the major research areas of today - and possibly also of tomorrow.

A conclusion is: we need the Work With Display Units conferences as a forum to discuss all this in a perspective which stresses health and well-being of the VDT worker.

An Alternative Perspective on the VDT Health Hazards Debate: Folk Hazards and Health Panics

Brian Pearce

HUSAT Research Institute, Loughborough University of Technology, Loughborough, Leicestershire, LE11 1RG, England

1. INTRODUCTION

The hypothesis examined in this contribution is that the use of a VDT has become a *folk hazard* associated with a series of ephemeral *health panics*. It is suggested that the health concerns associated with VDT use should be viewed more as a socio-political phenomenon rather than the consequence of evidence of harm. An alternative way of expressing this hypothesis is to suggest that the health concerns associated with VDT use have developed into a debate of vested interests, which has been influenced as much by social, political, economic and cultural factors as by the (lack of) scientific and medical evidence.

The health concerns associated with VDT use have their origins in complaints of discomfort and fatigue reportedly experienced by VDT users. However, it is the possibility of more permanent damage or a chronic disease process, such as cataracts, miscarriages, and latterly, so-called repetitive strain injuries (RSIs), arising from VDT use which has sporadically and significantly fuelled the debate. Many of these concerns were not, and are not, responded to adequately. It is clear that in some areas there is still an absence of evidence (lack of research), rather than an evidence of absence (negative findings), concerning the alleged health effects of VDT work. However, there are those who are more than willing to suggest that most of the problems are 'all in the mind' or the creation of the media.

This contribution does not seek to deny the legitimacy of the symptoms and conditions experienced in many cases, it must be noted, by a relatively small proportion of VDT users. Nor does this contribution seek to deny the legitimacy of particular health concerns which have been associated with VDT use. Rather, it attempts to examine why and how a wide variety of symptoms, adverse health outcomes and health concerns have been associated with VDT use. The intention is to step beyond the scientific and medical debate, to examine some of the other factors which may have caused these health concerns to flourish and sometimes to decline in different countries.

2. THE VDT HEALTH HAZARDS DEBATE

There are no statistical data which allow an international comparison of the prevalence of these alleged, occupational health problems. Even within any one country there is often a lack of reliable, occupational morbidity statistics. However, even if there were such statistics they would not necessarily reflect the level of concern about these alleged hazards to health. What has come to be known as the 'VDT health hazards debate' is more than simply a debate about what proportion of VDT users in a particular country experience which symptoms. The 'VDT Health Hazards Debate' can be defined as: *The evolving exchange of facts, opinions and propaganda and the actions and reactions associated with the alleged, actual or perceived effects upon the physical and mental well-being of those who work with or near computer terminals.*

The term 'debate' usually implies a dialogue between two opposing viewpoints. However, the VDT health hazards debate has not been an orderly exchange of views. While many contributions to the debate are the results of medical and scientific studies, others could be described as monologues of propaganda, which are reiterated, often unquestioned, in various media. The 'VDT health hazards debate' has been, and is, a contentious, evolving phenomenon. It has been, and is, a debate: about the interpretation and presentation of the available scientific and medical knowledge; about what research is needed; and about what actions to take in the absence of a scientific or medical consensus.

3. HISTORIC AND GEOGRAPHIC CONTEXT

Allegations that work at VDTs may present a hazard to health have been raised in many countries over the last two decades. However, the focus of concern appears to vary from country to country and in any one country the emphasis appears to vary over time. The words 'appears to vary' have to be used simply because one of the immediate problems encountered in trying to examine the health concerns associated with the use of VDTs is to find a way by which to quantify the level of concern about a particular allegation in any particular country at any particular time.

Even though it is extremely difficult to identify any valid metrics of the level of concern about these various health issues or to identify precisely what fuels the debate in any particular country it is possible to identify certain trends. Some of the earliest scientific papers concerning possible health effects of VDT work emanate from Scandinavia in the mid 1970s. The emphasis tended to be on visual problems and particularly ocular discomfort. The suggestion of more serious irreversible effects and the possible implication of electromagnetic radiation emissions e.g. cataracts and miscarriages, came later and appeared to become a particular issue in North America. Concerns about facial rashes which arose in the 1980s were almost exclusively Scandinavian in origin. Musculo-skeletal complaints among VDT users have been reported in many countries for many years but it was in Australia that the suggestion that these might be irreversible first rose to prominence in the early 1980s, in the guise of so-called repetitive strain injuries (RSIs).

With hindsight, it appears that at the peak of concern about a particular VDT related health problem in a particular country, the severity, if not the existence, of the next health problem to emerge in that particular country is usually not recognised. An observer might be forgiven for speculating that the 'health concerns' are contagious and transmitted most effectively at international conferences concerned with the alleged health problems of working with VDTs.

It is interesting to note how the component of the VDT which allegedly causes harm has changed over time. Originally it was the screen and its associated electronics, which were perceived as the 'cause' of health problems. The screen has given way to the keyboard and latterly to the mouse, with the emergence of the so-called 'mouse arm syndrome'. However, at the same time, there has been a growing recognition that it is not what the VDT is doing to the user, in terms of emissions or how the workstation is set up, but what the user is doing with the VDT, which is perhaps the source of the problems. The design of the VDT users' jobs and psycho-social factors in the work place have overtaken the VDT itself as the perceived source of 'hazard'.

4. FOLK HAZARDS AND HEALTH PANICS

The terms *folk hazard* and *health panics* have been derived, by this author, from the title of a seminal publication in sociology: *Folk Devils & Moral Panics*[1]. This book, which is an account of the social reaction to deviant behaviour among youths, in England, in the 1960s, contains some interesting observations on the rôle of the media in the development of social reactions, some of which are directly relevant to an examination of the factors which have contributed to the perception of VDT use as a potentially harmful activity.

The term *folk hazard* is not used in a pejorative sense and does not imply that a hazard does or does not exist. Other activities or agents which are suggested to have assumed the position of a *folk hazard* and have been associated with *health panics* at one time or another include: sexual intercourse (herpes, and AIDS); passive smoking (cardio-vascular disease and lung cancer); viewing television (damage to eyes and children's minds); masturbation (blindness); mining (nystagmus); writing (writer's cramp); eating beef (BSE), or raw eggs (salmonella); living near power lines (various cancers); and sun bathing (skin cancer). It will be noted that many of these, one-time *folk hazards* have been substantiated, some have faded into history, while others are still the subject of debate.

One of the underlying concepts of a *folk hazard* is that there is a difference, among the stakeholders in the debate, in the perception of the risk of undertaking an activity or of exposure to an agent, at a particular time. The stakeholders who first perceive the *folk hazard* may well be the health professionals or, in an occupational setting, trade union officials though the *health panics* are usually the prerogative of the media. One of the beneficial functions of these *health panics* is that they may well be the driving force for the necessary research to be undertaken. If, however, there is perceived or found to be no risk then those involved in the *health panic* are often considered to be scaremongers. It is possible to argue, particularly in the context of occupational health, that in some countries a *health panic* has been the only way in which to stimulate the necessary action and research given the intransigence of the stakeholders who do not subscribe to the *folk hazard*. Unfortunately, during this process there is often an extreme polarisation of views.

The factors which cause a *folk hazard* and the associated *health panics* to emerge are many and varied. However, it is suggested that essential ingredients for the existence of a *folk hazard* and the associated *health panics* are: a lack of scientific knowledge or a lack of consensus on the interpretation of the available scientific data concerning the causes of a perceived health problem; partial information or propaganda provided by those with often well intentioned but sometimes vested interests; access to and involvement of the media; and putative victims along with their vociferous champions.

5. FACTORS INFLUENCING THE VDT HEALTH HAZARDS DEBATE

It is suggested that the differences in the VDT health hazards debate in different countries, in part, reflect national differences in: attitudes to occupational health; the framework of health and safety legislation and compensation; and variations in the classification and attribution of the symptoms and conditions, rather than perhaps any major differences in the incidence of the problems. For example, legal actions by VDT users in the UK and the USA, alleging serious musculo-skeletal injuries, differ significantly. In the USA, VDT users are suing the keyboard manufacturers mostly, it would appear, for carpal tunnel syndrome, whereas in the UK, VDT users are suing their employer, mostly for tenosynovitis and so-called RSIs, but rarely for carpal tunnel syndrome.

The reactions to the health concerns associated with VDT use and the way the issues develop in any particular country can be influenced by a wide variety of different factors and stakeholders. These include: the health professions; the scientific community; the equipment manufacturers; the management in user organisations; organised labour, both at national and local level; and even advertising copy writers[2]. However, perhaps the most significant influence is the treatment the allegations receive in the trade and popular press. In passing, it is interesting to note the frequency with which some of the more serious alleged health problems have been identified among VDT users in newspapers: cataracts at the *New York Times*; adverse pregnancy outcomes at the *Toronto Star*; musculo-skeletal problems at the *Financial Times* and the *Los Angeles Times*. In their time, each of these events generated considerable publicity.

Beardsworth[3] describes the mechanisms through which a novel anxiety emerges, is transmitted to the public and then declines, with 'problem-amplifying' and subsequently, 'problem-dampening' feedback provided by the media. While this may explain much of the ontogeny of a health concern, it is also necessary to consider its conception, the point at which the novel anxiety is identified. For example, at the time, the question was: what caused the cataracts in the workers at the *New York Times*? The question now is: what, or perhaps who, caused the cataracts in the workers at the *New York Times* to be attributed to the use of VDTs?

All of the symptoms and medical conditions which have been attributed to VDT use occur within the population with a certain baseline frequency. Unless VDT use confers some form of immunity on a VDT user it would be surprising if VDT users did not experience everyday ailments, symptoms and adverse health outcomes with at least the same frequency as any other comparable group of workers. One of the major issues would appear to be whether VDT users actually experience significantly higher levels of ailments, symptoms and adverse health outcomes than any other comparable group of workers. Unfortunately, this was an issue which the vast majority of early studies failed to address adequately. These early studies also failed to consider the sometimes random occurrence of clusters of adverse health outcomes[4] and too readily attributed the cause of clustered events to VDT use.

It should be noted that the VDT health hazards debate co-exists with a number of other health debates concerned with: the quality of working life and stress; the effects of chronic exposure to electromagnetic radiation; the quality of the indoor environment, including passive smoking and electrical hypersensitivity; and the underlying causes of the gamut of apparently work-related upper limb disorders. These co-existing debates are not necessarily confined to occupational health matters. However, it appears that the 'apostles' of particular hazards or disputed medical conditions have, at times, hijacked the VDT health hazards debate for their own purposes. For example, it can be argued that the VDT was used as a convenient vehicle to draw attention to the hazards of chronic exposure to low levels of electromagnetic radiation and is currently seen by some as a convenient vehicle for promoting RSIs which present with no objective, clinical signs of abnormality.

Research has failed to provide conclusive evidence of permanent damage, such as cataracts or miscarriages, arising from VDT use. Research has, so far, also failed to provide conclusive evidence of a chronic disease process, such as so-called RSIs, arising from VDT use. Yet, the (mis)attribution of permanent damage or a chronic disease process to VDT use has sporadically and significantly fuelled the VDT health hazards debate.

The ever increasing number of new VDT users, some working in less than 'ideal' conditions, ensures that there is a background level of VDT users who experience mild symptoms of fatigue and discomfort. However, the emergence of hypotheses indicating that psychosocial modifiers might act to amplify and channel the expression of both the normally occurring background levels of non-specific symptoms that are present in any population and the symptoms associated with specific exposure to discomfort provoking agents[5-6], suggests that the existing models of causation of low grade symptoms associated with VDT use might be over-simplistic. Consideration might also need to be given to the possibility of 'sociogenic illness' in an occupational setting[7] given the localised nature of some health problems allegedly related to VDT use.

The (mis)attribution, to VDT use, of naturally occurring or pre-existing symptoms and medical conditions cannot, itself, be attributed solely to psychogenic factors or even the actions of the media, which might be termed mediagenic factors. Consideration also needs to be given to actions of the health professionals: the gatekeepers to the illness rôle and compensation systems. The very diagnosis of a so-called repetitive strain injury attributes the cause and implies culpability. Iatrogenic factors clearly play a part in the legitimisation of work related 'injuries' and can influence the perception of health concerns. For example, well intentioned advice by a medical practitioner to transfer a pregnant VDT user to alternative work to reduce anxiety, may be interpreted by other VDT users as legitimising their concerns that VDTs emit harmful radiation. Similarly, the casual remark by an eye care practitioner, to the effect that spectacles are needed because of the use of a VDT, may be interpreted by the VDT user as evidence that the VDT has somehow damaged his eyesight, whereas in reality, it has merely highlighted a naturally occurring deficiency.

The symptoms and the adverse health outcomes and the allegedly hazardous agents and activities associated with VDTs are the raw materials which form the foundations of the health concerns upon which the VDT health hazards debate has been built. To some the VDT health hazards debate is a mountain, to others a molehill. A *folk hazard* requires stakeholders with alternative perspectives.

6. CONCLUDING COMMENTS

The publication of the European Directive 90/270/EEC, in May 1990, "on the minimum safety and health requirements for work with display screen equipment" required the enactment of legislation in each Member State by the end of 1992. While it can be argued that, in the long term, this legislation may lead to a reduction in health problems, real or perceived, in the short term, it has fuelled the debate by drawing attention to, and increasing awareness of, the various health concerns. However, it should be noted that equivalent, some might argue better framed, legislation, enacted somewhat earlier in Sweden, does not seem to have diminished the problems, if the number of contributions by Swedish authors to the last four conferences on Work With Display Units is anything to go by. Attempts in the USA to legislate these problems away will be viewed by all observers of the VDT health hazards debate with interest.

A number of long term observers of, and sometime contributors to, the debate, including this author[8], have suggested that the level of publicity and concern regarding VDT health hazards - the perceived risks - far exceed the possible, actual risks. At various times over the last two decades these observers have (inaccurately) predicted the demise of the VDT health hazards debate. Despite nearly twenty years of investigation, numerous international scientific conferences, the publication of literally thousands of research studies and a dozen books, the VDT health hazards debate marches on. It could be argued that any attempt to place the VDT health hazards debate in its historical and sociological context would best be conducted when the debate is over. An obituary of the VDT health hazards debate would undoubtedly be premature. However, the very persistence of the debate and its ability to change focus go to make the use of a VDT a fascinating *folk hazard* worthy of further examination.

REFERENCES

1. Cohen, S. *Folk devils and moral panics: The creation of the Mods and Rockers.* Basil Blackwell Ltd, Oxford (1972).
2. Pearce, B. G. *Products to relieve or prevent VDU health problems: Exploitation, Placebos or Prophylaxis ?* In: Luczak, H., Cakir, A. & Cakir, G. (eds.) Work With Display Units 92. Elsevier Science Publishers B.V., Amsterdam (1993).
3. Beardsworth, A. D. *Trans-science and Moral Panics: Understanding Food Scares.* British Food Journal 5, pp. 11-16 (1992).
4. Wakeford, R. *Some problems in the interpretation of childhood leukaemia clusters.* In: Thomas, R. W. (ed.) Spatial Epidemiology. Pion, London (1990)
5. Simon, G. E., Katon, W. J. & Sparks, P. J. *Allergic to life: psychological factors in environmental illness.* American Journal of Psychiatry Vol. 147, pp. 901-906 (1990).
6. Howard, L. M. & Wessely, S. *The psychology of multiple allergy.* British Medical Journal Vol. 307, pp. 747-748 (1993).
7. Kerckhoff, A. D. & Back, K. W. *The June Bug: A study of hysterical contagion.* Appleton-Century-Crofts, New York (1968).
8. Pearce, B. G. *Health Hazards of VDTs ?* John Wiley & Sons, Chichester (1984).

Comparison of VDT workplaces in Australia and Sweden

A. Johansson and H. Shahnavaz

Department of Human Work Science, Division of Industrial Ergonomics,
University of Luleå, 971 87 Luleå, Sweden

This paper presents the results from ergonomic investigations performed at VDT workplaces in Australia and Sweden in order to study the prevailing situation for VDT operators at four selected workplaces.

1. BACKGROUND

During the last decades more and more people have been involved in VDT activities. VDTs are not only being used more extensively but also more intensively by more and more people. Computers can be found in almost every branch of society and are meant to be used to increase work efficiency and productivity. Computerised technology has the capability to enhance the jobs of office workers by reducing undesirable, repetitive tasks that require little thought and by increasing the content of jobs to provide greater task variety and meaning [1]. Meanwhile many studies have shown and still show that VDT operators have reported a wide range of health problems such as visual problems, psychosocial, and musculoskeletal problems [2]. Musculoskeletal symptoms may be of various types (pain, numbness, stiffness, fatigue, etc.), found in various parts of the body (neck, shoulder, back, arm, etc.), and occurring with varying frequency and intensity for each operator.

The studies presented in this paper started in Sweden where two workplaces with routine VDT work were selected for field studies. The Swedish study was conducted within the international project known as MEPS (Musculoskeletal, Visual, and Psychosocial Stress in VDT Operators in Optimised Environment). The aim of the MEPS project was to minimise stress amongst VDT operators by creating optimum working conditions through intervention measures at individual workstations [3]. The two workplaces selected for investigation were each chosen because of the management's great interest in the aims and ideas of the project. Investigation was done at an accounts centre within the Swedish Post where work was dominated by routine data-entry work, and at a telephone exchange within a large trading company where data-dialogue work predominated [4, 5]. In all, 36 female operators took part in the investigations (background data see table 1).

After completion of these studies, opportunities were given to perform similar studies in Australia. RSI (repetitive strain injury)-related symptoms associated with VDT work had been much discussed in Australia. A large body of literature and many reports were published in the past in this area, and RSI became a major social issue in the mid-1980s. RSI was broadly portrayed either as a work related injury (the 'standard view') or as one of four principal contrary views: that people with RSI are malingerers, that they have a conversion disorder, that the discomfort experienced is nothing but normal fatigue or that RSI is a form of compensation neurosis [6].

However, very little has been published in Australia during recent years which consequently has created a belief that RSI related symptoms are no longer a problem [7]. If pain and discomfort were no longer experienced by VDT operators in Australia, it would be interesting to find out what had then been done at different workplaces in terms of prevention.

Two workplaces, both with a large extent of their work force involved in repetitive VDT work, were selected for thorough investigation. Both of these workplaces were in the limelight during the 1980s because of the large extent of RSI-related cases and worker compensation claims. All together, 61 female operators participated in the Australian study (background data are given in table 1)

Table 1.
Background data to the investigated workplaces

	Sweden		Australia	
	Company A	Company B	Company C	Company D
Type of work	Data-entry	Data-dialogue	Data-entry	Data-dialogue
No. of subjects	25	11	24	37
Mean age (years)	39	44	29	38

2. METHOD

While doing ergonomic evaluations, it is important to collect both an objective as well as a subjective estimation of the work situation to be able to provide a comprehensive description of the actual situation and how it is perceived by the operators. Two questionnaires were used in these studies, one was completed by the VDT operators and the other by the ergonomic experts [3]. Operators having years of experience in their work are regarded as valuable resources for identifying work-related problems in their work environment, since they are facing the work environment daily. However, experts can contribute by identifying problems that have long term effects. It is also true that some operators can get used to a certain type of problem and are for that reason unable to identify it as a problem. In such cases, expert evaluations are a vital contribution [8]. Both questionnaires covered aspects like adjustability and usability of work station facilities, as well as ergonomic aspects of the general work environment, such as climate, lighting conditions, and noise level. Specific measurements were made by an expert in those cases where a condition in itself was not clear and did not allow for correct estimation. The lighting and available height and angular adjustment possibilities are examples of conditions that were measured [3]. The operators were also asked to assess their perceived pain/discomfort in several body regions during the last six months.

3. RESULTS

This section is divided into two parts. The first part presents results regarding operators' assessments of perceived pain/discomfort. The second part deals with some considerations concerning their work environment.

3.1 Operators' assessments of perceived pain/discomfort

Similar to other studies performed in this area [2], the studies presented in this paper have confirmed that several symptoms are prevalent among VDT operators. By looking at the responses concerning self-reported discomfort, it shows that the problems experienced in the two different countries are similar, although the number of operators that reported pain/discomfort is greater in Sweden. Problems in the neck/shoulder area were the most frequently reported problems in both countries (table 2). More than 90 % of the operators at "company A" have reported pain/discomfort in the neck and shoulder area. "Company C" reported the lowest frequency of musculoskeletal complaints. It is interesting to note that no one at "company B" was completely free of musculoskeletal discomfort. Among the data-entry operators at "company A", only 2 persons out of 25 reported no musculoskeletal discomfort at all. At the two Australian workplaces 4 out of 24 and 15 out of 37 operators reported no musculoskeletal problems.

Table 2
Prevalence rates of self-reported pain/discomfort experienced during previous six months (%).

	Sweden		Australia	
	Company A	Company B	Company C	Company D
Neck	91	72	41	46
Shoulder	91	60	30	58
Back	45	52	30	42
Head	73	64	19	17
Visual	45	52	16	37

Pain/discomfort can be experienced in many ways and no one can say that a minor problem experienced for a longer period of time is perceived as any less than an unbearable problem for a shorter period of time. Figure 1 indicate the distribution of intensity and frequency of pain/discomfort in the neck as reported at Company A and B (Sweden) and Company C and D (Australia).

No one at Company C or D reported unbearable problems. The Australian operators most frequently reported only minor discomfort. Most of the perceived pain/discomfort was experienced less than 30 days during the last six months period. The numbers of operators reporting daily pain/discomfort was limited to three persons. These persons suffered from daily pain/discomfort of moderate type in the neck area.

Seven Swedish operators reported daily problems in the neck area, and three of them reported unbearable pain. Seventeen operators reported moderately painful neck problems, and nine of them had experienced the pain/discomfort for more than 30 days during the last six months period.

Figure 1
Reported frequency and intensity of experienced pain/discomfort in the neck during previous six months amongst Swedish and Australian operators.

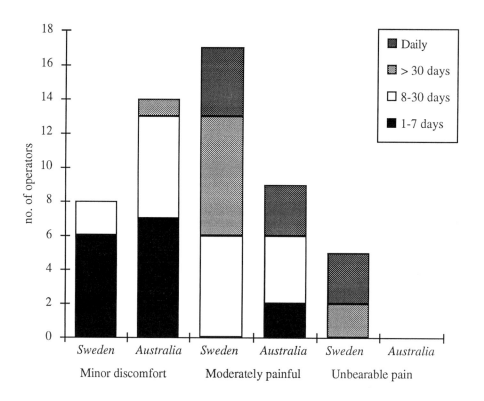

3.2 Work environment considerations

The general work environment was satisfactory at all studied workplaces, according to international standards and recommendations. The Swedish workplaces were even more well equipped and up to date in terms of computer equipment, adjustability, and usability of the furniture. There is a difference, however, in the operators' judgements of their situations [3, 9]. In many ways, the Swedish operators have judged their situation as poorer than the Australians. For example, by looking at the responses concerning the possibility for chair adjustments while seated, only a few Swedish operators have judged this possibility as good compared to almost 50 % of the Australian operators (figure 2).

Figure 2
Frequency distribution of operators' assessments of the possibility of making chair adjustments while seated.

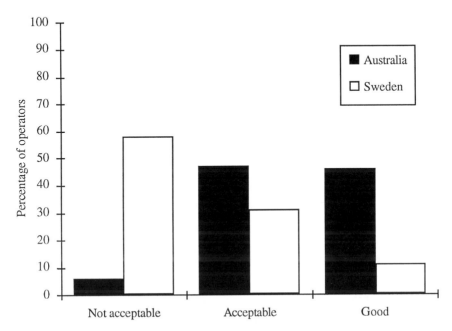

Most operators have their own ideas of how the workplace should be adjusted to suit their individual preferences and demands. The workstations should consequently allow these adjustments of furniture and equipment. All necessary adjustment facilities should be located within comfortable reach and should be easy to use, i.e. height and angular adjustments of chair, desk, VDT and other facilities needed to perform the work and to avoid harmful postures. Nevertheless many operators at the studied workplaces, both in Australia and Sweden, lacked necessary information on how to use the adjustments and how the equipment could be used to reduce the pain/discomfort experienced. At one of the Swedish workplaces, 16 out of 25 operators were unaware of how to use the adjustment facilities and how musculoskeletal problems could be reduced by the appropriate use of facilities provided. At Company C in Australia, 19 out of 24 operators had very limited knowledge of available adjustment possibilities and were therefore not adjusting available equipment and furniture. This is in line with earlier studies made by Koeffler [10] that showed that people tend to adjust their furniture only when it is easy to perform and when they have been taught how to do it.

4. DISCUSSION

Musculoskeletal problems were prevalent among the operators although their work stations were of good quality. The workplaces in Sweden were even regarded, by the experts, as having furniture and equipment of better quality. How come, if workplaces in Sweden were better equipped in terms of ergonomic facilities, that the operators have reported more severe discomfort symptoms than the Australian operators? An explanation might be that by only considering micro-ergonomic factors, it is possible that the influence of macro-ergonomic factors, such as social or organisational parameters may be overlooked.

The actual working time differed among the investigated companies although everyone was working full-time. Company A, B, and D regarded full-time work as 9 hours a day with approximately 8 hours of actual working time each day. Company C regarded full-time work as 6 hours and 40 minutes a day with approximately 5 hours of actual work each day. Company C is also the company that reported less complaints than other companies.

There was also a difference in the willingness of operators and management to talk about experienced pain/discomfort. In Sweden there existed a relatively open atmosphere for discussion about existing problems. In Australia, however, the management at both companies were afraid of a possible new "wave" of RSI related problems and the following compensation claims. The operators were afraid of talking about the problems, because of the fear of losing their job, of not being believed, or of confronting the argument that the problems were not work related. One respondent told the researchers, "If I tell you about all the pain/discomfort I have, they [the management] might fire me". Reid and colleagues [11] found in their studies that a dominant theme among RSI sufferers is their anxiety about being believed by their doctors, friends, families, and work mates. However, a problem will not disappear because it is neglected or ignored. It is much better to talk about small problems before they grow to large costly problems in terms of sick leave and compensations.

REFERENCES

1. Smith, M. J. (1984). Ergonomic Aspects of Health Problems in VDT Operators. In B. G. F. Cohen (Ed.) Human Aspects in Office Automation. Amsterdam: Elseiver Science Publishers B. V.
2. World Health Organisation. (1990). Update on Visual Display Terminals and Worker's Health. WHO/OCH/90.3. Geneva.
3. MEPS Trialplan no. 140. Project: Musculoskeletal, Visual, and Psychosocial Stress in VDT Operators in Optimised Environment: an International Study. (Co-ordinators: A. Aarås, O. Cho Nam, M. Dainoff, M. Konarska, M. Kumashiro, and H. Shahnavaz).
4. Johansson, A. (1992). Synthesis of experts' and users' knowledge for ergonomic improvements of VDU workplaces. Licentiate thesis, 1992:26L, Luleå University of Technology, Luleå.
5. Westlander, G., Shahnavaz, H., Johansson, A., & Viitasara, E. (1992). An Intervention-Oriented Study of VDT Operators in Routinized Work. Research report 1992:32, National Institute of Occupational Health, Solna. (In Swedish, summary in English)
6. Bammer, G. and Martin, B. (1988). The Arguments about RSI: an Examination. Community Health Studies, vol. 12, pp. 348-358.
7. Bammer, G. (1992). Current Issues on Musculo-Skeletal Problems of VDT workers: An International Perspective. Proceedings of the Third International Scientific Conference, Work with Display Units. Berlin, September 1-4, p. D-2.
8. Noro, K. (1991). Methods and people. In K. Noro & A. Imada (Eds.) Participatory Ergonomics. London:Taylor&Francis Ltd.
9. Johansson, A. (1994). RSI in Oz. Research Report, TULEA 1994:17. Luleå University of Technology, Luleå. (In Swedish)
10. Koeffler, R. P. (1986). Workstation Design Guidelines: Do We Need to Reconsider? Proceedings of the International Scientific Conference, Work with Display Units, Stockholm, May 12-15, p. 1042-1045.
11. Reid, J. Ewan, C, and Lowy, E. (1991). Pilgrimage of Pain: The Illness Experiences of Women with Repetition Strain Injury and the Search for Credibility. Social Science and Medicine, vol. 32, no. 5, pp. 601-612.

Skin symptoms and VDT work - Reports from three continents

B. Stenberg

Department of Dermatology
Umeå University, S-901 85 Umeå, Sweden

Facial skin symptoms related to VDT work appeared in Great Britain and Norway in the late 1970s.[1-5] Since the first Swedish cases were reported in 1986[6] this issue has become of major concern to local company health services and a topic of considerable controversy in Sweden. There are also cases reported from the US[7,8] and Japan.[9]

1. CASE REPORTS

In the case series facial skin complaints are commonest, with sensory symptoms, erythema and signs of rosacea.[3,5,6,8,9] In one case dryness and erythema of the hands and forearms was seen.[7]

2. OBSERVATIONAL STUDIES

The observational studies are summarized in Table 1. Three surveys of VDT-related skin complaints have been reported from the US and the UK. One showed an association between VDT use and the prevalence of skin symptom at one work site[10], two failed to show any such relation.[11,12] Three Swedish cross-sectional studies have been published and all reported an exposure-response relationship between the amount of VDT work and the occurrence of skin complaints.[13,14,15] In one survey,[13] people who complained of skin symptoms were examined by occupational dermatologists.[16] Subjects with seborrhoeic eczema, acne and rosacea were over-represented in the exposed group. However, in another study objective skin signs did not show this pattern.[14]

A longitudinal study, emanating from a prior cross-sectional study[13], showed an increased incidence of skin symptoms in VDT workers with intensive VDT work.[17] The effect was modified by company type, suggesting an impact from locale-specific factors such as indoor climate factors or job-specific factors such as stress. A recent Swedish cross-sectional study reported a tendency for increased occurrence of seborrhoeic eczema, nonspecific erythema and skin symptoms among VDT users compared with non-users. Psychosocial and organizational conditions were associated with skin symptoms and facial erythema while photosensitive skin type and low relative humidity were related to an increased prevalence of seborrhoeic eczema. No association was found between measured VDT-related electromagnetic fields and skin symptoms or signs.[18] In a Swedish case-referent study background electric fields and fluorescent tubes with plastic shielding (compared with metal shielding) and VDT-related magnetic fields in the ELF range were risk indicators in bivariate analysis.[19] The electric fields and the VDT-related magnetic fields showed a dose-response relationship with the risk of facial skin symptoms. The prevalence of skin complaints among plasma display users in Singapore was found to be similar to that found among those using cathode ray tubes.[20]

Table 1. Main features of and findings from observational studies on skin symptoms in visual display terminal users

OBSERVATIONAL STUDIES

Author Year of publication Country	Design Method	Return/ Participation rate	Control for confounding	Results
Murray et al 1981 (US)[10]	Selected work sites, questionnaire	37-51%	No	Skin symptoms were more prevalent among VDT users at one work site
Frank 1983 (US)[11]	Selected work sites, questionnaire	40%	No	No significant difference between VDT users and non-users
Knave et al 1985 (S)[13]	Selected work sites, questionnaire	91%	Yes	Skin symptoms were more prevalent among female VDT users
Lidén et al 1985 (S)[16]	Employees with symptoms invited, clinical examination	77%	No	Seborrhoeic eczema, acne, rosacea and perioral dermatitis as a group were more prevalent among VDT users
Berg et al 1990 (S)[14]	Random sample of employees in selected work sites, questionnaire, clinical examination	97% 92%	Yes	Facial skin complaints were more prevalent among VDT users, no difference in skin signs
Koh et al 1990 (SG)[20]	Selected work sites, questionnaire	97%	No	No significant difference between CRT and PD operators
Carmichael et al 1992 (UK)[12]	Selected work sites	41%	No	No significant difference between VDT users and non-users
Bergqvist et al 1992 (S)[17]	Selected work sites, follow up, questionnaire	82-97%	Yes	An increased incidence of skin problems was associated with extensive VDT work; the effect was modified by company type
Stenberg et al 1993 (S)[15]	Random sample, questionnaire	94%	Yes	Skin symptoms were more prevalent among VDT users
Bergqvist et al 1994 (S)[18]	Selected work sites, questionnaire, clinical examination, measures of electromagnetic fields	92% 85% 83%	Yes	Seborrhoeic eczema, erythema and skin symptoms tended to be more prevalent among VDT users; psychosocial and organizational factors were associated with symptom occurrence; photosensitive skin was associated with seborrhoeic eczema, no association between measured fields and symptoms
Sandström et al 1995 (S)[19]	Case-referent study	91%	Yes	Background electric fields and VDT-related magnetic fields (ELF) were risk indicators

CRT = Cathode Ray Tube   PD = Plasma Display   VDT = Visual Display Terminal

Table 2. Main features of and findings from experimental studies on skin problems in visual display terminal users

EXPERIMENTAL STUDIES

Author Year of publication Country	Design	Exposure	Outcome	Results
Cato Olsen 1981 (N) [25]	Open	ES fields	Deposition of particles onto face-mounted subtrates	Elevated ES potentials increased the deposition
Swanbeck et al 1989 (S) [26]	Randomized, double blind, referred VDT users	ES, B-VLF fields from VDTs, different levels of RH	Skin symptoms and signs	No significant difference between exposures
Sandström et al 1989 (S) [27]	Blinded, referred VDT users	E and B fields of VDT type, 50 Hz	Skin symptom reports	B-ELF and E-VLF increased symptom intensity in some patients
Hamnerius et al 1992 (S) [28]	Double blind, referred patients, with "hypersensitivity" to electrical equipment	E and B fields of VDT type	Skin symptoms, temperature, conductance, peripheral blood flow, pulse rate	No significant difference between exposures
Franzén et al 1992 (S) [29]	Double blind, selected subjects with "hypersensitivity" to electricial equipment	E and B fields	Detection of exposure	Two subjects detected exposure significantly more often than expected by chance
Berg et al 1992 (S) [30]	Open, invited VDT users with or without symptoms	VDT work, leisure	Itching behaviour, perceived mental strain, stress hormones	Symptomatic persons had higher itching frequency, perceived higher mental strain and had elevated stress hormones during work

B = Magnetic field E = Electric field ELF = Extremely Low Frequency (picture refreshment frequency) ES = Electrostatic
RH = Relative Humidity VDT = Visual Display Terminal VLF = Very Low Frequency (line frequency)

3. CLINICAL STUDIES

Clinical studies of referred patients have not shown any specific VDT-related skin disease.[21] Seborrhoeic dermatitis, acne and rosacea have been the most prevalent diagnoses observed[21,22] and routine histopathological examination of VDT exposed subjects have shown similar findings to those in a control group.[23] During the last years an increasing number of patients have reported aggravation of symptoms from different electric devices, the term "electric hypersensitivity" has come into use among those patients. These patients often preceive multiple symptoms. A psychological study of patients with isolated skin symptoms aggravated by VDT use and exposure to TV set and flourescent light, and a group of multisymptomatic patients with perceived "electric hypersensitivity" has shown that these patient groups represent different types of personality and that psychological factors of possible importance for the symptoms were more often found in the latter group.[24]

4. EXPERIMENTAL STUDIES

Experimental studies are shown in Table 2. An experiment has demonstrated that the deposition of particles onto the cheek of an operator increases with the intensity of the electrostatic field.[25] The investigator suggested that irritant aerosols cause the observed rashes. This hypothesis was not supported by an experiment performed on patients with VDT-related skin symptoms. The effect of exposure to VDTs with powerful or no electrostatic fields did not differ in a double blind provocation study. High relative humidity, which reduces the electrostatic charge, did not prevent reactions.[26]

Preliminary reports from double blind provocation tests with electromagnetic fields on VDT workers have so far not presented evidence for alternating fields as a cause of symptoms.[27-29] Stress has been studied as a cause for the skin reactions.[30] VDT users with skin symptoms had higher levels of stress-sensitive hormones during work and reported more occupational work strain compared with employees without symptoms. From these findings the investigators proposed a model, techno-stress, in which the working conditions rather than the VDT itself cause the symptoms.

5. CLINICAL EXPERIENCE

Since 1985 over 200 patients have been referred to our department for alleged VDT-related skin conditions. Nine out of ten patients are women and the symptoms have often started in relation to changes in working conditions. Sensory symptoms mimicking a sunburn with facial erythema are common, sometimes accompanied by eye irritation, periorbital swelling and facial eczema. One out of ten patients also report irritation on the back of the hands. The symptoms are aggravated during winter-time and 10-20% of the patients report worsening of the symptoms when being close to TV-sets, fluorescent tubes and other electric devices. Sun light is often reported to worsen the symptoms until a protective suntan is developed.

The most common conditions are rosacea, facial erythema and telangiectasia, seborrhoeic and atopic eczema and acne. Routine blood tests are normal as are photo tests on facial skin. Routine histopathology does not differ from that normally found in patients with similar, but non-VDT-related, conditions. Patients with isolated skin symptoms seem to have a good prognosis for work in the office environment. Most patients can continue with, or return to VDT work after some measures have been taken. In many cases shortening VDT work is enough. Many patients report that the application of filters reducing the alternating electric fields or the change to liquid crystal display (LCD) screens permits them to extend their VDT work before symptoms develop. Those reporting multiple systemic symptoms from electric devices are worse off and have difficulties in adapting to office work, even after measures have been taken.[31]

6. SUMMARY

With the exception of the Swedish studies, the cited surveys have had low response rates or no control for confounders. In studies with a strong design in these respects, there is a consistent pattern showing an exposure-response relation between the amount of VDT work and the prevalence of self-reported skin symptoms. Whether VDT work induces or aggravates skin diseases has not definitely been resolved. Reported skin symptoms and signs are predominantly localized to facial skin.

The cause of the symptoms is still obscure. Experiments with static electric fields have given inconsistent results. However, if skin symptoms are evoked by irritants in the ambient air of the workplace, and whose deposition onto the skin is influenced by the static electric field, experiments in clean air would not be expected to confirm this mechanism. Consequently such experiments should be conducted at the workplace where the symptoms started or in similar IAQ conditions. Until now there is only one observational study showing an association between measurement of electromagnetic fields and skin problems and experiments contradict such an association. Stress as a risk factor is not refuted by any study. Skin symptoms in VDT users, although reported from three continents, are most commonly reported from Sweden. No single factor serves as a good explanation for the geographic distribution of complaints and reports. It is suggested that isolated skin symptoms related to VDT work should be separated from so called "electric hypersensitivity" with multiple symptoms attributed to all kinds of electric devices.

REFERENCES

1. Pearce BG. Health hazards in perspective. In Pearce BG. (Ed) Health Hazards of VDT's? John Wiley & Sons, New York 1984, 5-12.
2. Lindén V, Rolfsen S. Video computer terminals and occupational dermatitis. *Scand J Work Environ Health* 1981; 7: 62-67.
3. Rycroft RJG, Calnan CD. Facial rashes among visual display unit (VDU) operators. In Pearce BG. (Ed) Health Hazards of VDT's? John Wiley & Sons, New York 1984, 13-16.
4. Tjonn HH. Report of facial rashes among VDU operators in Norway. In Pearce BG. (Ed) Health Hazards of VDT's? John Wiley & Sons, New York 1984, 17-23.
5. Nielsen A. Facial rash in visual display unit operators. *Contact Dermatitis* 1982; 8: 25-28.
6. Stenberg B. A rosacea-lika skin rash in VDU-operators. In Knave B. and Widebäck P-G. (Eds) Work with Display Units 86, Elsevier/North-Holland, Amsterdam, 1987, 160-64.
7. Feldman RL, Eaglstein WH. Terminal illness. *J Am Acad Dermatol* 1985; 12: 366.
8. Fisher AA. "Terminal" dermatitis due to computers (visual display units). *Cutis* 1986; 37: 153-54.
9. Matsunaga K, Hayakawa R, Ono Y, Hisinaga N. Facial rash in a visual display terminal operator. *Ann Rep Nagoya Univ Br Hosp* 1988; 22: 57-61 (in Japanese, summary in English).
10. Murray WE, Moss CE, Parr WH. et al. Potential health hazards of video display terminals. NIOSH Research Report 81-129. Public Health Service, Cincinnati, Ohio, 1981.
11. Frank AL. Effects on health following occupational exposure to video display terminals. Dept. of Preventive Medicine and Environmental Health, University of Kentucky, Lexington, Ky. 40536-0084,1983.

12. Carmichael AJ, Roberts DL. Visual display units and facial rashes. *Contact Dermatitis* 1992; 26: 63-64.
13. Knave, BG, Wibom RI, Voss M, Hedström LD, Bergqvist UOV. Work with video display terminals among office employees. I. Subjective symptoms and discomfort. *Scand J Work Environ Health* 1985; 11: 457-66.
14. Berg M, Lidén S, Axelson O. Facial skin complaints and work at visual display units; an epidemiologic study of office employees. *J Am Acad Dermatol* 1990; 22: 621-25.
15. Stenberg B, Hansson Mild K, Sandström M, Sundell J, Wall S. A prevalence study of the sick building syndrome (SBS) and facial skin symptoms in office workers. *Indoor Air* 1993; 3: 71-81.
16. Lidén C, Wahlberg JE. Work with video display terminals among office employees. V. Dermatologic factors. *Scand J Work Environ Health* 1985; 11: 489-93.
17. Bergqvist U, Knave B, Voss M, Wibom R. A longitudinal study of VDT work and health. *Int J Human Computer Interaction* 1992; 4: 197-219.
18. Bergqvist U, Wahlberg JE. Skin symptoms and disease during work with visual display terminals. *Contact Dermatitis* 1994; 30: 197-204.
19. Sandström M, Hansson Mild K, Stenberg B, Wall S. Skin symptoms among VDT workers related to electromagnetic fields - a case-referent study. *Indoor Air*, 1995. In press.
20. Koh D, Goh CL, Jeyaratnam J, Kee WC, Ong CN. Dermatological symptoms among visual display unit operators using plasma display and cathode ray tube screens. *Ann Acad Med* 1990, 19: 617-20.
21. Wahlberg JE, Stenberg B. Skin problems in the office environment. In Menné T, Maibach HI. (Eds) Exogenous Dermatoses: Environmental dermatitis. CRC Press, Boca Raton, 1991, 327-38.
22. Berg M. Skin problems in workers using visual display terminals. A study of 201 patients. *Contact Dermatitis* 1988; 19: 335-41.
23. Berg M, Hedblad M-A, Erhardt K. Facial skin complaints and work at visual display units: a histopathological study. *Acta Derm Venereol (Stockh)* 1990; 70: 216-20.
24. Bergdahl J. Psychological aspects of patients with symptoms presumed to be caused by electricity or visual display units. *Acta Odontol Scand*, 1995. In press.
25. Cato Olsen W. Electric field enhanced aerosol exposure in visual display unit environments. The Chr. Michelsen Institute, Dept. of Science and Technology, Bergen 1981, 1-40.
26. Swanbeck G, Bleeker T. Skin problems from visual display units. *Acta Derm Venereol (Stockh)* 1989; 69: 46-51.
27. Sandström M, Stenberg B, Hansson Mild K. Provocation tests with ELF and VLF electromagnetic fields on patients with skin problems asssociated with VDT work. Abstract to Work with Display Units 11-14 September 1989, Montreal, 117.
28. Hamnerius Y, Agrup G, Galt S, Nilsson R, Sandblom J, Lindgren R. Provocation study of hypersensitivity reactions associated with exposure to electromagnetic fields from VDUs. Abstract to Work with Display Units 1-4 September 1992, Berlin.
29. Franzén O, Paulsson L-E, Wennberg A. Human exposure to electrical and magnetic fields: an experimental detection study. Abstract to Work with Display Units 1-4 September 1992, Berlin.
30. Berg M, Arnetz B, Lidén S, Eneroth P, Kallner A. Techno-stress. A psychophysiological study of employees with VDU-associated skin complaints. *J Occup Med* 1992; 34: 698-701.
31. Stenberg B. Office Illness. The worker, the work and the workplace. Umeå University Medical Dissertation 1994.

The relationship between video display terminal use and pregnancy outcome

Fabio Parazzini[1,2], Laura Luchini[1] and Pier Giorgio Crosignani[2]

1. Istituto di Ricerche Farmacologiche "Mario Negri", via Eritrea 62, 20157 Milano, Italy
2. I Clinica Ostetrico-Ginecologica, Centro Medicina della Riproduzione, Università di Milano, Italy

In the recent years several concerns have been raised in scientific and lay press on the potential adverse effect of video display terminal (VDT) use on pregnancy outcome (1). Published series have however shown controversial results.

Further, considering the large number of women exposed to VDT, even a limited risk of adverse reproductive outcome may be a considerable public health issue. To obtain quantitative information on the potential association between VDT use and various reproductive outcomes, we have reviewed the results of published epidemiological studies on this topic.

1. METHODS

Results of published case-control studies (or cohort studies analysed as case-control) on the relation between VDT exposure and pregnancy outcome were sought by reviewing reference lists in relevant papers and by conducting manual and computer (MEDLINE) searches of the papes published in English (see (2) for more details). A total of eleven papers were retrieved (3-13), two of which were based on the same study (8,12). Most studies were initially designed in the early 80's as cohort investigations of pregnant women to evaluate the effect of several occupational exposures on reproductive outcomes. The definition of exposure was generally based on self-reporting. The level of exposure was defined in terms of the average number of working hours with VDT per week.

2. RESULTS

2.1. Spontaneous abortions

Nine studies analyzed the relation between VDT exposure in pregnancy and risk of miscarriages. The prevalence of exposure among controls varied widely from less than 20% (7) to more than 50% (4). The estimated odds ratio, OR, for spontaneous abortion ranged from 0.8 to 1.2 and the pooled OR was 1.0 (95% confidence interval, CI, 1.0-1.1, Table 1). Potential covariates were taken into account in most analysis: no marked differences were observed between crude and adjusted estimates.

Most studies failed to describe an increasing risk with duration of exposure to VDT: it was found only in two studies (5,7). Likewise, the pooled trend in risk was not statistically significant (χ^2_1 trend 0.455, Table 2).

2.2. Other pregnancy outcomes

Two studies analyzed the relation between VDT use and risk of low birth weight (defined as $\leq$2,500g) for a total of 1,565 cases and 21,996 controls (7, 11). The OR estimates in the individual studies ranged from 1.0 to 1.1, with a pooled OR of 1.0 (95% CI 0.9-1.2).

No relation emerged from five studies providing information on congenital malformation and VDT use (4,5,7,12,13): the pooled OR based on about 2,000 cases and 50,000 controls was 1.0 (95% CI 0.9-1.2). Increased risks of low birth weight (11) and of a specific malformation (4) with increasing exposure to VDT were described, but did not find confirmation in other studies. Table 3 considers the results from studies which considered the relationship between VDT exposure and risk of malformation.

Finally, no association emerged between preterm births, perinatal mortality and VDT exposure in pregnancy (4,7,11).

3. DISCUSSION

The present overview provides important reassuring evidence on the absence of any major risk of miscarriage, low birth weight and congenital malformations for exposure to VDT. No consistent trend in risk was observed with duration of exposure and no specific pattern of malformation emerged in women exposed to electromagnetic fields from VDT. Fewer data are available on the effect of VDT on preterm births and perinatal mortality, but the scanty figures showed no convinging relationship.

We considered only unadjusted estimates in the computation of the pooled OR. However, in the individual studies, multivariate estimates including terms for major potential covariates (such as smoking habits or socio-economic indicators) were in general consistent with crude ones.

Studies reviewed differ in terms of study population, type of exposure and methods of data collection. However, the OR estimates in individual studies were generally comparable, and, in any case, not statistically heterogeneous, giving strong evidence of the consistency of the pooled results.

Publication bias is a major issue in the interpretation of the results of meta-analysis, but it should not invalidate our results: unpublished negative epidemiological studies would tend to overestimate the true association.

Several studies have suggested that potential pregnancy risk of VDT exposure could be due to psychological stress associated with some occupations (1, 16-18). No difference emerged however in OR estimates from hospital based case-control or cohort studies including non working women.

Recall bias should not account for present results: any bias in exposure assessment tends to overestimate the true association, since cases may systematically better remember their potential sources of exposures.

The absence of information on subclinical miscarriages in published studies, do not allow us to do any inference on this field. However, early concern about the reproductive hazards of VDT was raised after identification of clusters of clinically recognized miscarriages. In general, any definition and hence risk assessment of chemical or physical risk factors for subclinical miscarriage is always extremely difficult.

It has been suggested that it is difficult to define exposure to VDT, since the ambient extremely-low-frequency fields in an office are per se a source of exposure to electromagnetic fields (19,20). Further, electromagnetic fields due to VDT exposure are minimal and generally not significantly above background levels (21). Other sources of electromagnetic fields may constitute a greater risks for reproduction (22) and the contribution of VDT may therefore be irrelevant.

In conclusion, the present overview do not allow us to exclude any potential effect on reproduction of other sources of electromagnetic fields, but it is largely or totally reassurance with reference to the effect of VDT use on prengnacy outcomes. In fact, considering the number of cases reviewed, it was possible to exclude an excess risk of 20% for spontaneous abortion, low birth weight and congenital malformation.

ACKNOWLEDGEMENTS - This work was conducted within the framework of the CNR (Italian National Research Council) Applied Project "Fattori di Rischio di Malattia" (sottoprogetto "Fattori di Malattia nella Patologia Materno Infantile") and of the ENEL-CNR Project "Interazione Energia e Salute" (sottoprogetto "Epidemiologia") - Roma. Laura Luchini had a fellowship by Lombardia Fondazione per l'Ambiente, Milan, Italy.

REFERENCES

1. U.O. Bergqvist. Video display terminals and health. A technical and medical appraisal of the state of the art. Scand. J. Work Environ. Health, 10 suppl 2 (1984) 1-87.
2. F. Parazzini, L. Luchini, C. La Vecchia, P.G. Crosignani. Videodisplay terminal use during pregnancy and reproductive outcome - a meta-analysis. J. Epidemiol. Community Health 47 (1993) 265-268.
3. H.E. Bryant, E.J. Love. Video display terminal use and spontaneous abortion risk. Int. J. Epidemiol. 18 (1989) 132-8.
4. A. Ericson, B. Kallen. An Epidemiological study of work with video sreens and pregnancy outcome: II. A case-control study. Am. J. Ind. Med. 9 (1986) 459-75.
5. M.K. Goldhaber, M.R. Polen, R.A. Hiatt. The risk of miscarriage and birth defects among women who use visual display terminals during pregnancy. Am. J. Ind. Med. 13 (1988) 695-706.
6. M.L. Lindbohm, M. Hietanen, P. Kyyronen et al. Magnetic fields of video display terminals and spontaneous abortion. Am. J. Epidemiol. 136 (1992) 1041-51.
7. A.D. McDonald, J.C. McDonald, B. Armstrong et al. Work with video display units in pregnancy. Br. J. Ind. Med. 45 (1988) 509-15.
8. C.V. Nielsen, L.P.A. Brandt. Spontaneous abortion among women using video display terminals. Scand. J. Work Environ. Health 16 (1990) 323-8.
9. E. Roman, V. Beral, M. Pelerin et al. Spontaneous abortion and work with visual display units. Br. J. Ind. Med. 49 (1992) 507-512.
10. T.M. Schnorr, B.A. Grajewsky, R.W. Hornung et al. Video display terminals and the risk of spontaneous abortion. N. Engl. J. Med. 324 (1991) 727-33.
11. G.C. Windham, L. Fenster, S.H. Swan et al. Use of video display terminals during pregnancy and the risk of spontaneous abortion, low birth weight, or intrauterine growth retardation. Am. J. Ind. Med. 18 (1990) 675-88.
12. L.P.A. Brandt, C.V. Nielsen. Congenital malformations among children of women using video display terminals. Scand. J. Work Environ. Health 16 (1990) 329-33.
13. K. Kurppa, P.C. Holmberg, K. Rantala et al. Birth defects and exposure to video display terminals during pregnancy. A Finnish case-referent study. Scand. J. Work Environ. Health 11 (1985) 353-56.
14. N. Mantel, W. Haenszel. Statistical aspects of the analysis of data from retrospective studies of disease. J. Natl. Cancer Inst. 22 (1959) 719-48.
15. N. Mantel. Chi-square test with one degree of freedom: extension of the Mantel-Haenszel procedure. J. Am. Stat. Assoc. 58 (1963) 690-700.
16. G. Johansson, G. Aronsson. Stress reactions in computerized administrative work. J. Occup. Behav. 5 (1980) 159-81.
17. M. Smith, B. Cohen, L. Sammerjohn. An investigation of health complaints and job stress in video display operations. Hum. Factors 23 (1981) 387-400.
18. T. Tenaka, T. Fukumoto. The effects of VDT work on urinary excretion of catecholamines. Ergonomics 31 (1988) 1753-63.
19. L. Slesin, M. Connelly. Video display terminals and spontaneous abortions. N. Engl. J. Med. 325 (1991) 811-2.
20. R. Tell. An investigation of electric and magnetic fields and operator exposure produced by VDTs: NIOSH VDT epidemiology study, final report. Cincinnati: National Institute for Occupational Safety and Health (1990) (NTIS publication no. PB91-500).
21. Bureau fo Radiologic Health. An evaluation of radiation emission from video display terminals. US Dept of Health and Human Services. HHS publ FDA 81 (1981) 8153.
22. N. Werthmeier, E. Leeper. Fetal loss associated with two seasonal sources of electromagnetic field exposure. Am. J. Epidemiol. 129 (1989) 220-4.

TABLE 1
Main results from selected studies on spontaneous abortion (SA) and VDT use.

Authors	SA exposed/total	Controls exposed/total	Odds Ratio (95% CI)	Comments
Bryant and Love (3)	140/334	151/314[a] 127/333[b]	0.8 (0.6-1.1) 1.2 (0.9-1.6)	No change after adjustment for covariates
Ericson and Kallen (4)	208/327	572/926	1.1 (0.8-1.4)	No change after taking into account major covariates
Goldhaber et al (5)	115/355	213/723	1.1 (0.9-1.5)	No change after adjustment for covariates
Lindbohm et al. (6)	87/191	172/394	1.1 (0.8-1.6)	No change after adjustment for covariates
McDonald et al (7)	361/1763	4711/24,614[c]	1.1 (1.0-1.2)	-
	415/4887	2164/22,517[d]	0.9 (0.8-1.0)	
Nielsen and Brandt (8)	353/666	421/764	0.9 (0.7-1.1)	No marked difference in OR in an analysis stratified for major potential covariates.
Roman et al. (9)	82/150	168/297	0.9 (0.6-1.4)	No change after adjustment for covariates.
Schnorr et al (13)	54/134[e]	312/742	0.9 (0.6-1.4)	No excess risk among women who used VDT in the first trimester of pregnancy.
Windham et al (14)	239/439	461/909	1.2 (0.9-1.5)	No change after adjustment for covariates. OR= 1.5 in the first trimester of pregnancy.
Total	2,054/9,246	9,345/52,200	1.0 (0.9-1.0)	

a) Prenatal controls, included in the pooled analysis; b) Postnatal controls, not included in the pooled analysis; c) Current pregnancies; d) Previous pregnancies; e) Estimated from percentages.

TABLE 2
Odds ratio (OR) of spontaneous abortions according to level of VDT exposure (defined as hours/week)

Authors	No VDT use		Level of exposure Low		High+		χ^2 trend
Bryant and Love (3)	1++	(191:175) ø, øø	0.8	(102:121)	1.0	(21:18)	0.72 (p= ns)
Ericson and Kaller (4)	1++	(119:354)	1.0	(125:360)	1.2	(73:177)	1.19 (p= ns)
Goldhaber et al (5)	1++	(240:510)	0.9	(63:148)	1.7	(52:65)	3.82 (p= 0.05)
Lindbohm et al. (6)	1++	(104:222)	1.0	(65:142)	1.6	(22:30)	1.01 (p=ns)
Mc Donald et al (7)	1++	(1402:18,501) a	1.0	(177:2243)	1.2	(184:2107) +++	2.96 (p=n.s.)
	1++	(4472:15,885) b	1.0	(249:859)	0.7	(166:890)	16.74 (p < 0.001) *
Nielsen and Brandt (8)	1++	(316:356)	1.0	(273:319)	1.0	(77:89)	0.07 (p= ns)
Roman et al. (9)	1++	(68:129)	1.0	(58:111)	0.8	(24:57)	0.47 (p=ns)
Schnorr et al (10)	1++	(78:421) øøø	1.1	(22:106)	1.0	(26:143) ++++	0.00 (p= ns)
Windham et al (11)	1++	(200:448)	1.2	(109:207)	1.1	(130:254)	1.18 (p=ns)
Total	1++	(7,190:37,001)	1.0	(1,243:4,616)	1.0	(775:3,830)	0.46 (p= ns)

+ >20 h/wk; ++ Reference category; +++ > 15 h/wk; ++++ >25 h/wk; a) Current pregnancies; b Previous pregnancies; ø Number of cases:controls; øø Prenatal controls; numbers estimated from percentages. They are generally consistent, but not exactly consistent with those published in Table 1; * In the original paper the trend was not significant after adjustment for year of conception.

TABLE 3
Main results form selected studies on congenital malformations (CM) and VDT use.

Authors	CM exposed/total	Controls exposed/total	Odds Ratio (95% CI)	Comments
Brandt and Nielsen (12)	137/421	456/1365	1.0 (0.8-1.2)	No change after adjustment for covariates. No trend in risk with increasing exposure. OR for hydrocephalus 12.0 (95% CI 1.4-104.0).
Ericson et al (4)	73/102	572/926	1.6 (1.0-2.4)	No specific pattern of CM; significant trend in risk with number of hours of exposure to VDT. OR 2.0 for 10h/week and 2.3 for >20h/week.
Goldhaber et al (5)	32/97	213/723	1.2 (0.7-1.9)	No change after adjustment for covariates. OR 1.4 for >25 h/wk exposure. No specific pattern of CM
Kurppa et al (13)	51/235	601/255	0.9 (0.6-1.4)	No trend in risk with increasing exposure. OR for cardiovascular defects 1.6 (95% CI 0.7-3.9)
McDonald et al (7)	103/627[a] 55/572[bc]	4628/26,755 1702/19,699	0.9 (0.8-1.2) 1.1 (0.8-1.5)	OR for renal/urinary organs 1.8 (p 0.02) in current pregnancies.
Total	451/2054	6330/49,723	1.0 (0.9-1.2)	

a) Current pregnancies; b) Previous pregnancies; c) In the birth defects groups the Authors included also few non-malformed died infants and very low birth weight infants (< 1500 g)

A longitudinal study of quality of working life among computer users: Preliminary results [*]

P. Carayon

Department of Industrial Engineering, University of Wisconsin-Madison, 1513 University Avenue, Madison WI 53706, USA

This study examines the stability of the relationship between job design and quality of working life in a group of 113 computer users from one public service organization. Two rounds of questionnaire data was collected at two different times separated by 1 to 1.5 years. Results suggest that the relationship between job design and quality of working life is not stable over time. The job design factors that are related to quality of working life at round 1 include task control and frequency of computer-related problems, while at round 2, they include task control, skill variety and supervisor social support.

1. INTRODUCTION

The objective of this study is to examine the stability of the relationship between job design and quality of working life among computer users. This study builds on previous longitudinal research studies conducted by the author and her colleagues (Carayon, 1992a; Carayon et al., 1993). Most studies of quality of working life among computer users have been cross-sectional (see Carayon, 1993a, for a review of longitudinal studies of computer use). In a three-year longitudinal study of computer users, Carayon and her colleagues (Carayon, 1992a; Carayon et al., 1993) found that the relationship between job design and worker stress was not stable over time. The job design factors that were related to worker stress vary over time. At time 1, they were quantitative workload, work pressure and supervisor social support, while at time 2, they were task clarity, supervisor social support and job future ambiguity, and at time 3, they were task clarity, attention and job future ambiguity. Lindstrom et al. (1994) collected 3 rounds of data on a group of 33 employees from an insurance company. They found that the relationship between VDT characteristics, job demands and well-being was not constant over time. This study was designed to test the stability of the relationship between job design and quality of working life in a population similar to the one used in the previous studies conducted by Carayon and her colleagues.

---

[*] Funding for this study was provided by the National Science Foundation (No. IRI-9109566).

2. METHODS

2.1 Study design

Two rounds of data were collected from a group of 113 computer users of one public service organization. The two rounds of data collection were separated by 1-1.5 years. A total of 171 employees participated in the first round of questionnaire survey (response rate = 85%), while 129 employees participated in the second round of the survey (response rate = 64%). A total of 113 employees participated in both rounds of questionnaire survey and were used as the source of data for this study.

2.2 Sample

The study participants were all volunteers. Lists of employee names were provided by management. The criteria of inclusion on the list were: heavy computer usage and clerical job. They were mainly female (86%) and performed a range of clerical tasks (e.g., data entry, processing, and receptionist). The average age was 43 years (S.D.=9 years), the average tenure with the employer was 14 years (S.D.=8 years), and the average experience with one's current position was 6 years (S.D.=5 years). The average daily computer use was 7.2 hours per day (S.D.=1.8 hours).

2.3 Measurement

A questionnaire survey was designed that asks questions on a range of job design factors and quality of working life. The measures of job design used in this study included: quantitative workload (Caplan et al., 1975), task control (McLaney and Hurrell, 1988), skill variety (Sims et al., 1976), frequency of computer-related problems (Carayon-Sainfort, 1992), supervisor social support (Caplan et al., 1975) and colleague social support (Caplan et al., 1975). The measures of quality of working life included 3 measures of mood states, tension-anxiety, anger and fatigue (McNair et al., 1971), a measure of anxiety (Sainfort and Carayon, 1994) and a measure of job satisfaction (Quinn and Staines, 1979). Table 1 shows the basic statistics of the study variables. Paired t-tests were used to compare the round 1 data to the round 2 data for each of the variables, and yielded significant results for frequency of computer-related problems ($p<.01$) and supervisor social support ($p<.01$). Cronbach-alpha scores for both rounds were very similar and showed that the scales had adequate reliability (see table 1 for the Cronbach-alpha scores for round 1).

2.4 Statistical analyses

Various correlational analyses were performed to examine the stability of the relationship between job design and quality of working life. First, the stability of each measure was examined by computing the correlation between the round 1 measure and the round 2 measure. Second, cross-sectional correlations between job design and quality of working life were computed for each of the two rounds. The comparison of these correlations is an indication of the stability of the relationship between job design and quality of working life. Finally, regression analyses were performed to examine the concomitant effect of the job design factors on each of the measures of quality of working life at both rounds.

Table 1
Basic statistics of the study variables

	Mean (S.D.) Round 1	Mean (S.D.) Round 2	Cronbach Round 1	Pearson correl. R1/R2
JOB DESIGN				
quantit. workload	3.7 (0.6)	3.6 (0.6)	0.84	0.68
task control	2.7 (0.7)	2.8 (0.7)	0.73	0.59
skill variety	2.7 (0.9)	2.7 (0.9)	0.84	0.69
comput. probs.	2.5 (0.6)	2.2 (0.5)	0.70	0.45
superv. support	2.6 (0.9)	2.9 (0.8)	0.90	0.51
colleague support	2.9 (0.6)	2.9 (0.6)	0.74	0.51
QWL				
tension-anxiety	7.5 (5.1)	7.2 (5.0)	0.85	0.65
anger	5.5 (5.8)	6.3 (7.3)	0.91	0.59
fatigue	7.2 (6.1)	7.4 (5.7)	0.93	0.64
anxiety	1.7 (0.5)	1.7 (0.5)	0.83	0.70
job satisfaction	3.4 (1.1)	3.4 (1.1)	0.82	0.69

3. RESULTS

The Pearson correlations between the two rounds for each of the measures are displayed in table 1 (last column). All these correlations are significant at the 0.001 level. This analysis shows that the study variables, except frequency of computer problems, are quite stable from round 1 to round 2.

Table 2
Pearson correlations between job design and quality of working life (QWL)

QWL		quantit. workload	task control	skill variety	comput. probs.	superv. support	colleague support
tension-	R1	.13	-.21*	-.13	.26**	-.08	-.10
anxiety	R2	.11	-.20*	-.22*	.18	-.25**	-.10
anger	R1	.09	-.15	-.09	.25*	-.15	-.12
	R2	.06	-.16	-.23*	.04	-.39***	-.15
fatigue	R1	.19*	-.15	-.16	.20*	-.11	.05
	R2	.15	-.12	-.21*	.17	-.29**	-.17
anxiety	R1	.18	-.18	-.07	.22*	-.05	-.13
	R2	.17	-.12	-.14	.21*	-.11	-.05
job	R1	-.12	.21*	.21*	-.10	.27**	.09
satisfaction	R2	-.08	.26**	.33***	-.07	.37***	.03

* p<.05, ** p<.01, *** p<.001

Table 2 shows the correlations between job design and quality of working life for each of the two rounds. In both rounds, quantitative workload and colleague social support were not related to quality of working life, task control was related to tension-anxiety and job satisfaction, and computer-related problems was related to anxiety. However, there were also differences between the two rounds. Computer-related problems was related to tension-anxiety, anger, and fatigue in round 1, but not in round 2. On the other hand, skill variety and supervisor social support were related to these same measures in round 2, but not in round 1. The correlations for job satisfaction were stable between the two rounds. Skill variety and supervisor social support were both related to job satisfaction in both rounds, while quantitative workload, computer-related problems and colleague support were not.

Table 3 shows the results of the regression analyses. Table 3 reports the adjusted R^2 for each of the regression analyses. The job design factors did not explain a significant amount of the variance of tension-anxiety at both rounds, of anger at round 1, and of anxiety at round 2. At round 1, increased quantitative workload was related to increased fatigue, and increased task control was related to decreased anxiety. At round 2, increased support from one's supervisor was related to decreased anger, and increased skill variety was related to decreased fatigue. The results of the regression analysis of job satisfaction were consistent between round 1 and round 2. Job design factors explained a significant amount of variance of job satisfaction (12% at round 1 and 18% at round 2). Both skill variety and supervisor social support were significant predictors of job satisfaction at both rounds.

Table 3
Regression analyses of quality of working life

QWL	ROUND 1	ROUND 2
tension-anxiety	adj. R^2=5%, n.s.	adj. R^2=6%, n.s.
anger	adj. R^2=5%, n.s.	adj. R^2=13% ** superv. social support: beta=-0.30 **
fatigue	adj. R^2=11% * quantit. workload: beta=0.34 **	adj. R^2=9% * skill variety: beta=-0.26 *
anxiety	adj. R^2=12% * task control: beta=-0.29 **	adj. R^2=1%, n.s.
job satisfaction	adj. R^2=12% * skill variety: beta=0.25 * superv. social support: beta=0.23 *	adj. R^2=18% *** skill variety: beta=0.27 * superv. social support: beta=0.22 *

Note: the table shows only the independent variables (i.e. job design factors) that are statistically significant predictors of the measures of quality of working life.

4. DISCUSSION

The results of this study confirm results of previous longitudinal studies (Carayon, 1992a; Carayon et al., 1993; Lindstrom et al., 1994). First, the measures of job design and quality of working life are relatively stable over time. The cross-lagged correlations vary from 0.45 to 0.69 for job design, and from 0.59 to 0.70 for quality of working life. Second, the relationship between job design and quality of working life varies over time. The job design factors that are correlated to quality of working life in round 1 are not the same in round 2. This is true for all measures of quality of working life, except job satisfaction. In round 1, the major determinants of quality of working life are task control and computer-related problems, while in round 2 they are task control, skill variety and supervisor social support. It is possible that frequency of computer-related problems was a major determinant of quality of working life at round 1, but not at round 2, because of the greater significance of the problem at round 1. Actually, the paired t-test shows that employees report more computer-related problems at round 1 than at round 2.

The results of the correlational and regression analyses show that the only consistent relationship is between job satisfaction and the job design factors. Both skill variety and supervisor social support were significant predictors of job satisfaction at rounds 1 and 2. The relationship between the other measures of quality of working life (tension-anxiety, anger, fatigue and anxiety) and job design factors is not stable over time.

The results of this study and previous studies (Carayon, 1992a; Carayon et al., 1993; Lindstrom et al., 1994) confirm that results of cross-sectional studies may not be reliable because the job design factors that influence quality of working life may vary over time. Therefore, it is important to understand the temporal dimensions of the dynamic relationship between people and work (Carayon, 1993a, 1993b). Various temporal dimensions of the relationship between people and work have been studied. For instance, Carayon (1992b) examines the "chronic" effects of three job stressors, lack of job control, lack of supervisor social support and work pressure, on various measures of stress in a group of office workers. In this longitudinal study, both the strength and duration of the stressors were examined. Job control and supervisor social support were both found to have a "chronic" effect on stress. Other temporal dimensions of the relationship between people and work have been suggested by Carayon (1993a, 1993b) and Frese and Zapf (1988).

Furthermore, it is important to study the effect of multiple job design factors and their interactions on multiple quality of working life responses. Most studies of job design and quality of working life have examined "simple" linear relationships between the independent variables and the dependent variables. Carayon (1994) has found that certain jobs tend to have an "accumulation" of job stressors, while other jobs have a more "balanced" set of characteristics. The lack of over-time stability of the relationship between job design and quality of working life found in this study of computer users may be due to the fact that "simple" linear relationships were tested. Therefore, other models need to be developed to capture the multitude of job design factors that can potentially affect people. The Balance Theory of Smith and Carayon-Sainfort (1989) is such a model.

REFERENCES

Caplan, R.D., Cobb, S., French, J.R.P. Jr., Van Harrison, R. and Pinneau, S.R. Jr. (1975). Job Demands and Worker Health. U.S. DHEW, NIOSH, Washington, D.C..

Carayon, P. (1992a). A longitudinal study of job design and worker strain: Preliminary results. In J.C. Quick, L.R. Murphy and J.J. Hurrell Jr. (Eds.) Stress and Well-Being at Work: Assessments and Interventions for Occupational Mental Health, APA, Washington, D.C., pp.19-32.

Carayon, P. (1992b). Chronic effect of job control, work pressure and supervisor social support on office worker stress. APA/NIOSH Conference on Occupational Stress, Washington, D.C., (to be published in Job Stress 2,000: Emergent Issues).

Carayon-Sainfort, P. (1992). The use of computer in offices: Impact on task characteristics and worker stress. The International Journal of Human-Computer Interaction, 4(3): 245-261.

Carayon, P. (1993a). Longitudinal studies of job design and VDT use: Overview and synthesis. In H. Luczak, A.E. Cakir and G. Cakir (Eds.) Work With Display Units 92, North-Holland, Amsterdam, The Netherlands, pp.390-394.

Carayon, P. (1993b). Automation and the design of work: Stress problems and research needs. Workshop on Stress in New Occupations, Tilburg University, The Netherlands.

Carayon, P. (1994). Stressful jobs and non-stressful jobs: A cluster analysis of office jobs. Ergonomics, 37(2): 311-323.

Carayon, P., Yang, C.-L. and Lim, S.-Y. (1993). Examining the relationship between job design and worker strain over time: A longitudinal study of office workers. to be published in Ergonomics.

Frese, M. and Zapf, D. (1989). Methodological issues in the study of work stress: Objective vs subjective measurement of work stress and the question of longitudinal studies. In Causes, Coping and Consequences of Stress at Work, edited by C.L. Cooper and R. Payne, John Wiley & Sons, New York, pp.375-411.

Lindstrom, K., Leino, T., Puhakainen, M. and Torstila, I. (1994). Follow-up of job stress and its relation to characteristics of VDT user among insurance employees. In A. Grieco, G. Molteni, E. Occhipinti and B. Piccoli (Eds.) Fourth International Scientific Conference - WWDU'94 - Book of Short Papers, volume 1, pp.F17-F18.

McLaney, M.A. and Hurrell, J.J. Jr. (1988). Control, stress, and job satisfaction in Canadian nurses. Work and Stress, 2(3): 217-224.

McNair, D.M., Lorr, M. and Droppleman, L.F. (1971). EITS Manual for the Profile of Mood States. Educational and Industrial Testing Service, San Diego, CA.

Quinn, R., Seashore, S., Kahn, R., Mangione, T., Campbell, D., Staines, G. and McCullough, M. (1971). Survey of Working Conditions: Final Report on Univariate and Bivariate Tables. U.S. Govt. Printing Office, Washington, D.C.

Sainfort, F. and Carayon, P. (1994). Self-assessment of VDT operator health: Validity analysis of a health checklist. International Journal of Human-Computer Interaction, 6(3): 235-252.

Sims, H.P., Szilagyi, A.D. and Keller, R.T. (1976). The measurement of job characteristics. Academy of Management Journal, 19: 195-212.

Smith, M.J. and Carayon-Sainfort, P. (1989). A balance theory of job design for stress reduction. International Journal of Industrial Ergonomics, 4: 67-79.

Follow-up of job stress and its relation to characteristics of VDT use among insurance employees

K. Lindström[a], T. Leino[a], M. Puhakainen[b] and I. Torstila[b]

[a]Department of Psychology, Finnish Insitute of Occupational Health, Topeliuksenkatu 41 a A, FIN-00250 Helsinki, Finland

[b]Pohjola Insurance Company, Lapinmäentie 1, FIN-00300 Helsinki, Finland

1. OBJECTIVES

In the mid-1980s a new integrated and flexible data system for handling life insurance policies was implemented in a Finnish Insurance Company. We had an opportunity to follow this technical, social and individual change process. The first stage of this longitudinal study was conducted before the implementation of the more advanced system; the second phase took place one year after the transition, and the third one six years later. Follow-up studies of this kind are rare, however [3]. In cross-sectional studies, the problems associated with the functioning of new data systems and a great amount of daily VDT work have been found to be associated with psychic and somatic strain symptoms [1-2]. The preliminary analysis of office and customer service employees in this follow-up indicated qualitative differences between the study phases, but the effects of selection were difficult to control [4].

The objective of the study was to follow up a group of employees in an insurance company and see how the characteristics of VDT use, job demands and stressors, as well as the well-being of employees changed during a seven-year period. Special attention was paid to how the characteristics of VDT work were related to job demands and stressors and to indicators of well-being at three consecutive time points.

2. SUBJECTS AND METHODS

The study group consisted of employees from the head office and branch offices of a Finnish insurance company. 146 employees, both men and women, participated in all of the three questionnaire surveys, and their results are reported here. Their mean age was 38.0 years (sd 7.7) in 1985, 39.9 (sd 7.7) in 1987 and 45.2 (sd 7.7) in 1993. 2/3 were women and 1/3 men. In the first study phase 30% were in customer service and office work, 12% were supervisors and managers and 15% marketing personnel, and the rest were in other occupations. During the follow-up, the distinction between customer service and other office employees was no longer so clear, because nearly all employees had direct contacts with customers.

The method applied was a structured questionnaire including questions about the characteristics of VDT work, cognitive and social work demands, sensory and motor work demands, and psychological strain symptoms and job satisfaction [2].

3. RESULTS

During the follow-up, the total amount of time spent daily in VDT work has increased gradually. In 1985 27% of the respondents did more than four hours of VDT work daily, and in 1993 the percentage was 47%. The access to VDT or to certain applications affecting the scheduling of work was a problem rather or very often for 10% in 1993, as compared to 11% and 6% in the two earlier study phases. The breakdowns and slow response times of the data system were a problem rather or very often for 27% in 1985 but only for 15% in 1993. The mastery of the used VDT application was clearly better in 1993 than in the two earlier study phases.

Table 1
Job stressors and mental work load in 1985, 1987 and 1993. % of employees who perceived it rather or very often (n=146)

	1985 %	1987 %	1993 %
Haste at work	63	72	51
Poor coworker relations	13	8	9
Poor supervisory practices	12	6	11
Low content variety of work	6	3	1
Mental work load, overall	50	64	49

Haste at work and the overall perception of mental work load were maximal after the implementation of the new data system in 1987, but decreased gradually (Table 1). The variety in job content increased continuously, and the content was not perceived as monotonous in the last study phase. The interpersonal relations between coworkers had improved. The social and cognitive job demands as well as sensory and motor demands remain high and quite stable during the follow-up.

Job satisfaction was better in the last study phase than in the first. 8% were dissatisfied in the first phase, but only 3% reported dissatisfaction in the last study phase. The reported excessive fatigue decreased also (Table 2).

Table 2
Job dissatisfaction, strain symptoms and difficulties to cope with job demands

	1985 %	1987 %	1993 %
Job dissatisfaction	8	9	3
Excessive fatigue	33	23	19
Nervousness	8	12	4
Lack of competence	13	6	10
Difficulties to cope with job demands	-[1]	28	28

[1] data lacking

The relationships between VDT characteristics and job demands and well-being were the most interesting.

The high amount of daily VDT work related to high sensory and motor job demands at all three time points, but to low social and cognitive demands especially just after the major change in the data system, but not after the long-term follow-up (Table 3). This might indicate that the use of the new advanced system itself is more flexible, but that VDT use in itself demands better finger dexterity and vision. This can be due to the higher age of the employees too. The high daily amount of VDT work was related to low content variety in the job.

The disturbances and problems related to VDT use were also related to job demands and stress. The breakdowns and slow response times of VDT use were related to high sensory and motor demands at each phase of assessment. However, the scheduling of work dependent on access to VDT or to data system was no longer related to high sensory and motor demands after the long-term follow-up (Table 4). The disturbances and problems related to VDT work were only very slightly correlated to job stressors or strain after the major change in VDT systems in 1987.

Table 3
Relationships of amount of VDT use to job demands and stressors, and well-being in 1985, 1987 and 1993. Pearsons' r.

	Amount of daily VDT work		
	1985	1987	1993
Social and cognitive job demands			
- good memory		.22**	
- independent decisions	-.34***	-.31***	
- rapid decision making	-.22***	-.20*	
- reasoning			
- initiativeness			
- getting along with clients		-.22*	
- organizing ability		-.24**	
Sensory and motor job demands			
- specific precision	.36***	.27**	.48***
- specific concentration			.25**
- finger dexterity	.44***	.51***	.52***
- good eye sight	.44***	.42***	.47***
- good concentration	.27**		.33***
Job stressors			
- haste at work			
- poor coworker relations			
- poor supervisory practices			
- lack of content variety	.23**		.32**
- mental work load		-.17*	-.20*
Well-being			
- job dissatisfaction			
- excessive fatigue			
- nervousness			
- lack of competence	-.26**	-.19*	
- difficulties to cope with job demands			

* $p<0.05$, ** $p<0.01$, *** $p<0.001$

Table 4
Relationships of disturbances in VDT use to job demands in 1985, 1987 and 1993. Pearson's r.

	Breakdowns and slow response times			Scheduling of work dependent on		
	1985	1987	1993	1985	1987	1993
Social and cognitive job demands						
- good memory			-.21**			
- independent decisions						
- rapid decision making	.17*	.20*				
- reasoning			-.19*			-.22**
- initiativeness						
- getting along with clients				.18*	.33***	
- organizing ability						
Sensory and motor job demands						
- specific precision	-.28***		-.32***	-.36***		-.19*
- specific concentration			-.21*	-.24**		
- finger dexterity	-.26**	-.31***	-.20*	-.38***	-.23**	
- good eye sight	-.29***	-.41***	-.18*	-.33***	-.28***	
- good concentration	-.29***		-.22**	-.17*		-.16*

* p<0.05, ** p<0.01, *** p<0.001

4. DISCUSSION

During the follow-up in 1985-93, the amount of daily VDT work increased gradually and breakdowns and slow response times decreased, whereas the cognitive and social demands as well as sensory and motor demands remained stable. Time pressure and mental work load were highest just after the implementation of the new data systems in 1987.

The amount of VDT use, both before and after the major change in the data system, was related to low cognitive demands and high sensory and motor demands. In the long-term follow-up, only high sensory and motor demands were related to the amount of VDT work. Before the major changes, both breakdowns and dependence of work on VDT functioning were related to high sensory and motor demands, but in the follow-up only the breakdowns were related to these demands. Perhaps it has become an irrelevant problem as the VDT systems applied have advanced.

Because the follow-up period was quite long, other simultaneous changes, such as the redesign of jobs and reorganization of units occurred. The results from the third study phase illustrate the situation when the VDT applications used were numerous, and their mastery was already good. The selection that had taken place in the study group implied that those who had participated in all three study phases were probably the ones with originally better working and adaptation capacity.

REFERENCES

1 G. Aronson, Work content, stress and health in computer-mediated work. A seven-year follow-up study. Proceedings of the International Scientific Conference on Work with Display Units. National Board of Occupational Safety and Health, Stockholm 1986, 401-404.
2 K. Lindström, Well-Being and Computer-Mediated Work of Various Occupational Groups in Banking and Insurance. International Journal of Human-Computer Interaction 3 (1991) 339-361.
3 K. Lindström, Finnish Longitudinal Studies of Job Design and VDT work. In: Human-Computer Interaction: Applications and Case Studies. Ed. by M.J. Smith & G. Salvendy. Elsevier, New York, 1993, 697-702.
4 K. Lindström, T. Leino and M. Puhakainen, Follow-up of job demands and strain symptoms after implementation of new VDT applications in an insurance company. In: Human-Computer Interaction: Applications and Case Studies. Ed. by M.J. Smith & G. Salvendy. Elsevier, New York, 1993, 1005-1010.

Gender and Computing: Is change occurring?

A. Durndell and P. Lightbody

Dept. of Psychology, Glasgow Caledonian University, Cowcaddens Road, Glasgow G4 0BA, Scotland.

1. ABSTRACT

Targetted 16-18 year olds in 1992 were compared to similar groups in 1989 and 1986. Reported use of computers, knowledge about IT and reasons for not studying computing were assessed. Reported use of computers in school had risen to a non gender differentiated high level. However, reported domestic use of computers remained highly gendered, with males retaining a higher level of use of their own computers. Social computing appeared to be still a male oriented phenomenon. Knowledge about IT concepts had not increased over the last 3 years, nor had males apparently lost their advantage over females in this knowledge. Analysis, both open ended and statistical, of responses to questions about choosing not to study computing indicated a considerable stability over time. Working extensively with a computer was not attractive to most of these students. It is concluded that gender related changes over time in the UK are occurring but are limited.

2. INTRODUCTION

Durndell [1] reported on a study which compared the responses of a targetted group of natural science and business studies students to a number of questions about their experience of computers, knowledge about IT (Information Technology) and reasons for their choice of study subject. Overall both knowledge about IT and reported use of computers increased between 1986 and 1989, but males retained an advantage in knowledge over females and in general reported more use of computers than females. Both males and females when answering questions about their choice of subject produced rather negative views about computer specialists.

It was decided to follow up this study in 1992, extending the comparison period from 3 to 6 years, using the same defined subject group and the same data collection method to facilitate comparisons. Would knowledge about IT and reported use of computers continue to increase over time, would males continue to have an advantage in both these areas, and would reported factors in course choice remain similar over time?

3. METHOD

The method of Durndell [1] was followed. All samples comprised students enrolling for their first year at a Scottish university. They were targetted because they had selected to study business or natural science degree subjects and would provide reasonable numbers of male and female students who might be qualified to study computing under the Scottish system. 16-18 year olds were extracted from the samples so that recent school leavers were identified. This yielded 52 males and 85 females in 1986, 53 males and 105 females in 1989, and 50 males and 84 females in 1992.

All subjects in 1986, 1989, and 1992 were presented with a questionnaire as part of their enrolment programme, administered in a group situation by a researcher who was not to be one of their tutors. A promise of confidentiality was given and an assurance that this was a research exercise and that no information on an individual would be passed on to the course organiser. Filling in the questionnaire took about a half an hour.

The questionnaire used in 1992 was the same as that used in 1989. This initially requested background information on age and sex, and asked an open ended question - 'why did you choose to study on this course?', followed by a request that subjects write in their answer on the front page. Page 2 consisted of an IT quiz. Respondents were asked to match 12 items (such as 'bit', 'cursor', 'ROM', 'modem', 'word processor') with the appropriate definitions out of 17 presented (such as 'the physical devices which comprise a computer', 'a method of logging incoming data', 'a device used to interface a digital computer to a telephone line' 'a distinctive marker moving on a video screen indicating the next point at which a symbol can be entered', 'a basic unit of data as handled internally by a computer', etc.). The first example was completed in advance, and the respondents were invited to omit items that they could not answer.

On the third page of the questionnaire respondents were asked whether they had ever considered studying a course comprising mainly of computer studies, and then presented with a subsequent open ended question 'if yes, why are you not intending to study computer studies now?', or 'if no, why do you think that you never considered this?'.

After allowing space for the above answer, respondents were asked various questions about their use and experience of computers in the last two years. Finally on page 4 they were presented with a 5 point scale going from 1 - of no importance to me - through to 5 - very important to me. They were then asked how important to them were a series of items in their decision not to study computing, each item to be evaluated for themselves using the 5 point scale.

4. RESULTS

4.1 Reported use of computers and the IT quiz:

Data for 1986, 1989 and 1992, by gender, are shown in tables 1 and 2. χ^2 analysis was carried out on the reported use data for 1992 (the analysis of the 1986 and 1989 data was reported in [1]). In 1992 males reported significantly more use than females of their own computer ($\chi^2 = 18.3$, p<.001) and of a friend's computer ($\chi^2 = 15.49$, p<.001). In addition the responses for each reported use were compared over time. Analyses were done for males and females together, for females alone and for males alone. Total reported use of a computer at school increased significantly over time, ($\chi^2 = 28.10$, p<.001), with both the female increase ($\chi^2 = 13.60$, p<.01) and the male increase ($\chi^2 = 14.47$, p<.001) being significant. Total reported use of a family computer increased significantly over time, ($\chi^2 = 13.53$, p<.01), the female increase being non significant, whilst the male increase was significant ($\chi^2 = 14.86$, p<.001). Total reported use of a friends computer varied in an unclear fashion over time, ($\chi^2 = 7.26$, p<.05), with the female decrease significant ($\chi^2 = 6.56$, p<.05). Total reported use of ones own computer increased significantly over time ($\chi^2 = 18.13$, p<.001), with only the male increase being significant ($\chi^2 = 15.18$, p<.001). Anova of the IT quiz data for 1992 by gender and course type (the 1986 and 1989 results were reported in [1]) produced a significant male advantage (f = 43.83, p<.01).

Table 1
% reporting experience of computing in previous two years, 16-18 year old university entrants, by gender and year of intake

	1986			1989			1992		
	M	F	total	M	F	total	M	F	total
used computer at school	42	52	48	67	61	63	80	80	80
used own computer	24*	9*	14	49*	18*	29	61*	22*	37
used family computer	24	29	27	26	38	34	58	46	50
used friend's computer	65*	46*	53	50*	31*	38	66*	29*	43

* Gender difference p< 0.05, M=male, F=female

Table 2
IT quiz score, 16-18 year old university entrants, by gender and year of intake

	Female mean	Male mean	Male-female difference
1986	2.54*	4.60*	2.06
1989	4.10*	6.02*	1.92
1992	4.06*	5.77*	1.71

* Gender difference p< 0.01

4.2 Open ended material concerning reasons for *not studying computing*:

These were categorised by an independent judge. Apart from comments about lack of interest in computing, two responses were volunteered at quite a high level: 20% of respondents wrote that they had insufficient experience to choose to follow a computer based course, and 18% commented that computing courses were too specialised and narrow vis a vis future careers. Individual comments included 'I would rather work with people than a monitor', 'I don't envisage myself sitting in front of a computer all day', and 'I don't fancy the idea of staring at a screen for the rest of my life'.

4.3 Statistical results of suggested items in student choice not to study computer studies:

Full details are available in [2]. These results were only available for 1989 and 1992. The 4 most important items were *I do not want to be sitting in front of a terminal all day; the subject matter would not be interesting; I am more interested in people than objects; I don't mind using computers, but they are not an end in themselves to me.* The four least important items were *males can be hostile to females with abilities in computing; I was advised not to study computing; the prospect of being in nearly all male groups is offputting; computing has a rather unfeminine image.*

Each item was individually analysed by Anova for gender and year of testing. The following items produced significant results: Females gave more importance than males to '*I am not qualified to study computing*', f = 3.94, p<.05, ' *I would have difficulty getting a job with a computer qualification*', f = 6.97, p<.01, '*I don't mind using computers but they are not an end in themselves to me*', f = 4.12, p<.05, and '*computing has a rather unfeminine image*', f = 5.93, p<.05. Males gave significantly more weight than females to '*the prospect of being in nearly all male groups is offputting*', f = 14.86, p<.001. Only one year of testing result was significant, with the 1992 sample giving more importance to '*I am not qualified to study computing*', f = 4.72, p<.05 (in fact thay all were qualified to study computing). Whether the subjects had considered studying computing or not produced no significant effects.

Reference to [2] shows that even when the results were significant, the size of the effects were very small.

5. DISCUSSION

The data presented here do show evidence of some change over time. Reported use of computers by recent school leavers continued in general to increase over time and reported computer use in school had become very high, with no gender differentiation. However the comments indicated that the frequency of this use may be rather limited, although this would be an improvement on the reports in the past which were often of no use at all. Reported use of a family computer also tended to have increased over time, with little consistent gender differentiation. On the other hand, reported ownership of computers continued to increase, but mainly as a male phenomenon, whilst reported social computing with a friend showed an unclear general trend, but a gender difference was retained with female use of this sort gently declining.

Instead of increasing, IT knowledge has plateauxed according to the measure used here. It was tempting to alter the test to update it, but then the comparative aspect of the study would be lost. The gender effect, with males outscoring females, remained however, even if it declined slightly in absolute terms.

The reasons given for choosing not to study computing have remained very consistent over time, and have also remained very little gender differentiated. The student perception is still of a computer specialist hunched over their terminal all day having little contact with human beings and restricted in their future career patterns. Whether this is a realistic stereotype or not, it is not something that is attractive to these students. Their comments also seemed to imply that many of them, whilst having at least some contact with computers in their last two years at school, still experienced this contact as too limited to give a realistic appreciation of what computing would require. Thus the next problem having ensured almost complete computer contact at school is to make this contact more substantial and meaningful, which of course requires investment in computers and teacher training. It was also notable that one of the few items to produce a significant gender effect whenever investigated [3] [1] was the finding that the prospect of being in nearly all male groups was always more offputting for males than for females, the converse of what might be predicted if fear of male domination was an important feature for females.

Returning to the questions posed in the introduction, in summary knowledge about IT has not increased further since 1989, reported use of computers has continued to increase, and males have retained an advantage in both areas. The perception of computing revealed in investigating the choice not to study computing has remained constant and non gendered.

It would be unrealistic to expect the same trends to be visible throughout the world, and studies in S. E. Asia have shown females to be in the majority in some undergraduate computing courses [4] [5]. In the U.S.A. there is some evidence that the female percentage of enrolments in computing courses peaked in the late 1980's and is now dropping, with the same happening in engineering [6] [7]. The position in the U.K. is uncertain. Archer [8] was optimistic in arguing that he had evidence that gender stereotyping in course choice in schools was decreasing. He thought that the newly introduced National Curriculum would decrease gender stereotyping of courses in the longer term. However, the technology component of the National Curriculum, which includes computing, has been subject to much debate and is likely to be revised. The University entrance figures in Britain for the percentage of computing students that are female, 13% in 1991, has also recently increased slightly from a very low base [9]. On the other hand the present study fits with Shotton's [10] data from the mid 1980's about the male dominance of computer purchases, and Provenzo's [11] semi academic discussion of the male orientation of the very popular computer game market. Neither of these sources provide evidence of increased female participation in computing. Robertson and Stark [12] also failed to find evidence of a reduction in subject stereotyping at school in Scotland over the last 10 years, using government figures. Finally there are researchers who question the necessary attractiveness of computing as presently conceived as a career for women [13].

Overall, the results of the present study and related work in Britain would seem to point to a small and limited change over time in female as compared with male involvement with computing, with very slightly greater female participation developing.

Finally, this paper is intended to report changes over time, rather than to offer any particular theoretical insights. However, the results do seem to be compatible with a number of contemporary ideas: Computing has become linked in Britain to physics and engineering to be part of a male oriented domain concerned with machines rather than with living things (see [14] for a contemporary feminist analysis of this). Bem [15] has described her idea of a gender polarisation lens, which is a process which amplifies any small gender variations by culturally stereotyping certain behaviours as suitable for males or females. This seems a powerful idea in the gender and computing arena. Many of the polarisation effects appear to be most marked in the early teens [16] when the most marked gender variations in attitudes towards and use of computers are often found. This also leads to the classic 'we can I can't' (eg [17]) formulation, or perhaps rather to the 'we can I do not want to' [18] version of it: Teenage females believe that females in general can cope with computers, but most individual teenage females also choose themselves not to spend much time with computers, perhaps for good reasons [13].

REFERENCES

1. A. Durndell, 'The persistence of the gender gap in computing.' *Computers and Education,* **16** (1991), 283-287.
2. A. Durndell and P. Lightbody, 'Gender and Computing: Change over time?' *Computers and Education*, **21** (1993), 331-336.
3. A. Durndell, 'Why do female students avoid computer studies?' *Research in Science and Technological Education*, **8** (1990), 163-170.
4. L. Kheng, 'The Singaporean way'. *Computer Bulletin*, 2 (1990), 18-21.
5. G. Lim & M. Wang, 'A study of academic performance of male and female students on a computer studies course.' In L. Rennie, L. Parker & G. Hildebrand (Eds.), *Action For Equity: The Second Decade, Volume 2: Beyond Schooling*, Perth, Australia, National Key Centre for School Science and Maths, Curtin University of Technology, 1991.
6. L. Moses, 'The status of women in computing: The USA.' In B. Bank, H. Buxton et al, *Teaching Computing: Context and Method*, Keele, England, WIC/Dept Computer Science, Keele University, 1992.
7. R. Carter and G. Kirkup, 'Why do we still have so few women engineers in Europe and the U.S.A.?' In A. Alting, M. Brand et al (Eds.), *GASAT 92: East and West European Conference,* GASAT/Eindhoven Technical University, Eindhoven, Holland, 1992.
8. J. Archer, 'Gender stereotyping of school subjects.' *The Psychologist*, **15** (1992), 66-69.
9. UCCA, *29th Annual Report 1990/1991*. Cheltenham, England, UCCA, 1992.
10. M. Shotton, *Computer Addiction: a study of computer dependency.* London, Taylor and Francis, 1989.
11. E. Provenzo, *Video Kids: Making Sense of Nintendo*. Cambridge, Mass., USA, Harvard University Press, 1991.
12. I. Robertson & R. Stark, 'Performance in science: Is gender an issue?' paper presented to *Scottish Educational Research Association*, University of Dundee, 1992. Manuscript (in press) available from the authors at Jordanhill College of Education, Glasgow, Scotland.
13. P. Newton, 'Computing: An ideal occupation for Women?' in J. Firth- Cozens & M. West (Eds.), *Women at Work,* Milton Keynes, England, Open University Press, 1991.
14. G. Kirkup & L. Keller (Eds), *Inventing Women: Science, Gender and Technology*. London, Polity Press, 1992.
15. S. Bem, *The Lenses of Gender*, New Haven, Yale University Press, 1993.
16 A. Durndell, P. Glissov & G. Siann, 'Gender and computing: Persisting differences.' *Educational Research*, in press.
17. V. Makrakis, 'Gender and computing in schools in Japan: The we can I can't paradox.' *Computers and Education*, **20** (1993), 191-198.
18. P. Lightbody & A. Durndell, 'Senior school pupils' career aspirations: Is gender an issue?' *Proceedings of the British Psychological Society*, **2** (1994), 51.

Psychosocial Work Factors and Upper Extremity Musculoskeletal Discomfort Among Office Workers

Soo-Yee Lim* and Pascale Carayon[a]

[a] Department of Industrial Engineering, University of Wisconsin-Madison, 1513 University Avenue, Madison, WI 53706 U.S.A.

1. INTRODUCTION

In the last decade, research studies have shown the importance of musculoskeletal problems among office workers (Smith et al., 1992; NIOSH, 1989; and Smith et al., 1981). This raises some concerns on the characteristics of office work environment and its impact on workers' health. The majority of research studies on musculoskeletal health have been conducted in the industrial/manufacturing environment with a specific focus on ergonomic risk factors such as repetition, posture, and force (see for example, Silverstein et al., 1986 and 1987). In addition to the role of ergonomic factors, there is evidence that psychosocial work factors can also contribute to the development of musculoskeletal health problems.

1.1 The role of psychosocial work factors

An extensive review of literature conducted by Bongers et al. (1993) showed that the role of psychosocial work factors in cumulative trauma disorders cannot be disregarded. Smith and Carayon (1993) proposed a model that depicts various mechanisms linking psychosocial work factors to musculoskeletal health problems. Research studies conducted by Lim and Carayon (1993, 1994) indicated that psychosocial work factors have indirect effects on musculoskeletal discomfort in a group of office workers. Thus, a multi-factorial perspective of the study of musculoskeletal health problems must be considered.

The purpose of this study is to further investigate the effects of psychosocial work factors on upper extremity musculoskeletal discomfort (UEMD) by integrating the roles of psychosocial work factors and ergonomic risk factors. Figure 1 shows the relationships among psychosocial work factors,

---

* National Institute of Occupational Safety and Health. 4676 Columbia Parkway MS C-24, Cincinnati, OH 45226 U.S.A. This work was conducted while the author was at University of Wisconsin-Madison.

ergonomic factors, and UEMD. The model shows that psychosocial work factors can be related to ergonomic risk factors which in turn can be related to UEMD.

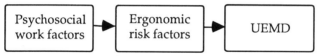

Figure 1. Relationships among psychosocial work factors, ergonomic factors, and upper extremity musculoskeletal discomfort

2. METHODS

The subjects of this field study came from an on-going longitudinal study of office automation. A total of 129 office workers who performed a wide range of office activities participated in the study. The majority of the study participants were female office workers (87%) and the average age was 44 years old (standard deviation (std. dev.) = 9.2 years). The average job tenure was 7.4 years (std. dev. = 5.5 years) and the average computer use was 7.1 hours per day (std. dev. = 1.7 hours).

2.1 Measures

A questionnaire survey was administered to gather information on psychosocial work factors, ergonomic risk factors, and worker health. The psychosocial work factors used in this study were work pressure, a 6-item scale, defined as the extent to which time is critical in getting work done, for example, a deadline to be met and the extent to which there is a backlog of work (Sainfort, 1990); task control, a 7-item scale, defined as the amount of control one has on the tasks performed (McLaney and Hurrell, 1987); and production standards/quotas, a single measure of having to meet a set production quota or standard.

The ergonomic measures were repetition, defined as repetitiveness of office duties or activities; postures, which included awkward work postures, a 3-item scale, defined as the extent to which one has to reach and/or twist to reach for work materials and the extent that one has to use awkward work motions; and dynamic work postures, a 4-item scale, defined as the extent to which one is able to move around at work and the extent that one has to work in a constrained work position for a period of time (Lim, 1994); and contact stress, which is defined as the extent to which one has to rest their wrist and forearm on the edge of a table and/or their elbow on the arm of a chair.

Self-reports of musculoskeletal discomfort of the upper extremity (neck, shoulder, elbow, and hand) were used in this study. The discomfort measures were very similar to those used in the NIOSH (1989) study. The discomfort score is a standardized score of the intensity, frequency, and duration of discomfort experienced for each of the upper extremity regions. Additionally, an index of the total musculoskeletal discomfort was used, which is the summation of the discomfort scores for the neck, shoulder, elbow, and hand.

3. RESULTS

Table 1 shows the results of the Pearson correlations and the regression analyses. Pearson correlation analyses showed that two psychosocial work factors, task control and production standard/quotas, were significantly correlated with repetition. Production standard/quotas was also significantly correlated with dynamic work postures, and work pressure is significantly correlated with awkward work postures. The correlation analyses of ergonomic factors and UEMD showed that repetition was significantly correlated with neck and total discomfort, while awkward work postures were significantly correlated with all of the discomfort outcomes (neck, shoulder, elbow, hand, and total discomfort); and dynamic work postures were significantly correlated with the neck, shoulder, and total discomfort. Only one measure of contact stress, the exposure to elbow contact stress, was significantly correlated with elbow discomfort.

Results of the regression analyses indicated that psychosocial work factors are related to ergonomic factors. Task control was negatively related to repetition: having more task control was related to less repetition. Production quotas/standards was significantly related to repetition and negatively related to dynamic work postures. An increase in production quotas/standards was related to more repetition and less ability to move around (i.e. dynamic work postures).

Regression results between the relationship of ergonomic factors and UEMD indicated that awkward working postures was a consistent predictor for all of the measures of upper extremity discomfort. Only one measure of contact stress, exposure to elbow contact stress, was significantly related to elbow discomfort.

Additional analyses were conducted to examine the direct effect of psychosocial work factors on UEMD. Pearson correlations indicated that psychosocial work factors were not significantly correlated with any of the UEMD outcomes. Demographic factors, such as age, gender, job tenure, and amount of computer use per day, were examined in relation to the UEMD outcomes. Only age was shown to be related to hand discomfort. Older employees tended to report more hand discomfort.

4. DISCUSSION AND CONCLUSION

This study showed that psychosocial work factors are related to upper extremity musculoskeletal discomfort via ergonomic factors. This suggests that psychosocial work factors have an indirect effect on upper extremity musculoskeletal discomfort. Findings of this study also suggested that psychosocial work factors can have an influence on ergonomic factors. For example, if one has more control on the task performed then he/she may experience less repetitive office activities or duties.

Table 1. Pearson correlations and regression results on psychosocial work factors, ergonomic risk factors, and upper extremity musculoskeletal discomfort.

	Ergonomic risk factors						Musculoskeletal discomfort				
	REPET	AWKP	DYNAP	WRISC	FOREC	ELBOC	NECK	SHOUL	ELBO	HAND	TOTAL
PRESS	r=0.01 b=-0.12	r=0.22* b=0.25	r=-0.12 b=0.03	r=0.05 b=-0.00	r=0.05 b=0.02	r=0.04 b=0.15	r=-0.00 b=-0.11	r=0.11 b=0.07	r=0.09 b=-0.05	r=0.00 b=-0.11	r=0.07 b=-0.07
TASKC	r=-0.28** b=-0.24**	r=-0.07 b=-0.08	r=0.16 b=0.10	r=0.14 b=0.17	r=0.05 b=0.00	r=0.01 b=-0.03	r=0.01 b=0.09	r=-0.02 b=-0.01	r=0.03 b=0.08	r=-0.00 b=0.06	r=0.02 b=0.14
QUOTA	r=0.21* b=0.22*	r=0.11 b=-0.06	r=-0.28** b=-0.27**	r=0.07 b=0.12	r=-0.04 b=0.08	r=-0.10 b=-0.19	r=0.07 b=0.05	r=0.05 b=-0.06	r=0.17 b=0.14	r=0.05 b=0.11	r=0.11 b=0.13
REPET							r=0.20* b=0.06	r=0.08 b=-0.03	r=0.12 b=0.04	r=0.14 b=0.01	r=0.18* b=0.02
AWKP							r=0.32*** b=0.27**	r=0.34*** b=0.30**	r=0.28** b=0.26**	r=0.31*** b=0.31**	r=0.41*** b=0.36***
DYNAP							r=-0.30** b=-0.17	r=-0.21* b=-0.13	r=-0.16 b=-0.03	r=-0.19 b=-0.06	r=-0.28** b=-0.15
WRISC										r=-0.02 b=-0.00	r=-0.10 b=-0.09
FOREC									r=-0.12 b=-0.01	r=-0.04 b=-0.05	r=-0.08 b=-0.11
ELBOC									r=-0.22* b=-0.18		r=-0.02 b=0.10
ADJ. R²	9%***	3% (p=0.07)	6%*	1%	1%	2%	12%***	9%**	8%*	6% (p=0.06)	17%***

*p<0.05   **p<0.01   ***p<0.001   r=correlation coefficient   b=beta coefficient
PRESS: Work pressure   TASKC: task control   QUOTA: production quotas/standards
REPET: repetition   AWKP: awkward work postures   DYNAP: dynamic work postures   WRISC: exposure to wrist contact stress
FOREC : exposure to forearm contact stress   ELBOC: exposure to elbow contact stress   SHOUL: shoulder discomfort   ELBO: elbow discomfort

The existence of the relationship found between psychosocial work factors and ergonomic factors suggests that the psychosocial work environment can either exacerbate or improve the ergonomic working conditions in the workplace. Thus, in addition to making ergonomic changes in the workplace to reduce musculoskeletal health problems, it is also important to look at aspects of the psychosocial work environment to reduce musculoskeletal health problems. From this study, psychosocial work factors, such as task control and production quotas/standards, are important elements to consider for the reduction of musculoskeletal discomfort. Both factors have an impact on repetition, while production standards/quotas also affects dynamic work postures. Additionally, awkward work postures is an important factor to consider since it is a significant and consistent predictor of all types of upper extremity musculoskeletal discomfort (neck, shoulder, elbow, hand, and total discomfort) examined. This shows that the way work is being organized can influence the ergonomic working conditions in the workplace.

This study proposed a mechanism linking psychosocial work factors and UEMD. Musculoskeletal health (cumulative trauma disorders or musculoskeletal discomfort) is a multi-factorial problem and a broader perspective must be adopted to study this issue. While it has been established in the literature that ergonomic factors, such as repetition, posture, and force, can contribute to the development of musculoskeletal problems, the characteristics of the psychosocial work environment that can contribute to the development of musculoskeletal health must also be recognized. Accordingly, the different mechanisms by which psychosocial work factors can be related to musculoskeletal health must be further explored.

4.1. Limitations and future research

Since this is a cross-sectional study with data being collected at one point in time, results of this study cannot imply any causal relationships. In addition, the small amount of variance explained in the study limits the generalization of results. The small percentages of variance explained between psychosocial work factors and ergonomic factors suggests that other psychosocial work factors may need to be considered.

The office work environment is different from the industrial working environment. Some of the traditional ergonomic risk factors that were found in previous research studies may not necessarily apply to office settings. For example, force may not be a major issue in office work especially for those who use a computer to conduct their work. It may also be possible that the kind of posture used may not be as "extreme" as what can be found in industry. Much research still needs to be conducted in the office work environment to validate traditional ergonomic risk factors in the office setting. In addition, the role of psychosocial work factors must be explored. Multiple psychosocial work factors should be considered.

REFERENCES

Bongers, P.M., Winter, C.R. de, Kompier, M.A.J., Hildebrandt, V.H. (1993). Psychosocial factors at work and musculoskeletal disease: a review of the literature. Scand J Work Environment Health, vol. 19, no. 5.

Lim, S.Y. and Carayon, P. (1993). An Integrated Approach to Cumulative Trauma Disorders in the Office Environment : The Role of Psychosocial Work Factors, Psychological Stress, and Ergonomic Risk Factors. In M.J. Smith and G. Salvendy (eds), Human-Computer Interaction : Applications and Case Studies, proceedings of the 5th International Conference on Human-Computer Interaction, Elsevier, pp. 880-885.

Lim, S.Y. and Carayon, P. (1994). Relationship between physical and psychosocial work factors and upper extremity symptoms in a group of office workers. Proceedings of the 12th Triaennial Congress, International Ergonomics Association Conference, vol. 6, pp. 132-134.

Lim, S.Y. (1994). An Integrated Approach to Cumulative Trauma Disorders in the Office Environment : The Role of Psychosocial Work Factors, Psychological Stress, and Ergonomic Risk Factors. Ph.D. Dissertation.

McLaney, M. A., and Hurrell, J.J. Jr. (1988). Control, stress, and job satisfaction in Canadian nurses. Work and Stress, 2(3), 217-224.

National Institute of Occupational Safety and Health (NIOSH) (1989). HETA 89-299-2230, US West Communictions (Phoenix, Arizona; Minneapolis, Minnesota; and Denver, Colorado). U.S. Department of Health and Human Services, Public Health Service, Centers for Disease Control, National Institute for Occupational Safety and Health.

Sainfort, P. C. (1990). Job design predictors of stress in automated offices. Behaviour and Information Technology, 9(1), 3-16.

Silerstein, B. A., Fine, L.J., and Armstrong, T.J. (1986). Hand wrist cumulative trauma disorders in industry. British Journal of Industrial Medicine, 43, 779-784.

Silerstein, B. A., Fine, L.J., and Armstrong, T.J. (1987). Occupational factors and carpal tunnel syndrome. American Journal of Industrial Medicine, 11, 343-358.

Smith, M. J., Cohen, B.G.F., Stammerjohn, L., and Happ, A. (1981). An investigation of health complaints and job stress in video display operations. Human Factors, 23, 389-400.

Smith, M. J., Carayon, P., Sanders, K.J., Lim, S-Y. and LeGrande, D. (1992). Employee stress and health complaints in jobs with and without electronic performance monitoring. Applied Ergonomics

Smith, M. J. and Carayon, P. (1993). Work Organization, stress, and cumulative trauma disorders. Presented at the conference on Psychosocial Influence in Office Work CTD. Duke University, Nov. 11-12, 1993. (To be published as a chapter in Psychosocial Aspects of Musculoskeletal Disorders in Office Work. Edited by S.L. Sauter and S.D. Moon).

Psychosocial and Physiological Effects of Reorganizing Data-Entry Work - a longitudinal study

C. Åborg (1,2), E. Fernström (1,3), M. O. Ericson (3)

1. Stiftelsen Statshälsan, Karlskrona, Sweden

2. Department of Human Work Science, Luleå University of Technology, Luleå, Sweden

3. Department of Environmental Technology and Work Science, Royal Institute of Technology, Stockholm, Sweden

1. INTRODUCTION

The consequences of computerization and visual display unit (VDU)-work vary among occupational groups. The data entry group reports more somatic and mental symptoms than other groups of users (1). The prevalence of neck- and- shoulder disorders is high among people working with repetitive VDU work . The occupational "low"- exposure risk factors for shoulder-neck complaints have been described as: monotonous work tasks, poor psychosocial work environment, high work/production intensity, lack of breaks and lack of alternative tasks offering a different exposure pattern during working hours (2). To decrease the level of symptoms work organization needs to be changed and job tasks redistributed.

2. OBJECTIVES

The project reported in this paper was designed to study the psychosocial and physical effects of the reorganization of data entry work at a public authority in Sweden.
The aims of the reorganization were to redistribute the repetitive data entry work, provide the staff with new tasks and increase the variety of the work. It was hoped that this would involve less risk of prolonged static work and of health problems.

3. MATERIAL AND METHODS

Our subjects were employed by a Swedish State authority. Their main work was computer entry of statistical data, and their neck- and- shoulder pain was severe.

We used questionnaires, individual interviews, diaries, video recordings, physiological measurements and physical examination to describe the subjects psychosocial and physiological states on two occasions - before and after the organisational change.

The entire personnel of the data processing unit (N=150) were asked to answer the questionnaires, before the start of the reorganization and 18 months later. The questions concerned physical and psychosocial work environment and mental and somatic health symptoms.

Twenty-two female VDU workers volunteered to take part in the entire study, and were followed for two years. They were examined with all the methods mentioned above, before the reorganization (1991). Eighteen months later (1992), 18 of them were still employed at the same authority.

Seventeen participated in the follow- up interview and 16 in the entire reexamination. One subject did not want to participate in 1992 and one could not, for medical reasons. The mean age of the final group (n=16) was 39.6 years, and mean length of employment was 9.8 years.

The interviews were semi-structured and concerned work content, work load, work development, influence, contact and collaboration. Upper- arm elevation was measured with the Abduflex inclinometer measuring device. Fixed to the upper arm, the Abduflex records upper- arm position in terms of angle intervals, seconds and percentage of measured time within each interval. Shoulder muscular activity was measured with surface amplitude EMG (ME3000) from the trapezius. The subjects wore a lightweight data collecting unit in a girdle belt, during a whole working day including lunch and breaks. They could move freely and perform their work without any risk of disturbing the measurements. The subjects activities were videotaped during the test days both in 1991 and in 1992.

They also kept a diary on three different days during three weeks, both in 1991 and in 1992, where they recorded the time they worked with a number of predetermined main tasks.

4. RESULTS

During the study period the data entry work was totally restructured. The data processing unit was closed down and the personnel transferred to a number of other units, most to groups dealing with more varied and qualified tasks. The interviews, diaries and video recordings show large individual differences in the effects of this restructuring on job content. Some subjects in the sub-group (n=17) perceived their new job as more qualified, interesting and satisfying, while others found it even more repetitive and boring than before. Most of the subjects wanted more demanding jobs and more chances to acquire new skills. They did not feel that they had been sufficiently involved in the change process. In 1992 the subjects still had data entry as their main task although the time spent on desk work without the computer had increased. They also changed work tasks more often in 1992 than in 1991. Still we found no change in the subjects neck- and- shoulder problems.

Mean trapezius muscle activity during the whole working day as well as during different tasks was analysed. For the subjects participating on both occasions, mean left shoulder muscular activity was 7.7 MVC in 1991 and 8.8 %MVC in 1992 (n=15). For the right shoulder it was 7.3 % MVC in 1991 and 6.8 %MVC in 1992 (n=16). The differences for the pairs are not statistically significant.

Concerning mean muscular activity measured in different work tasks, data entry required 7.2% MVC and 6% MVC in the left and right trapezius muscles respectively. The corresponding values for desk work were 9.1 and 9% MVC.

The mean values for upper-arm elevation were calculated for all the seven angle intervals. At the 30-degree level the left side elevation increased significantly from 1991 to 1992, while there was no statistical difference on the right side or at the 45-degree level.

For the total group(N=150) the results of the questionnaire study show only small changes in work satisfaction and health complaints. In 1991 the response rate was 86%, and in 1992 63%. In both years the results show high frequencies of psychological and psychosomatic complaints (30-43%) and of neck/shoulder complaints (1991:40% last week, 81% last year, and no significant change 1992). Both before and after the reorganization a majority of the subjects answering the questionnaires reported repetitive movements and constrained work postures. The number of subjects reporting lack of influence over work situation decreased from 57% 1991 to 44% 1992.

5. DISCUSSION

Work environment and health aspects were not stressed by the management, and therefore lost significance during the reorganization period.

Our subjects were transferred to new workinggroups, but most retained almost the same job content. The work changes did not seem to be far-reaching enough to influence the shoulder muscular load or the health complaints.

Many studies have shown a relation between upper-arm elevation and shoulder muscular load and also that working with raised arms implies a risk of neck- and-shoulder disorders. In Sweden it has been ruled that upper-arm elevation below 30° does not imply this risk. Although our subjects were working below 30 degrees of elevation, they still had neck- and-shoulder disorders and also relatively high whole-day mean muscular loads (7-8%). The mean level of muscular activity does not seem to be as important for the risk of muscular disorders as is the muscular variation in load, frequency and duration. The more dynamic the working technique, the less the neck/shoulder symptoms (3). Consequently, work should allow enough pauses and dynamic changes in muscular load. Work content and mix of tasks seem to be very important factors for the risk of musculoskeletal disorders.

The change in work organization studied was not great enough and did not focus enough on providing employees with variation in work load.

6. SCIENTIFIC AND PRACTICAL CONCLUSIONS

A systems approach, where the VDU is only one element, is needed in studies of reorganization of VDUwork. We need to follow the changes over a long period. Data entry work can be organized to avoid negative effects on quality of working life, such as: repetitive, boring work, lack of control of work situation, lack of social support, bad task design, constrained postures, eye strain, musculoskeletal strain. If work environmental aspects are not taken into account a reorganization may increase such negative effects.

A strategy for prevention should use both a "macro ergonomics" and a "micro ergonomics" approach. "Macro- ergonomics" as an overall systems approach to the design of organizations and work systems, and "micro-ergonomics" as an approach to the design of specific jobs and work- stations.

To improve health and satisfaction, as well as the effectiveness of work, by an organizational change, user-participation and an interested management are needed.

ACKNOWLEDGEMENT

Financial support was obtained from the Swedish Work Environment Fund.

REFERENCES

1. Åborg,C., Aronsson,G., Dallner,M.: Work organization and health aspects of work with VDU:s. In: Luczak, Cakir, Cakir (eds.): Work with display units -92, Elsevier Science Publishers, Amsterdam, 1993.

2. Winkel,J., Westgaard,R.: Occupational and individual risk factors for shoulder-neck complaints: Part 1 - Guidelines for the practitioner. International Journal of Industrial Ergonomics 1992:10:79-83.

3. Kilbom,Å., Persson,J., Jonsson,B.G.: Risk factors for work-related disorders of the neck and shoulder - with special emphasis on working postures and movements. In : Corlett, Wilson, Mahenica (eds) : The Ergonomics of Working Postures, Taylor & Francis, 1986.

Musculoskeletal disorders, working posture, psychosocial environment in female VDU operators and conventional office workers

D. Camerino, P. Lavano, M. Ferrario, G. Ferretti and G. Molteni

Ergonomics Research Unit, Institute of Occupational Health, University of Milan, Via S. Barnaba 8, 20122 Milan, Italy.

1. INTRODUCTION

Musculoskeletal disorders are very diffuse among sedentary workers; moreover, recent literature indicates a higher prevalence of spine disorders in VDU operators than in conventional office workers (1). The aetiology is not yet clear since task related factors and psychosocial conditions can both be taken into consideration.

Aims of the present study are to compare prevalence of cervical and lumbar spine disorders in VDU operators and conventional office workers with a gender- and age-specific control group, and to investigate the relationships between self-reported spine disorders and working or psychosocial conditions.

2. METHODS

2.1 Subjects and workplaces

A sample of 106 female office workers (47 VDU operators and 59 conventional office workers) was recruited into the study, in the age range 26-45, to allow direct age-specific comparisons. The overall participation rate was 86%.

In this sample the educational level was not very high (50% without a high school degree), the actual job seniority mean was 7.08 (S.D. 5.18) years, but 75.5% of the population had previous work exposure to prolonged fixed posture for more than 5 years, without relevant differences in the two exposed groups.

Prior to the investigation, a procedure to evaluate the degree of fixity of the different spine segments was applied in order to verify the substantial identity in working posture of the two groups under study (2).

This procedure describes and evaluates fixed working postures taking into account the following parameters:
- job organization, with particular regard to working time, pauses and work shift,
- position of different body segments (head, trunk and limbs) during work, and time duration.
- ergonomic quality of furniture, with particular attention to working area, VDU, chair, desk, document holder, foot rest, etc.

The weighted integration of the three parameters gives a postural risk index for each body segment. The index final score is subdivided into four risk categories: slight (0-10), moderate (11-40), marked (41-70), extreme (71-100). The score of the synthetic risk index for fixed working posture was moderate in both groups under study, indicating a substantial identity in working posture.

The control group selected from different companies and composed of 236 females, in same age range as the experimental groups, was not occupationally exposed to prolonged fixed posture (sitting and/or standing less than 4 hours/day), heavy manual handling and whole body vibration.

2.2 Measurements

Musculoskeletal disorders were investigated by administering a standardised questionnaire to collect information on job duration, past exposure to risk factors for the spine and previous and/or actual spine complaints.

The main characteristics of the questionnaire are:
- availability of an occupational history specially focused on the existence of one or more risk factors for the spine in the present job; past exposure to spine risk factors is collected only on jobs lasting for more than one year and is judged as significant only when there is at least a five year exposure to a specific risk, independent of the number of jobs held;
- availability of detailed, clear replies: for this purpose the questionnaire included illustrations and wording was clearly comprehensible; there are three sections concerning respectively the cervical, the thoracic and the lumbosacral spine;
- availability of a precisely defined reading grid allowing the examiner to classify the data on both occupational exposure and past disorders according to a positive negative type logic;
- use of criteria for the classification of spinal disorders similar to those recommended in the most authoritative international literature.

In previous evaluations the questionnaire demonstrated excellent intra and inter observer reproducibility and good validity in comparison to a more complex protocol for clinical examination of the spine (3).

The annual prevalence of cervical and lumbar spine disorders was calculated adopting the "threshold criteria" proposed by Nachemson and Andersson (4). Spine disorders that did not satisfy the "threshold criteria" were classified "below threshold" and not considered positive.

Psychological variables were assessed by means of the Depression Questionnaire developed by Krug and Laughlin (5), and the Mood Scale proposed by Kjelberg & Ivaiwski (6):

The Depression Questionnaire, validated for the Italian population, is a widely used tool in psychiatric and clinical psychology research. It is composed of 40 assertions on depressive feeling and behaviour. It is preferable that subjects answer either "yes" or "no", rather than "I don't know". As our female group was homogeneous, the score (range 0-50) was not standardised.

The Mood Scale translated from the Swedish battery of computerized neuropsychological tests (SPES) proved to be a sensitive, rapid, repeatable tool. It concerns two basic mood dimensions, resulting from factor analysis: arousal and stress. The check list is constructed on six items for each dimension with a six step response scale. In our case, it was administered with the specific indication to answer on the basis of how one feels at work. The results are entered as separate sums for arousal scale (range 0-30) and stress scale (0-30).

The three questionnaires were correctly filled out in the presence of expert personnel.

Psychosocial characteristics were evaluated using a semistructured interview aimed to explore incongruities in the following areas: workload/workplace, work schedule, job content, control/participation, home/work interface, interpersonal relationships at work, role in organization, career development, organizational culture and function. Each question was assigned a score according to whether a problem was present (=1), or absent (=0).

2.3 Statistical analysis

Comparison of risk prevalence of spine disorders between exposed and control groups was estimated by calculating age-specific prevalence ratios (PR). Statistically significant differences were tested by calculating 95% confidence intervals (95% Cl) of prevalence ratios.

The age-stratified approach (age groups 26-35 and 36-45) was preferred since statistically significant interactions in a prevalence of spine disorders have been detected between age-and exposure-strata (Breslow and Day test).

Due to the skewness of the distribution and to the small sample size available, non parametric statistical tests (U-Mann Whitney test and Chi square test) were used to evaluate differences in work-related and psychological variables between the two exposed groups.

For analogous considerations, non parametric tests have been used to assess associations among spine disorders, working conditions, psychosocial variables and self-reported assessments of the working environment (Kendall's Tau).

3. RESULTS

Age-specific prevalence ratios and 95% confidence intervals for each of the two exposed groups and for the two combined are reported in the following table.

Table 1
Age-specific prevalence rations (PR) and 95% confidence intervals (95% Cl) for VDU operators and office workers and for the two combined groups

SPINE DISORDERS	CERVICAL				LUMBAR			
Age groups	26-35 years		36-45 years		26-35 years		36-45 years	
	PR	95% Cl	PR	95% Cl	PR	95% Cl	PR	95% Cl
VDU operators	1.88	1.03-3.40	0.91	0.26-3.17	2.57	1.40-4.73	0.89	0.25-3.10
Office workers	1.25	0.61-2.56	0.58	0.20-1.72	1.58	0.75-3.33	0.97	0.42-2.13
Combined group	1.56	0.92-2.64	0.68	0.29-2.64	2.08	1.19-3.62	0.93	0.46-1.87

Prevalence of cervical and lumbar disorders in the combined group exposed to prolonged fixed posture was found to be higher than in the control group in the younger age class (26% lumbar segments; excess of risk was found statistically significant for the lumbar segment only (95% CI= 1.19,3.62). No statistically significant PRs were found in the older age class.

Considering exposed groups separately, in comparison with the control group, statistically significant risk excess for both cervical and lumbar segments was observed in the younger VDU operators: PR = 1.88; 95% CI = 1.04-3.41; PR = 2.58; 95% CI = 1.40-4.73, respectively. Direct comparisons between the two exposed groups did not show any statistically signficant differences, even if higher PRs for both spine segments were detected in the VDU group.

In VDU operators more monotonous work (z 2.82 p .004), poor work content (z. 2.70 p .006), less responsibility (z 2.10 p .03) and fewer needs for social relationships with colleagues and supervisors (z 2.70 p .006) were found than in conventional office workers.

Statistically significant positive correlations were found between length of exposure to fixed posture and cervical disorders in the younger age class (τ .33 p .001), and between length of exposure and depression score (τ.13 p .03), poor work content (τ .23 p .005) and monotonous work in both age classes. The objective evaluation of workplace inadequacy was positively correlated with lumbar disorders among younger VDU operators (τ .24 p .007).

A high percentage (49.1%) of subjects was found to exceed the 70th percentile value of the reference Italian population depression scale. On the other hand, prevalence of subjects under strain was low: 13.2%). Moreover, both depression and stress scores were correlated to educational level, job title seniority, poor work content and poor social support.

No relationship was found between spinal disorders, depression and stress. Instead significant relationships were found between spine disorders and constrictive aspects of the job, and between spine disorders and psychosocial conditions in the areas of social support (table 2).

Table 2
Relationships between spine disorders, working and psychosocial conditions, Chi Square and p value.

item	cervical		lumbar	
	X^2	p.	X^2	p.
Insufficient personnel	3.80	.05		
Indifferent colleagues	5.23	.02		
Aggressive clients	5.81	.01		
No internal meetings	4.37	.03		
Lack of communication	4.27	.03		
No support from colleagues	10.92	.0009		
Time constraints			16.36	.0001
Organizational obstacles			4.55	.03

4. CONCLUSIONS

The availability of a control group not occupationally exposed to prolonged fixed posture (sitting and/or standing less than 4 hours/day), heavy manual handling and whole body vibration is of primary importance in epidemiological investigations on office workers since studies on the mechanism of nutrition of intervertebral discs and paravertebral soft tissues have hypothesized that postural fixity plays an important role as a risk factor for the spinal segments, in addition to causing discomfort (7).

Moreover, in the case where a significant excess of disorders is demonstrated in the exposed compared with the non exposed, this could lay the grounds for speculation concerning the aetiology of the link between occupational risk and disorders of the spine. However, with cross-sectional studies it will be not possible, except in particular cases, to come to definite conclusions on such links, which should normally be obtained from longitudinal studies.

Finally, the use of threshold criteria, in regard to the severity of spinal disorders limits the possibility to classify as "positive" subjects suffering from only slight, temporary complaints.

In our female office workers, a significantly higher prevalence of spinal disorders (cervical and lumbar) were found in the younger age class, as literature also indicates (8). The absence of any risk excess in the older age groups may be due to the higher turnover as well as the higher prevalence of spine disorders in this age class, even in the control group. On the other hand, it may be possible that young workers have less experience in choosing adequate working conditions and have a higher work load and poor job satisfaction.

Fixity seems to be particularly relevant to cervical disorders, while work place inadequacy seems more relevant to lumbar disorders.

Working and psychosocial conditions were found to be related to spinal disorders and are related to an elevated percentage of depressed cases and a general feeling of discomfort. Contrary to Japanese cases (10,11), no diffuse overload and time pressure conditions were pointed out, but repetitive work, poor work content and low discretionality were present.

We observed, at an individual level, many objective difficulties in looking for more acceptable working conditions which led to depressive ideation. At the organisational level, no adequate policy was applied to training, career and rewards. Where flexibility to satisfy disfunctions/problems was lacking, relationships among subjects became formal.

The use of "threshold" criteria, might facilitate the observation of relationships among ergonomic design, working - psychosocial variables and muscoloskeletal disorders, thus eliminating some confounding elements.

REFERENCES

1. E. Occhipinti, D. Colombini, E. Cervi, N. Santini, A. Borrelli and A. Petri, Alterazioni del Rachide In Collettività Lavorative: Dati Preliminari su un Gruppo Femminile di Controllo e sui Valori di Riferimento per la Motilità del Rachide nel Sesso Femminile; Proceedings Of "Atti Seminario Nazionale Lavoro e Patologia del Rachide", Milan 1988, 29-30 maggio, 209-214.
2. D. Colombini, E. Occhipinti, Messa a Punto e Prime Sperimentazioni di una Procedura per l'espressione di Indici Sintetici di Rischio nella Valutazione delle Posture Fisse Prolungate. Proceedings of "53° Congresso Nazionale della Società Italiana di Medicina del Lavoro ed Igiene Industriale" Stresa, 10-13 ottobre 1990, Ed. Monduzzi Bologna, Italy 1990, 663-666.
3. G. Molteni, E. Occhipinti, D. Colombini, A. Grieco, Questionnaire and Clinical Functional Procedures for the Screening of Spinal Disorders in Working Communities. In: The Ergonomics of Manual Work. Ed. W.S. Marras, W. Karwowski, J.L. Smith and L. Pacholski. Taylor and Francis, 295-298 (1993).

4. A. Nachemson and G.B. Andersson; Classification of low-pain. Scand. J. Work Environ. Health., 1982, 8, 134-136.
5. E. S. Krug and J.E. Laughlin, Questionario di autovalutazione C.D.Q. (Ipat Depression Scale), Organizzazioni Speciali, Firenze 1979.
6. F.Gamberale and A. Iregren, A. Kjellberg: Swedish Performance Evaluation System. Background, Critical Issues, Empirical data, and Users' Manual . Arbete och Halsa, 1989, 6, 28-29.
7. A.Grieco, Sitting Posture: an Old Problem and a New One. Ergonomics, 1986, 29:3, 345-362.
8. Ong, Technological Change and Work Related Muscoskeletal Disorder. A Study of VDU Operators. In: Toward Human Work. Ed. Kumashiro M. and Megaw. E. Taylor and Francis (1991).
9. P.M. Bongers, C.R. De Winter, M.A.J. Kompier and V.H. Hildebrandt, Psychosocial Factors at Work and Musculoskeletal Disease, Scand.J. Work Health, No. 19 (1993) 297-312.
10. E. Satoko, A. Shunichi, O, Yataka, K. Norito and M. Katsuyuki, Work Stress in Japanese Computer Engineers: Effects of Computer Work on Bioeducational Factors. Environ. Research, 1993, 63, 148-156.
11. M. Yoshio, T. Toshihide et al. : Depressive States in Workers Using Computers. Environmental Research, 1993, 63, 64-59.

VDU workplace: experimentation in an electronics firm of a methodology of clinical functional evaluation of the spine.

A. Malcangi[a], M. Fregoso[a], G. Galletta[a], G. Ferretti[a], F. De Marco[b], D.Colombini [b], E. Occhipinti[b]

[a] Environment Health and Safety Service - ITALTEL SIT SPA (IRI-STET)
[b] Research Unit EPM - Milan

1. INTRODUCTION

At the end of the eighties, Italtel* and O.S.L.s (Workers Trade-Union Organizations) reached a Integrated Factory Agreement, establishing the intent to deal with the issues of VDU workers in a methodical way, in accordance to the EEC Directive 90/270.

In view of the computer units installed (about 5000) and of the employees operating them (about 8000), it was felt the need to obtain reliable data on which to base daily management and future planning in terms of their location, organization and health implications.

Let's remember that at the time, in spite of the extensive scientific studies that demonstrated the absence of specific "pathologies" definitively related to VDU activities, there were rumors suggesting to the contrary, coming also from the authorities in the field, creating videoterminal anxiety in the public. The danger was that of dismissing the problem and leave open an issue likely to increase the existing tension.

There was then the need to device a comprehensive approach, technically correct and scientifically reliable. Widely shared and supported within our company, this approach would have permitted to put an end the unfounded speculations and address the problem in a rational way, necessity for the management of a company policy.

---

* **Italtel** (part of IRI-STET Group) is Italy's largest telecommunications manufacturer. It designs, manufactures and markets systems and equipment for public and private telecommunications, and realizes telecommunications networks and installations both in Italy and abroad.
Italtel main italian facilities are located in Milan, Settimo Milanese (Milan), Terni, Rome, L'Aquila, Santa Maria Capua Vetere (near Naples), Carini (near Palermo) and employs a total of about 15,000 people, half of which regularly use VDU in their work.

In summary, the work plan was defined in the following terms:
- Training and information for all VDU users.
- Assessment of the existing workstation ergonomic requirements, establishing the company standards for corrective measures and the creation of the future VDU workplaces.
- Opportunity for users to receive a medical examination, evaluating the visual and musculoskeletal functions.

This report documents the first results of the assessment (still in progress) of the spinal function, performed on about 2000 workers with different postural activities.

2. RESEARCH SUBJECTS AND METHODS

In total, 1921 subjects have been examined, 1268 males constituting 66% (average age 39.6 ± 8.5 years), and 653 females, amounting to 34% (average age 37.6 ± 9.3 years). The sample was divided by age group, work activity and postural involvement. Of the employees examined, 1697 subjects, representing 88.3%, were using VDU, while 224, amounting to 11.7%, were involved in other work activities implying visual strain (magnifying glass, microscope, oscilloscope, etc.). The sample group, in regard to the postural requirements, was divided by four classifications: permanently seated (PS), constantly standing (CS), free posture (FP), and weight shifting (WS). The posture was considered significant when maintained for a daily total of 4 hours or more (not necessarily continuous). The clinical investigation is based on a protocol devised by EPM (Postural and Movement Ergonomy Study Center) for the analysis of spinal clinico-functional alterations (1, 2, 3). The examinations were performed in the company ambulatory, established for the purpose by medical personnel (work medicine experts or specialization students) in each ITALTEL plant. The medical staff was specifically trained and assisted by specialized nurses. The data gathered have been processed through a procedure created by ASPHI[+] - ANASTASIS (ANASTASIS is a cooperative created by ASPHI in 1986 of Bologna). To compare the data obtained to the average values, a control group was chosen, similar for sex and age, examined with the same clinical procedures in alike conditions (3, 4). The data has been statistically analyzed on the base of square-who and assigned to the corresponding range of statistical significance.

[+] A.S.P.H.I. - Information Handicap Project Development Association, established in 1980 in Bologna

3. RESULTS AND CONCLUSIONS

Figure 1 shows graphically the occurrence of cervical, thoracic and lumbosacral spondylarthropathy in each sex and age group, amongst the VDU operators.

The totality of the data obtained shows the tendency to a dramatic increment (also in comparison to the control group) of clinico-functional positive results in relation to age, more pronounced in the female population and for the cervical spinal tract. Statistically significant differences, in comparison to the control group, have emerged in both sexes. The presence of SAP in the spinal tract is particularly high in the females. In their case, the differences were statistically (P constantly <0.01) relevant in all age groups, except for the youngest (<26 years of age), while absent in the male population.

Also the lumbo-sacral spinal tract, in the older age group (36-45 and 46-55), the data shows substantial differences (P<0.01) between sexes. A comparison between the workers in the constantly-seated postural group demonstrates results that overlap the previous ones.

In conclusion, given the preliminary aspect of the research and the partial data analysis (still temporary and relative to the results so far obtained), the sample examined has shown a greater tendency to spinal disorders, especially in the thoracic tract of the female population. Overall, the disorder is associated to work activities performed with unsupported upper extremities or in activities that impose a leaning posture. Being such prevalence common to all the individual observed, it isn't possible at this time, to elaborate an hypothesis about the relationship between exposure to postural risks and vertebral pathology degree. Anyhow, the study has shown that the percentage of spinal disorders is far more than negligible, therefore requiring farther investigation and exam.

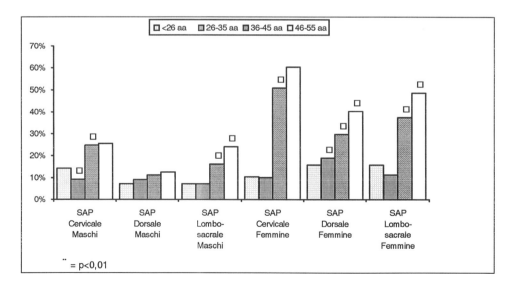

Figure 1. Percentage of spondyoloarthropathy in either sex by age group, in employees assigned to the VDU activities.

REFERENCES

1. D. Colombini , E. Occhipinti , O. Menoni e A. Grieco, Ulteriori esperienze su un nuovo metodo per la valutazione dei rischi e dei danni connessi con le posture di lavoro. Med. Lav., 1981; 72:128-161.
2. D. Colombini, E. Occhipinti, A. Grieco, S. Boccardi, O. Menoni, Posture di lavoro e artropatie. Metodi di indagine e principi di prevenzione. Ed. Comune di Milano, 1986; 63-91.
3. EPM Unità di ricerca Ergonomia della postura e del movimento, Atti del Seminario Nazionale "Lavoro e patologia del rachide". Milano, 29-30 maggio 1989.
4. E. Occhipinti , D. Colombini , O. Menoni e A. Grieco, Alterazioni del rachide in popolazioni lavorative: i dati su un gruppo maschile di controllo.
Med. Lav., 1985; 76: 387-398.

Symptoms and Reading Performance with Peripheral Glare Sources

J. E. Sheedy and I. L. Bailey

University of California, School of Optometry, Berkeley, CA 94720

Abstract

Most of the research into discomfort glare has dealt with studying the effects of luminous objects within 45 degrees of fixation. In this study we investigate effects of a parabolic louvered fixture which created a luminous glare source in the superior visual field extending from 45 degrees to the superior field limit. Thirty subjects each performed thirty minute reading trials on a computer screen under 4 different luminance levels of the glare source, tested in a randomized order. Filtered visors changed the glare luminance without affecting task lighting. Outcome measures were reading speed (words/minute) and symptoms rated on a continuous scale. The symptoms rated were asthenopic (tired eyes, sore eyes, headache), ocular (itchy eyes, dry eyes, watery eyes), visual (blurred vision, double vision), musculoskeletal (neck pain, back pain, shoulder pain) and discomfort from light. Subject rating of light discomfort was strongly related to the luminance level of the glare source (p<0.0001). The glare magnitude was also significantly related to asthenopic symptoms (p=0.012). Glare magnitude had a significant effect upon asthenopia (p=0.004) and musculoskeletal (p=0.017) symptoms in the high symptom group but not in the low symptom group, indicating that only those subjects who are more likely to experience and/or report symptoms have such glare induced effects. Accumulated reading time was positively related to asthenopia (p<0.0001) and musculoskeletal symptoms (p<0.0001), indicating a fatigue effect. This effect was significant for both the high and low symptom groups, indicating a more universal effect of fatigue on these symptoms in contrast to the effects of glare which are more pronounced in those subjects who report more symptoms.

1. Introduction

It is well established that highly luminous sources in the field of view can create discomfort glare. Discomfort glare is the sensation of discomfort that is induced by glare sources, not to be confused with disability glare which is a measure of reduced visual function caused by glare. Many of the luminance parameters which induce discomfort glare have been studied and quantified[1]. The physiological mechanism by which discomfort is produced is not understood but it has been suggested that it might be related to pupillary fluctuations in size[2,3].

It is clear from published research that glare sources closer to the line of sight contribute more to discomfort[4]. Most of the research into discomfort glare, however, has concentrated on studying the effects of luminous objects within 45 degrees of fixation. The effects of discomfort glare from sources between 45 and 90 degrees from the line of sight have received scant attention.

Many office fluorescent lighting systems are designed to reduce or eliminate the discomfort glare. One method is down lighting - usually accomplished by using baffles or louvers to direct the light straight down within a fairly restricted (narrow) angle from perpendicular. The restricted angle of light emergence from the fixture results in areas of high luminance which are more peripheral in the field of view of the room occupants. If, for example, a down lighting fixture were to have an angle of emergence which extended to 30 degrees from the perpendicular, a room occupant with a horizontal gaze could have a glare source 60 degrees from fixation. Although down lighting serves to place the glare source more peripheral to the line of sight compared to more conventional (wide angle) light fixtures, it is possible that it causes discomfort.

In order to test effects of peripheral glare sources upon visual comfort, we established a laboratory environment in which subjects performed a reading task on a computer screen under a large peripheral glare source located from 45 to 90 degrees superior to the line of sight. The luminance of the glare source was controlled by having subjects wear filtered visors.

2. Methods

The reading task was displayed on a Macintosh IIsi computer with a 12" color monitor. The furniture and computer screen were arranged so that the average eye to screen distance was 60 cm and the center of the screen was located to require about a 12 degree depression of the eyes. The following elements of the computer workstation environment were fixed for all testing: chair and table positions, chair and table height, monitor position, and location of the over head luminaire. Table top illumination of 860 lux (80 fc) was provided by a 2' x 4' 2PMO 332 Optimax Parabolic light control system. The luminaire had 3 four foot fluorescent lamps (GE Trimline 32T8 SP35 RS) with 2900 lumens/lamp output. The luminaire was 8 feet from the floor and oriented with the 4 foot dimension orthogonal to the line of sight of the subjects. With a design eye height of 47 inches, the far and near edges of the fixture were located to be 45 and 60.3 degrees respectively from the horizontal eye level of the average subject, or 57 to 72.3 degrees from the line of sight when looking at the center of the screen. The width of the luminaire subtended 36 degrees at the subjects eyes. From the subject viewing position, the fixture luminance appeared as a series of horizontal strips of differing luminances due to the structural details of the fixture. The spatially averaged luminance of the fixture was 4500 cd/m^2. Other luminances of relevant objects in the field of view were: screen - 150 cd/m^2, bezel - 80 cd/m^2, immediate visual background (provided by an off-white cloth backdrop) - 50 cd/m^2. Except for the glare source, all luminance ratios were within the lighting guidelines of the Illuminating Engineering Society[5].

The luminance of the overhead glare source was varied without changing other luminances in the working area by having the subjects wear visors that were opaque, gray (5% and 27% transmittance) and clear (91%). The resulting spatially averaged luminances of the glare source were 4095, 1215, and 225 cd/m^2 for the gray and clear visors. The luminance of the underside of the opaque visor was 6 cd/m^2. Since the background luminance was 50 cd/m^2 and the background and underside of the visor each occupied about half of visual space, the baseline glare level used for this condition was the average of the two, or 28 cd/m^2 . The visors were supported by headbands which were adjusted to the subject so that they were comfortable and so that the tip of the visor was midway visually between the top of the computer and the bottom of the glare source.

For each trial, subjects read selected stories from the Complete Text of Sherlock Holmes Stories as obtained on a CD-ROM disc (Creative Multimedia Corporation, Portland, OR, 1992) and transferred to Microsoft Word files. Since each subject performed 4 thirty-minute reading trials (one under each peripheral luminance condition), 4 sets of 2 stories each were established for testing purposes. Stories were selected for relative equality in story type, interest level, and length. Stories were displayed in 10 point New York font and 1.5 line spacing. The keyboard was covered with black felt to avoid reflections. Page advance was by depression of a single key which was exposed through a hole in the felt.

Thirty subjects, ages 21 - 39 were screened to have visual acuity of at least 20/20 either without correction or with spectacle correction. Contact lenses were not allowed as a correction during testing. The order of glare level and story set were systematically altered across subjects so that their orders were evenly distributed. Each 30 minute trial was divided into two 15 minute sub-trials for which all physical conditions were identical. All outcome measures, including symptom questionnaire, were obtained after each 15 minute sub-trial. The purpose of the sub-trials was to help mask the intent of the study and to help establish reliability of reading speed and symptoms under each condition After the first 15 minute sub-trial, and before the beginning of the second sub-trial, a meaningless but obvious mechanical switch was switched. The subjects had previously been told, in the protection of human subjects protocol, that effects of light flicker were being tested.

The outcome measures at the end of each sub-trial were the number of words read during each sub-trial and a symptom assessment recorded on a one page score sheet. Twelve named symptoms were on the questionnaire, each with a "0" that could be circled and with a 10 cm horizontal line with "Just Noticeable" and "Very Intense" labeled on either end of the line. Instructions were to "Please indicate which of the following symptoms you are experiencing now by circling 0 for "None" or drawing a vertical line through the horizontal line to rate the intensity of the symptom between the two extremes of "Just Noticeable" and "Very Intense". Symptoms were scored on a scale of 0 to 100 based upon the millimeter location of the vertical slash for each symptom. The symptoms were: tired eyes, sore eyes, itchy eyes, dry eyes, watery eyes, blurred vision, double vision, headache, neck pain, back pain, shoulder pain, and discomfort from lighting. The discomfort from lighting question was not asked of the first 8 subjects. For analysis, tired eyes, sore eyes, and headaches were combined into a group of "asthenopia"; itchy eyes, dry eyes, and watery eyes were combined into a group of "ocular symptoms", blurry vision and double vision were combined into a group of "visual symptoms"; back pain, neck pain, and shoulder pain were combined into a "musculoskeletal symptoms" group.

3. Results

Statistical analysis of the data was by analysis of covariance. The analysis included the following independent variables: subjects (30), trial order # (4), sub-trial # (2), glare level in log luminance (4), and story set (4). The reading speed (words/minute), each of the individual symptoms and each grouped symptom scores were separately treated as dependent variables.

These analyses were performed on the entire subject population (n=30) and also on the 10 subjects with the highest mean symptom ratings across all trials as well as the 10 subjects with the lowest mean symptom ratings.

The log of the glare source did not have a statistically significant effect upon the reading rate. However, it did have statistically significant effects upon reports of light discomfort and upon asthenopic symptoms, shown in Table 1. It can also be seen that the glare luminance had a significant effect upon asthenopia and musculoskeletal symptoms for the high symptom group, but not for the low symptom group. This indicates that those individuals who are more sensitive to reporting symptoms are the ones for whom glare causes these symptoms.

Table 2 shows the effects of elapsed reading time upon symptom reports. Asthenopia and musculoskeletal symptoms both increase with greater elapsed reading times, and this occurs in both the high and low symptom groups. Elapsed reading time has no effect upon reports of light discomfort.

Table 1.
Statistical significance of the effect of log glare luminance upon symptom categories (NS = not significant)

Symptom Category	All Subjects	Hi Symp Group	Lo Symp Group
Asthenopia	$p < 0.0001$	$p = 0.0035$	NS
Ocular	NS	NS	NS
Visual	NS	NS	NS
Musculoskeletal	NS	$p = 0.0169$	NS
Light Discomfort	$p < 0.0001$	$p < 0.0001$	$p = 0.0036$

Table 2.
Statistical significance of the effect of elapsed reading time upon symptom categories (NS = not significant)

Symptom Category	All Subjects	Hi Symp Group	Lo Symp Group
Asthenopia	$p < 0.0001$	$p = 0.0110$	$p = 0.0002$
Ocular	NS	NS	NS
Visual	NS	NS	NS
Musculoskeletal	$p < 0.0001$	$p = 0.0018$	$p = 0.0005$
Light Discomfort	NS	NS	NS

4. Discussion

It is clear that glare sources located beyond 45 degrees from fixation cause discomfort. Subject assessment of light discomfort is strongly related to the luminance level of the glare source. This was particularly true for individuals who reported greater levels of symptoms across all categories.

Glare magnitude had a significant effect upon asthenopic symptoms. It is reasonable to expect that glare would create symptoms associated with the eyes, although the exact mechanism of such a relationship is not known. This effect was significant in the high symptom group but not in the low symptom group. This indicates that subjects who are more prone to report symptoms, or are more sensitive to experiencing symptoms, are the ones who experience glare induced asthenopia.

The high symptom group, and, again, not the low symptom group, also showed a significant increase in musculoskeletal symptoms with increased glare level. The mechanism by which glare has an effect upon musculoskeletal symptoms may be by increased muscular tension, induced posture change, or light discomfort may be a potentiator upon other areas of discomfort.

Not unsurprisingly, the longer the subjects read, the more symptoms they had. Asthenopic and musculoskeletal symptoms were both significantly related to elapsed reading time. This is most likely an effect of fatigue associated with having read for a longer period of time. However, the effect of elapsed reading time was significant for both the high and low symptom groups of subjects. This indicates a more universal effect of elapsed reading time upon symptoms, whereas the symptom inducing effects of glare are much stronger in those who are more sensitive to experiencing symptoms.

5. Acknowledgment

This project was supported by a grant from the Peerless Lighting Corporation.

References

1. Guth, S.M. (1981). Prentice Memorial Lecture: The science of seeing - a search for criteria. American Journal of Optometry and Physiological Optics, 58, 870-884.
2. Fugate, J.M., and Fry, G.A. (1956). Relation of changes in pupil size to visual discomfort. Illuminating Engineering, 537-549.
3. Fry, G.A. and King, V.M. (1975). The pupillary response and discomfort glare. Journal of the Illuminating Engineering Society, July, 307-324.
4. Luckiesh, M., and Guth, S.K. (1946). Discomfort glare and angular distance of glare source. Illuminating Engineering, June, 485-492.
5. Illuminating Engineering Society (1989). VDT Lighting - IES Recommended Practice for Lighting Offices Containing Computer Visual Display Terminals. Illuminating Engineering Society of America, New York, New York.

Eye discomforts during work with visual display terminals

Ulf Bergqvist, Bengt Knave and Roger Wibom

Department of Neuromedicine, National Institute of Occupational Health, S-171 84 Solna Sweden

1. INTRODUCTION

During the middle 1970-ies, reports of eye discomforts began to appear about adverse health reactions among office workers using visual display terminals (VDUs) [1]. A study has been conducted at the Swedish National Institute of Occupational Health, in order to investigate a group of office workers, the majority of whom used a VDU. In a cross-sectional part of this study, we investigated the relationships between eye discomforts and the extent of VDU work as well as the impact of various visual ergonomic factors.

2. MATERIALS AND METHODS

2.1 Selection of subjects and data aquisition

361 individuals working in travel agencies, newspapers, postal offices and an insurance company were selected for study, with 353 agreeing to take part. In a first investigation in 1987, 327 (91%) of them responded to a questionnaire on discomforts and work conditions and 292 (81%) of them were examined as to positional ergonomic situations, relative humidity etc. (Results of these data have been reported by Bergqvist and Knave [2].) In that earlier investigation, 260 workers were identified as VDU workers. These 260 individuals form the basis for the present investigation.

At a later occasion (in 1989), 216 (83%) of these 260 VDT users' work-stations were examined for various visual ergonomic factors, and these individuals also responded to a questionnaire describing current eye discomforts as well as some work situation details.

2.2 Eye discomforts

Eye discomforts were noted as the occurrence of any of eight different eye discomfort symptoms. "Any" discomfort was affirmed by the answer "yes" to at least one of them, while "moderate" discomforts was the same, provided that the respondent had indicated that at least one of them occurred to a least a moderate severity and/or had a frequent occurrence. The individual occurrences of specific symptoms (smarting, gritty feeling and redness as well as itching, aches, sensitivity to light, tearness, or dryness) were also used in the analysis, except that the first three were combined as "SGR" symptoms.

2.3 VDU work and some individual factors

The reported hours per day at the VDU work station were used as a measure, together with an estimate of the hours actually viewing the VDU. This latter variable was based on the assumption that the work types data entry or word processing involved viewing the screen for 20% of the time, while other types of work such as data aquisition, interactive work, mixed work and/or programming involved viewing the screen for about 50% of the time. (See [3-6] for the basis for these assumptions.) In this manner, the individual´s reporting of the hours working with the VDU (which could be less than the hours spent at the VDU work station) were combined with the reported worktypes (if more than one work type, percent of time at each work type were reported) into an estimate of that individual's viewing time.

Age, gender, use of spectacles ("glasses") during VDU work and company type were also ascertained.

2.4 Visual ergonomic factors - the screen

During the worksite visit, the display was photographed together with a mm template, in order to measure pixel and character descriptors (character height, character width, stroke width and pixel size, character vertical format, pixel type) and text descriptors (between character spacing, between word spacing, between line spacing). The measured distance between the VDU user's eyes and the VDU (center) was used in order to compute the angular subtence of the character height, stroke width and pixel size, which in turn were used as comparisons for other measures [7]. Direct observations by the investigator provided data on image polarity, visible background lines and whether the text readability was decreased when the luminance setting was increased. For edge sharpness evaluation, a template with different display edge sharpness texts was used. The VDU user - and independently also the investigator - reported in the questionnaire subjective frontal and peripheral flicker.

The display background luminance and hence luminance non-uniformity were measured using a Hagner Universal Photometer S1. In the photograph, a grey scale was included. This greyscale was used to evaluate the character luminance, calibrated by actual readings on the endpoints of the greyscale obtained at the work station with the actual and recorded illumination situation. The luminance contrast ratio was obtained as the ratio between the bright character and the dark background luminance.

The screen image quality factors for which associations with relevant eye discomforts were found are further described in table 1. Relevant eye discomforts are -here - those for which an association with VDU work extent was found. Certain factors were not ascertained for all VDU work stations - some reasons are given in table 1 (see "comments").

Table 1
Prevalences of certain screen image quality factors

Variable	Categories	Prevalences	Comments
Between line spacing (ISO 6.12) n=174	Narrow (<2 S) **Adequate** (≥2 S)	18% 82%	Not measured on VDUs not displaying running text
Peripheral flicker n=196	Yes **No**	11% 89%	Subjective evaluation by operator
Image polarity (ISO 6.19) n=210	Negative polarity Positive polarity Colour capability	40% 50% 10%	Colour screens normally used negative polarity
Luminance non-uniformity (ISO 6.20), n=215	**Small** (<20%) Large (≥20%)	47% 53%	Actual luminance setting
Edge sharpness n=215	Not sharp **Sharp**	76% 24%	Evaluated by investigator using a template

ISO=refers to specification in ISO standard 9241 part 3 [7]. n=number of VDU work stations examined. Categorization of continuous variables as given by Bergqvist and Berns [8], or by categories of the template (edge sharpness). Reference categories ("unexposed") are shown in **bold** letters. S=stroke width or pixel size, whichever was smallest. In addition to the variables shown here - because of relationships described below - a number of additional screen image quality factors were examined (see the text).

2.5 Visual ergonomic factors - the office environment and the manuscript

A Brüel & Kjær Luminance Contrast meter (type 1100) was used to determine the highest luminance of the screen, the manuscript, the surrounding field (beyond the screen and manuscript but within some ±30° from the screen), and the periphery (beyond the surrounding field but within some ±90° from the screen). Measurements were made as averages over ±12°. These luminance levels were used to determine the general luminance level as well as the luminance balance between manuscript and screen.

If the subjects reported an increased readability of the screen when other luminant sources in the visual field was screened off, then this was considered an indication of the presence of disability glare. This observation was verified by an observation that the subject´s pupil size changed accordingly. Specular glare and use of filters were noted by the investigator.

The character height in mm was measured on the manuscript and expressed in minutes of arch by using the measured distance between the user´s eyes and the manuscript. The contrast reduction was measured by a Luminance Contrast meter. Type of manuscript and manuscript quality were noted by the investigator.

For added details, see table 2.

Table 2
Prevalences of certain office lighting and manuscript ergonomic factors

Variable	Categories	Prevalences	Comments
Luminance balance: manuscript/screen n=189	**<5:1** 5:1-10:1 >10:1	65% 21% 15%	Using measured data on screen and manuscripts.
Disability glare n=199	**No** Yes, some a/ Yes, much a/	21% 69% 10%	From manuscript, surrounding, periphery or specific light sources
Manuscript type n=182	Hand written Mixed **Machine written**	1% a/ 68% 31%	Note that some work stations did not involve manuscripts

n=number of VDU work stations examined. Categorization of continuous variables as given by Bergqvist and Berns [8]. Reference categories ("unexposed") are shown in **bold** letters. a/ Combined with "mixed" in the analysis. In addition to the variables shown here - because of relationships described below - a number of additional lighting and manuscript factors were examined (see the text).

2.5 Analysis

These variables (VDU work extent, individual and visual ergonomic factors) were subjected to multivariate logistic regression analyses, resulting in odds ratio estimates for relevant factors, with 95% confidence intervals. Categories involving less than 10% of the subjects were either excluded or combined with other categories in the analysis. Variables that did not retain a substantial association within models were eliminated - provided that their elimination did not affect the odds ratios of other variables. In order to avoid multicolinearity problems [9], the final models included only one of the VDU use variables - this was simplified by the finding that normally only one of them were indicated as important (see below). Crude (univariate) and stratum-specific odds ratios and their 95% precision-based confidence intervals were obtained by the FREQ procedure in the SAS programme. The multivariate logistic regression analysis resulted in unconditional maximum likelihood estimates by the use of the CATMOD procedure in the SAS System [10]. When the number of individuals in a subgroup was small, the results were verified by the use of Fishers' exact method.

3. RESULTS
3.1. Associations between eye discomforts and extent of VDU work

Some exposure-response relationships were found between the extent of VDU work - expressed as time normally spent at the VDU work station, or estimated time actually viewing the screen - and any or moderate discomforts, sensitivity to light, itching, dryness, and SGR (see table 3). In some contrast, results for tearness and aches did not indicate any relationship with the extent of VDU work (not shown), these two eye discomforts are not examined further here.

Table 3
Associations between extent of VDU work and eye discomforts

Discomfort	Prevalence	Odds ratio a/	Adjusted for
Any discomforts	67% (n=179)	2.0 (0.9-4.6)	gender
Moderate discomforts	30% (n=182)	2.0 (0.9-4.4)	gender
Dryness	24% (n=184)	2.1 (0.9-5.1)	gender, age
Itching	27% (n=181)	2.2 (0.9-5.4)	gender, company
Sensitivity to light	39% (n=178)	2.2 (1.0-4.6) a/	gender, glasses
SGR symptoms	51% (n=173)	4.2 (1.9-9.5)	gender, glasses

a/ see text below. Odds ratios with 95% confidence intervals are shown.

These odds ratios compare those with ≥1 estimated hours/day viewing the VDU with those with less. For sensitivity to light, however, the comparison was based on whether they were at the VDU work station more than 6 hour/day or not. Both VDU work extent variables were attempted in multivariate logistic regression, where essentially only the one shown exhibited a substantial increase in odds ratio. For e.g. SGR, the crude odds ratios were 1.5 (0.7-3.0) for "at VDU station" and 3.4 (1.6-7.1) for "VDU viewing". In a first multivariate model, the SGR odds ratios for these two variables (both were present in the same model) were 0.7 (0.3-1.9) and 5.4 (2.1-13.9), respectively. Retaining only the variable "VDU viewing", and further refining the multivariate model, resulted in an odds ratio between SGR and "VDU viewing" of 4.2 (1.9-9.5), as shown in table 3.

The variables shown under "adjusted for" were those retained in the multivariate analysis (others were eliminated - see methods).

3.2 Associations between eye discomforts and visual ergonomic factors

Furthermore, certain visual ergonomic variables were associated with - or showed a tendency for an association with - some eye discomfort symptoms. Only those eye discomforts showing an association with VDU work extent (table 1 above) are included in the results presented here.

The following display image quality factors were so indicated: *Flicker* with moderate eye discomforts (OR=2.7; 0.8-9.3), dryness (OR=3.1; 0.9-10.3), sensitivity to light (OR=3.4; 1.1-11.0) and SGR (OR=3.2; 0.9-10.6). *Non sharp character edges* with any discomforts (OR=2.3; 1.0-5.2) and SGR (OR=2.0; 0.8-4.8). *Colour capability* with SGR (OR=4.0; 1.1-14.3). *Luminance non-uniformity* with moderate discomforts (OR=2.0; 0.9-4.4). *Narrow between line spacing* with itching (OR=4.4; 1.5-12.9).

Lighting conditions associated with certain eye discomfort symptoms were: Some *disability glare* with any discomforts (OR=2.8; 1.2-6.3), moderate discomforts (OR=1.6; 0.6-4.3), SGR (OR=2.5; 1.1-5.9) and sensitivity to light (OR=5.8; 2.0-16.5) and much disability glare with any discomforts (OR=3.5; 0.7-16.8), moderate discomforts (OR=3.8; 0.8-17.0), SGR (OR= 1.3; 0.3-6.4) and sensitivity to light (OR=8.8; 1.8- 43.2). *Luminance balance* with sensitivity to light (OR=1.5 (0.5-4.0 for 5:1-10:1 compared to <5:1, and OR=2.7; 0.9-8.3 for >10:1 compared to <5:1).

In addition, there was a tentative association between *manuscript type* and moderate discomforts (OR=2.4; 0.8-6.1).

In addition to the findings reported here, other findings on the same investigated group were based on the results of questionnaires and work-site investigation in 1987 - as opposed to the 1989 examination results as reported here. In brief, these results suggested - apart from similar results on relationships between VDU work duration and eye discomforts - that having the VDU placed at about eye level (especially if combined with long VDU working or viewing hours), having the VDU or keyboard at a short distance, or having visual task objects at different distances (especially if using monofocal glasses) were all associated with certain symptoms. In addition, using lenses at VDU work in low relative humidity environment appeared to be a problem in conjunction with dryness symptoms. (See further Bergvist and Knave [2].)

For comparison purposes, it should be noted that about 3/4 of all individuals gave the same response in 1987 and 1989 to the question whether they had a specific eye discomfort symptom - this was fairly stable across all eye discomforts (67-83%). The similarity in VDU use between 1987 and 1989 was somewhat lower - only 49% of the individuals reported in 1989 the same working hours/day at a VDU as they had in 1987. Of the remainder, the majority (32%) reported less work with a VDU in 1989, while 19% reported more work with a VDU in 1989.

4. DISCUSSION

Taken together, these findings clearly argue for a causal role of VDU use regarding certain eye discomforts, and also include some suggestions as to some visual ergonomic factors that could contribute to this.

4.1 VDU work and eye discomforts

Despite the differences in reporting of eye discomforts and extent of VDU work between 1987 and 1989 among individuals (see above), the associations found here between a VDU work variable and discomforts were generally consistent with the findings of the 1987 analysis. Thus, despite these variations, the associations between VDT working hours and some eye discomfort were stable across two years within this closed but aging cohort - lending, as we see it, further support to the hypothesis of a causal connection between VDT work and these eye discomforts.

We have earlier made an analysis of eye discomforts and VDT work between 1981 and 1987. Within that analysis, the group of individuals who changed from non-VDU work to VDU work, did also experience a change in eye discomfort prevalences from "non-VDU" to "VDU levels" [11]. These associations between VDU work and eye discomforts are also consistent with the majority of other studies. For a review, see [2].

We consider the odds ratios with "at VDU stations" or "VDU viewing" in table 3 as being the best description based on our data, but would like to consider the preference of one or the other VDU use variable as exploratory only, pending further studies. Nevertheless, the preference for e.g. the "at VDU station" variable for sensitivity to light is consistent with the ergonomic variables associated with that discomfort; flicker and disability glare - both are relevant also when the operator is not looking directly at the VDU. Likewise, the preference for the "VDU viewing" variable for e.g. SGR is in line with some of the ergonomic variables - blurred edge and colour capability - associated with SGR, both should be relevant only when the operator is viewing the screen.

4.1 Eye discomforts and visual ergonomic

Some of the suggested factors have been indicated or discussed by others.

For example, in some experimental studies, decreased reading speed with small line spacing [12, 13] have been noted. The association between eye discomforts and low edge sharpness on the display characters, which may be of relevance to accommodation has been discussed in [14-17]. In other investigations of actual work situations, subjective flicker [18] or objective determinants of flicker [19] were found to be associated with eye discomforts.

In an experimental study by Radl [20], relationships between a high luminance source in the visual field and discomforts were found - similar to our finding of disability glare and discomforts. Our findings are further supported by the existence of dose-response relationships (except for SGR), see above. Some other studies have shown increased reports of eye discomforts [19] or measured over-accommodation [21] after work in situations with large luminance imbalances.

REFERENCES

1. Hultgren GV, Knave B, Werner M. Eye discomfort when reading microfilm in different enlargers. Appl Ergon 5 (1974) 194-200.
2. Bergqvist U, Knave B. Eye discomforts and work with visual display terminals. Scand J Work Environ Health 20 (1994) 27-33.
3. Bergqvist U. Video display terminals and health. Scand J Work Environ Health 10 suppl 2 (1984) 1-87.
4. De Groot JP, Kamphuis A. Eyestrain in VDU Users: Physical Correlates and Long-Term Effects. Hum Factors 25 (1983) 409-413.
5. Delvolve N, Queinnec Y. Operators activities at CRT terminals: a behavioural approach. Ergonomics 26 (1983) 329-340.
6. Knave B, Wibom R, Voss M, Hedström L, Bergqvist U. Work with video display terminals among office employees. I. Subjective symptoms and discomfort. Scand J Work Environ Health 11 (1985) 457-466.
7. ISO, Visual Display Terminals (VDTs) Used for Office Tasks - Ergonomic Requirements - Part 3: Visual Displays. 1992 (Berlin, International Organization for Standardization)
8. Bergqvist U, Berns T. Bildkvalitet på bildskärmar (Image quality on VDUs, in Swedish). 1988 (National Institute of Occupational Health, Solna, Sweden), report U88:11.
9. Checkoway H, Pearce NE, Crawford-Brown DJ. Research Methods in Occupational Epidemiology, 1989 (New York, Oxford University Press).
10. SAS Users Guide. Statistics, 5th edition. 1985 (Cary, NC, SAS Institute Inc).
11. Bergqvist U, Knave B, Voss M, Wibom R. A longitudinal study of VDT work and health. Int J Hum Comp Interact 4 (1992) 197-219.
12. Kolers PA, Duchnicky RL, Ferguson DC. Eye movement measurement of readability of CRT displays. Hum Factors 23 (1981) 517-527.
13. Kruk RS, Muter P. Reading of Continuous Text on Video Screens. Hum Factors 26 (1984) 339-345.
14. Harpster JL, Freivalds A, Shulman GL, Leibowitz HW. Visual Performance on CRT Screens and Hard-Copy Displays. Hum Factors 31 (1989) 247-257.
15. Korge A, Krueger H. Influence of edge sharpness on the accommodation of the human eye. Graefes Arch Clin Exp Ophthalmol 222 (1984) 26-28.
16. Lunn R, Banks WP. Visual fatigue and spatial frequency adaptation to video displays of text. Hum Factors 28 (1986) 457-464.
17. Schmidt MJ, Camisa JM. Display parameters for improved performance and reduced fatigue: An experimental study, in Grandjean, E. (ed), Ergonomics and Health in Modern Offices, 1984 (Taylor & Francis, London) p. 265-269.
18. Rechichi C, Scullica L. Asthénopie et écran de visualisation. J Fr Ophtalmol 13 (1990) 456-460.
19. Läubli T, Hünting W, Grandjean E. Postural and visual loads at VDT workplaces. II. Lighting conditions and visual impairments. Ergonomics 24 (1981) 933-944.
20. Radl GW. Experimental investigations for optimal presentation mode and colors of symbols on the CRT screen, in Grandjean and E. Vigliani, E. (eds), Ergonomic Aspects of Visual Display Terminals, 1982 (Taylor and Francis, London) p. 127-135.
21. Shahnavaz H, Hedman L. Visual accommodation changes in VDU-operators related to environmental lighting and screen quality. Ergonomics 27 (1984) 1071-1082.

ASTHENOPIA, ANXIETY AND NEUROPSYCHOLOGICAL FUNCTIONS IN VDU WORKERS

P. Apostoli, R. Lucchini, C. Frontali and L. Alessio

Institute of Occupational Health of the University of Brescia
P.le Spedali Civili 1, 25125 Brescia, Italy

1. INTRODUCTION

Office work tasks requiring prolonged visual effort "at near point", such as visual display unit (VDU) work can cause asthenopia (Bergqvist et al., 1990). This syndrome includes ocular signs and symptoms (burning, heaviness, sensitivity to light, itching, teariness, blinking, redness), general symptoms (headache, nausea) and visual symptoms (visual acuity reduction, unfocused vision, split vision) (Bergqvist, 1986). Asthenopic disturbances appear to be related to different factors involving visual function, several type of job tasks and environmental condition of the workplace. In this context, attention has also been focused on the possible involvement of neurobehavioral functions and mood state, which can be affected by intensive VDU use (Murata et al., 1991; Goldoni et al., 1992; Bergqvist and Knave, 1994). In this study we assessed these central nervous system functions by means of psychometric testing and questionnaires.

2. METHODS

Target population
    Two groups of office workers were examined:
a) Group A composed of 30 office workers (17 females and 13 males) whose daily VDU use was more than 4 hours;
b) Group B composed of 30 office workers (16 males and 14 males) whose daily VDU use was less or equal to 4 hours.
    These two groups consisted of bank and hospital administration employees who took part in health surveillance programs at the Institute of Occupational Health of the University of Brescia, Italy. Out of the total number of subjects, 90% of them volunteered to participate.
    All subjects were screened for smoking habits, alcohol, coffee and CNS drugs consumption, exposure to neurotoxic substances, visual and neurological pathologies. In addition, data regarding the number of school years and work seniority were collected. This information was gathered with the aid of questionnaires.

Ergophtalmological assessment

The incidence of asthenopic symptoms was assessed by a questionnaire proposed by the Italian Group for the Study of Work/Vision Relationships (Piccoli B. Et al., 1993). This questionnaire indicates the prevalence for each symptom and also includes a total score which is the sum of the individual symptoms' scores.

Refraction power was measured using the auto-refractometer Takagi AR-10.

Neuropshychological testing

The anxiety profile was tested with the aid of the Inventory Profile of Anxiety Trait (IPAT) scale (Cattel et al., 1968).

Neurobehavioral functions were examined using the following 4 tasks selected from the Swedish Performance Evaluation System (SPES) Ver.5 battery (Gamberale et al., 1990);

- Simple Reaction Time (SRT), a 6 minute sustained attention task measuring response speed to an easily discriminated but temporally uncertain visual signal. The task is to press a key on the keyboard as quickly as possible when a bright square is presented on the display. Performance level is evaluated as the mean latency of 80 stimuli, and the variability is calculated as the standard deviation of these latencies;
- Choice Reaction Time (CRT), a four-choice reaction time task similar to SRT, with the addition of response selection requirements;
- Digit Classification (DC), a continuous choice reaction time task. Digits ranging from 1 to 8 are presented one at a time on the screen and the subject is asked to determine whether it is odd or even by pressing one of two appropriately marked keys;
- Additions (ADD) measures speed of simple mental arithmetic operations. Three horizontally placed digits are presented on the screen, and the task is to add them as quickly as possible and enter the sum on the key board.

Statistical analyses

The frequency distribution of each variable was controlled with the Kolmogoroff-Smirnoff test and the skewed variables were transformed in the logarithmic form, to obtain a log-normal distribution. The Student's t test for unpaired values and the χ^2 tests were used to compare the results between the two groups and the Pearson's correlation coefficient was calculated between the test results and VDU usage parameters.

3. RESULTS

The general portrait of the population characteristics is illustrated in table 1. The two groups show similar characteristics except for VDU daily use. In table 2 the results of the refraction examination are reported, which is not significantly different between the two groups.

The percentage of asthenopic symptoms in group A and B and in the entire population is reported in table 3. Group B workers reported a significantly higher percentage of ocular symptoms (burning and teariness), of general symptoms (headache), and of visual symptoms (far unfocused vision and split vision). The same workers also exhibited a higher total score on the symptom's questionnaire (table 4).

Group B workers showed significantly higher anxiety levels compared to group A workers (table 5). Finally, the neurobehavioral tests did not show any differences between the groups, except for the SRT test (table 6).

The test results were not influenced by the other non-occupational factors such as age, scholarization, alcohol consumption and smoking habits.

The analysis of correlations between the different tests' scores and between the test scores and the VDU usage parameters did not show any association.

4. DISCUSSION

This cross-sectional study examined office workers with different degree of daily VDU usage. The workers with more than 4 hours of average daily VDU usage reported a higher frequency of asthenopic symptoms, exhibited a higher anxiety level and a poorer performance at response speed test compared to office workers with less than 4 hours of VDU work. Intensive VDU usage caused a higher prevalence of eye burning and headache followed by far unfocused vision, eye teariness, and to a lesser extent split vision too.

Since no associations were evident between this different kind of alterations, it is rather difficult to interpret the pathogenetical sequence of the different alterations. In other words it is not clear if anxiety is directly caused by intensive VDU use and then therefore the other asthenopic and neurobehavioral deteriorations occur. On the other hand, this impairment could represent a whole syndrome, which is connected to an intensive visual effort and consequently also affects emotional state and psychomotor performance.

Since VDU use will definitely increase among the office job tasks, attention should be focused on the organizational and psychological work aspects connected with this type of job. In fact, these factors can influence the general "well-being" of VDU workers and should be properly regulated to avoid future disturbances of visual, emotional and behavioral functions.

5. REFERENCES

U. Bergqvist. Video display terminals and health. A technical and medical appraisal of the state of the art. Scand J Work Environ Health (1986) 10 (suppl 2): 1-87.

U. Bergqvist, B. Nilsson, M. Voss et al. Discomforts and disorders among office workers using visual display terminals. A longitudinal study. In: L. Berlinguet and D. Berthelette (eds.) Work with display units '89. Elsevier Science Publisher, Amsterdam (1990) 1-11.

U. Bergqvist, B. Knave. Eye discomfort and work with visual display terminals. Scand. J. Work Environ. Health (1994) 20: 27-33.

RB. Cattel, IH. Scheier, EM. Madge. Manual for the IPAT Anxiety Scale Questionnaire. Pretoria, South Africa: National Bureau of Educational and Social Research, 1968.

F. Gamberale, A. Iregren, A. Kjellberg. SPES: Assessing the effects of the work environment with computerized performance testing. In: Computer-Aided Ergonomics. A Researchers

Guide. Eds: W. Karnowski, AM. Genaidy & SS. Asfour. Taylor & Francis, London (1990) 381-396.

J. Goldoni, J. Bobic, M. Saric. Psychological and ergonomic aspects of work with video display terminals. Arh. hig. rada toksikol. (1992) 43: 219-226.

K. Murata, S. Araki, N. Kawakami, Y. Saito, E. Hino. Central nervous system effects and visual fatigue in VDT workers. Int. Arch. Occup. Environ. Health (1991) 63: 109-113.

B. Piccoli et al. Work/vision relationship in a preventive medicine context: initial guidelines for a correct ergophtalmologic approach proposed by the Italian Group for the Sutdy of Work/Vision Relationships. Part 2: Methods. Med. Lav. (1993) 84; 4: 324-331.

6. TABLES

Table 1: General charachteristics of group A and B and of the entire population

N°	AGE (years)		SEX (%)		ALCOHOL (%)		SMOKE (index)		SCHOOL (index)		VDT USE (h/day)		VDT USE (years)	
	Mean	SD	Male	Fem.	Drink.	Non D.	Mean	SD	Mean	SD	Mean	SD	Mean	SD
GROUP A														
43	34,1	6,3	28	72	19	80	0,7	1,2	3	0,6	2,9	1	5,4	3,7
GROUP B												(*)		
54	31,7	6,2	26	74	20	78	1,1	1,2	2,9	0,4	6,3	1	6,5	4,2
GROUP TOTAL (A+B)														
97	32,8	6,3	27	73	19	78	0,9	1,2	2,9	0,6	4,7	1,9	6	4

(*): p = 0.0001, Group A vs. Group B

Table 2: Refraction power in the group A and B and in the entire population

N°	RIGHT EYE				LEFT EYE			
	(sf)		(cyl)		(sf)		(cyl)	
	Mean	SD	Mean	SD	Mean	SD	Mean	SD
GROUP A								
43	-1,4	2,5	-0,3	0,5	-1,4	2,1	-0,3	0,4
GROUP B								
54	-1,1	2,4	-0,2	0,6	-0,9	2,2	-0,2	0,5
GROUP TOTAL (A+B)								
97	-1,2	2,4	-0,2	0,5	-1,1	2,1	-0,2	0,5

Table 3: Percentage of asthenopic symptoms in group A and B

	REDNESS	BURNING	TEARINESS	SENSITIVITY TO LIGHT
GROUP A	62	44 (*)	21(*)	44
GROUP B	74	65	41	42
	DRYNESS	HEAVINESS	BLINKING	HEADACHE	FATIGUE
GROUP A	12	60	16	37 (*)	72
GROUP B	19	63	22	63	74
	FAR UNFOCUSED VISION		NEAR UNFOCUSED VISION		SPLIT VISION
GROUP A	32 (*)		28		5 (*)
GROUP B	54		33		13

(*) = P<0.05 Group A vs. Group B

Table 4: Total score for the asthenopic symtpms in group A and group B

	MEAN	SD	p	T unpaired
GROUP A	4,1	2,8	0,04	2,1
GROUP B	5,5	3,7		

Table 5: Total score for the anxiety profile in group A and group B

	MEAN	SD	p	T unpaired
GROUP A	25	6,8	0.001	5,1
GROUP B	31,8	6,4		

Table 6: Neurobehavioral test scores in group A and group B

	GROUP A		GROUP B		p	T unpaired
	MEAN	SD	MEAN	SD		
SRT	250,3	14,1	268,7	19,1	0.001	3,5
CRT	724	8,9	745	11	1,05	0,3
DC	478	12,3	490	15,3	0,4	0,7
ADD	1.910	8,5	2.150	10,3	1,2	0,2

Relationship between vertical gaze direction and tear volume

Satoru Abe[a], Midori Sotoyama[b], Sasitorn Taptagaporn[c], Shin Saito[d],
Maria Beatriz G. Villanueva[e], Susumu Saito[b]

[a]The Second Tokyo National Hospital, 2-5-1, Higashigaoka, Meguro-ku, Tokyo 152, Japan
[b]National Institute of Industrial Health, 6-21-1, Nagao, Tama-ku, Kawasaki-shi, Kanagawa 214, Japan
[c]Ministry of Public Health, Devavesm Palace, Samsen RD., Bangkok 10200, Thailand
[d]Aichi Mizuho College, 86-1, Namiiwa, Hiratobashi-cho, Toyota-shi, Aichi 470-03, Japan
[e]Nagoya University, Turumai-cho, Shouwa-ku, Nagoya-shi, Nagoya, 466, Japan

Abstract

In our previous study we found that vertical gaze direction was closely related to ocular surface area (OSA). These factors, vertical gaze direction and OSA, may affect tear evaporation. We conducted two experiments on ten subjects to confirm the relationship between vertical gaze direction and tear volume, and the relationship between eye movement and tear volume. The first experiment concerned vertical eye movement and tear volume. Downward gaze tear volume was greater than upward gaze tear volume. We used the phenol red thread test to measure tear volume. The second experiment concerned eye movement and tear volume. Tear volume during horizontal eye movement was less than during fixation or vertical eye movement. Based on the results we propose that a comfortable VDT workstation be designed to avoid upward gaze and to decrease eye movement.

1. OBJECTIVE

Recently many workers have been complaining of ocular symptoms because of the increasingly widespread use of visual display terminals (VDTs). Lacrimation is said to decrease during VDT operation [1,2], and this is related to ocular symptoms, such as dry eye, eye irritation, etc.[3]. In a previous study, we found that during VDT operation subjects tended to gaze upward more than during traditional desk work [4] and to exhibit more frequent eye movements. We therefore conducted two experiments to determine the relationship between vertical gaze direction and tear volume and the relationship between eye movements and tear volume.

2. EXPERIMENT 1: RELATIONSHIP BETWEEN VERTICAL GAZE DIRECTION AND TEAR VOLUME

2.1. Methods

In experiment 1 the apparatus was set up so that the three gaze targets were placed 50 cm in front of the eye and at 0 degrees, and 15 degrees below, 30 degrees below Reid's line. We used Reid's line as a horizontal reference instead of the traditional Frankfurt plane, because Reid's line is easy to measure for video analysis. Reid's line extends between the external canthus and the center of the ear canal, that is about ten degrees above the Frankfurt Plane. In this study, Reid's line is defined as 0 degrees (Fig.1).

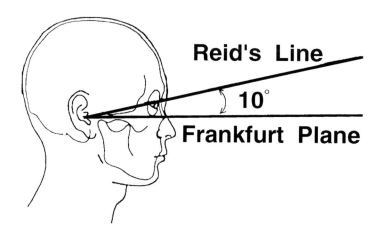

Figure.1. Reid's line

Tear volume was measured after gazing at the fixation target for three minutes. We used cotton thread to measure tear volume in this study. The yellow thread turns red when it comes into contact with tears [5,6]. The length of the thread that turns red is proportional to tear volume.

The fine thread was inserted into the inferolateral conjunctival sac of the left eye without anesthesia. The length of the thread which turned red during one minute with eye closed after three minutes fixation was measured in millimeters. Measurements were repeated three times at each of the three fixation targets, 0 degrees, -15 degrees, -30 degrees and we averaged the data.

2.2. Results

Figure 2 shows a typical example of the relationship between vertical gaze direction and tear volume. The average tear volume measurements were 21.5 ± 10.7 mm at 0 degrees, 21.8 ± 10.3 mm at -15 degrees, 26.5 ± 8.5 mm at -30 degrees. ANOVA showed significant differences in tear volume among the vertical gaze directions and the subjects ($p<0.001$).

The average tear volume at -30 degrees was significantly greater than at -15 and 0 degrees (between 0 degrees and -30 degrees : $p<0.05$, between -15 degrees and -30 degrees : $p<0.01$) .

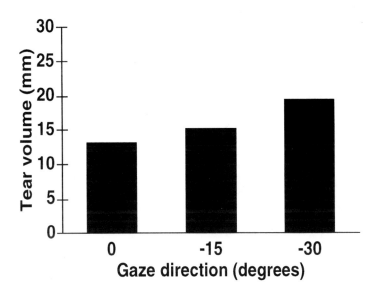

Figure 2. Relationship between vertical gaze direction and tear volume.

3. EXPERIMENT 2: RELATIONSHIP BETWEEN EYE MOVEMENT AND TEAR VOLUME

3.1. Methods

In experiment 2, we examined the effect of eye movement on tear volume. We measured tear volume with fine thread under each condition, horizontally and vertically. Two gaze targets were placed horizontally 50 cm from the eye and the distance of each target from the center was 20 degrees. The subject was asked to look at each target, alternating from one to the other every second. In the vertical eye movement experiment, two gaze targets were placed 50 cm from the eye and 0 degrees and 30 degrees below Reid's line. The subject was asked to alternately gaze at the two targets every second. As in the control study, we examined tear volume while fixating on the target 5 degrees below Reid's line. We measured tear volume after three minute periods, three times under each condition, horizontal eye movement, vertical eye movement, and fixation.

3.2. Results

Figure 3 shows a typical example of the relationship between eye movement and tear volume. The tear volume was 23.3 ± 11.2 mm during fixation, 16.7 ± 9.31 mm after horizontal eye movement, and 21.6 ± 8.7 mm after vertical eye movement. ANOVA showed significant differences in tear volume under the three experimental conditions and among the ten subjects. The average tear volume after horizontal eye movement was significantly less than after vertical eye movement and fixation (between fixation and horizontal eye movement : $p<0.001$, between horizontal and vertical eye movement : $p<0.01$).

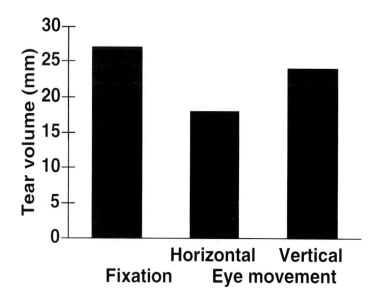

Figure 3. Relationship between eye movement and tear volume

4. DISCUSSION

As shown in the first experiment, the more upward the gaze induces the lower the tear volume. The reason that tear volume decreased during upward gaze is believed to be that ocular surface area (OSA) is larger in this gaze direction. OSA is the area of exposed eye surface. Our previous study on the relationship between gaze direction and OSA showed that OSA is larger during upward gaze than downward gaze [7]. Enlargement of OSA must increase tear evaporation and influences tear volume, and thus tear volume during VDT operation decreases more than during traditional desk work.

There is a report on the relationship between OSA and tear evaporation [8] showing that the large OSA during upward gaze direction increases tear evaporation. A large amount of tear evaporation decreases tear volume. As shown in our experiments, upward gaze decreased tear volume. Therefore, we think that the decrease in tear volume during upward gaze is related to dry eye, foreign body sensation, and asthenopia.

In the second experiment, the horizontal and vertical eye movements in our study simulated ordinary VDT operation. Tear volume during horizontal and vertical eye movement tended to decrease more than during fixation.

5. CONCLUSIONS

In this study, we investigated the relationship between vertical gaze direction and tear volume, and the relationship between eye movement and tear volume. We believe that adequate tear volume prevents dry eye and ocular symptoms. We propose that the display be set lower to provide a comfortable VDT workstation which prevents upward gaze and frequent eye movement.

REFERENCES

1. Y. Yaginuma, H. Yamada and H. Nagai, Ergonomics, vol.33 No.6 (1990) 799
2. T. Tanishima and M. Ochiai, Nihon no ganka, vol.58 No.9 (1987) 866
3. T. Iwasaki, S. Kurimoto and K. Okubo, Jpn. J. Clin. Opthalmol., vol.39 No.2 (1985) 172
4. S. Saito, S.Taptagaporn, Sh. Saito, M. Sotoyama and T. Suzuki, Work With Display Units 92, H. Luzak, A. Cakir and G.Cakir (eds.), North-Holland, Amsterdam, (1993) 110
5. K. Kurihashi, N. Yanagihara and Y. Honda, J. Ped. Opthalmol., vol.14 No.6 (1977) 390
6. T. Hamano, Folia Opthalmol. Jpn. vol. 42 No.5 (1991) 719
7. M. Sotoyama, Sh. Saito, S. Taptagaporn, T. Suzuki and S. Saito, Human-Computer Interaction 19 A: Applications and Case Studies, M.J.Smith and G.Salvendy (eds.), Elsevier Sci. Publ., Amsterdam (1993) 750
8. K.Tsubota and M.Yamada, Investigative Ophthalmology & Visual Science, vol.33, No.10 (1992) 2942

Vision Screening for Display Screen Users

T.J. Horberry, A.G. Gale and S.P. Taylor

Applied Vision Research Unit, University of Derby,
Derby DE3 5GX, U.K.

The research presented here compared six types of vision screening systems for display screen users to each other and to a full Optometric eye examination. The screeners were: the Titmus, Keystone, Optec, Ergovision, City and Vutest. The aim was to determine measures of visual function, using each of the screeners, and then to compare these both across the systems as well as to objective data obtained from the Optometric examinations.

The results found no statistical difference between the overall pass rates for the six vision screeners tested at intermediate range. Comparison with the Optometric data found:
-A significant correlation between the stereopsis tests performed by five of the screeners and the Frisby Stereo Acuity test.
-No significant correlations between eye health and overall pass rates for any of the six screeners.
-All the screeners that tested acuity at distance have a significant association with the results obtained through standard Optometric tests.
-A significant correlation between the overall pass/fail rates of the Optometric examination and the overall pass rate of the Optec, Keystone and Titmus systems. The data from the other three screeners were all positively correlated with the Optometric data, but not significantly.

The implications of these results are discussed in terms of the cost/benefits for testing the vision of display screen users.

1. INTRODUCTION

Adequate visual function is essential for an individual's overall task performance, safety and job satisfaction. For a task such as display screen use it is important therefore both to establish an acceptable visual 'standard' and to have the tools and techniques to measure the required visual functions. Vision screeners are devices intended to identify individuals with defective vision who require a full sight test. Thus they can be used to measure whether individuals have adequate vision for certain tasks, ie work with display screens.

Little previous research has compared the data obtained from the use of different vision screeners either to each other or to open field Optometric examinations (c.f. McAlister and Peters, 1). Thus an objective assessment of the accuracy and reliability of different screener systems has yet to have been systematically undertaken.

The introduction of European Community Directive (90/270/EEC) and the subsequent Health and Safety Executive (2) guidance on display regulations in the U.K. have made it the employer's responsibility to provide regular display screen equipment users with appropriate eye sight tests. This provision for vision screening has resulted in a rapid increase in demand for screening equipment and has, in part, led to the development of new dedicated products in the U.K.

The work carried out here aimed to screen a group of volunteers using the currently available main vision screeners and also to subject these volunteers to a full optometric examination. The vision performance measures obtained from all the screening systems could then be compared to one another as well as to the optometric data. The overall objective being to establish the suitability of each system for screening VDU users

The research therefore tested four screeners, ie the Vutest, the City screening system, the Titmus 2 and the Keystone VS-II. In addition two other systems were subsequently included in the research- the Optec 2500 and the Ergovision. All subjects were tested on the four initial screeners. A sample were tested on the Ergovision and on the Optec 2500.

The Titmus, Keystone, Ergovision and Optec are stand alone units that the user looks into and a tester controls the slides shown to the individual being tested. The Vutest and City screeners are newer software based products that test a user at his/her own machine and monitor. They are intended to be a direct assessment of whether a user's sight is adequate for the computer system as used in the workplace. See Horberry, Gale and Taylor (3) for a more extensive summary of the different screening systems.

2. METHOD

2.1. Subjects

Over 200 regular VDU users were recruited as volunteers. Subjects were selected to approximately represent the age, gender and skills level of the U.K. display screen users as a whole.

2.2. Equipment

A laboratory with the light level set at between 300 and 500 lux. together with the four stand alone screening systems (Keystone, Titmus, Ergovision and Optec). A 386 PC computer with Windows 3.1.and MS-DOS 6 was used to run the Vutest and City Screeners.

2.3. Procedure

The research was in two main parts. Firstly, the laboratory session where each subject was tested on the vision screeners presented in a random order. Secondly, a full eye examination - all subjects were given the examination on site by an Optometrist within several weeks of the laboratory based session. This took place as soon as possible after the laboratory based session to prevent any possible changes in an individual's eyesight affecting the accuracy of the results.

3. RESULTS

3.1. Overall pass rate comparison between the screeners.

An overall pass/fail figure was obtained for individuals for each of the screeners (ie whether, according to each screener's instructions, an individual had 'acceptable' vision for display screen work). Statistical analysis of the four main systems showed no significant difference between their overall pass rates (Cochran Q = 5.35, p < 0.15).

If all six tests are included (with a smaller sample as all subjects were not tested on the Ergovision and Optec 2500) the statistical analysis still reveals no significant difference in their overall pass rates (Cochran Q = 8.83, p < 0.12).

Therefore the null hypothesis (that no significant difference exists between the overall pass rates of the different screeners) has to be accepted.

3.2. Stereopsis

All the screeners, except the Vutest, had a measure of depth perception. The results were correlated against the Optometric results (using Frisby Stereotest plates) again on a pass/fail basis for each subject.

Table 1
Comparison of the Screeners' and Clinical Stereotests

	Screener				
	City	Keystone	Optec	Titmus	Ergovision
Coefficient	.57	.32	.42	.36	.49
Subject Number	196	194	23	194	59
p =	<.01	<.01	.02	<.01	<.01

(Spearman/1-tailed Significance)

Thus all the stereotests had a significant association with the Optometric results. At 1% all were significant except the Optec, which was significant at 5% (due to lower sample size).

3.3 Eye Health

A comparison was made between the Optometrists' opinions of subjects' eye health and the overall pass rate of the screeners (both on a pass/fail basis). The screeners stress that they do not detect eye health, thus the low correlations presented over the page do not directly reflect badly on the systems.

Table 2
Comparison of eye health and overall passes on the screeners.

	Screener					
	City	Vutest	Keystone	Optec	Titmus	Ergovision
Coefficient	.11	.09	.12	.32	.08	-.05
Subject Number	196	196	194	23	194	59
p =	.13	.23	.10	.13	.29	.70

(Spearman/2-tailed Significance)

As none of the correlations are significant, the above results allows it to be concluded that there is no significant link between overall pass rates of any of the screeners and eye health (as defined by the Optometrist).

Table 3
Distance acuity results for each eye.

	left eye			
	Screener			
	Ergovision	Keystone	Optec	Titmus
Coefficient	.29	.48	.47	.48
Subject Number	59	194	23	194
p =	.01	<.01	.01	<.01

	right eye			
	Screener			
	Ergovision	Keystone	Optec	Titmus
Coefficient	.57	.48	.39	.53
Subject Number	59	194	23	194
p =	<.01	<.01	.03	<.01

3.4 Distance Acuity

The four stand alone screeners all tested acuity at distance. The monocular results were compared to those obtained by the Optometric examination using a Pearson Correlation Coefficient (1 tailed) as shown in Table 3.

Thus all the coefficients are significant at 0.05 (and most at 0.01). Therefore all these screeners have a significant association with the results obtained through the standard Optometric tests on this particular visual function.

3.5 Overall pass rate comparison of screeners and Optometrist

The Optometrist produced an assessment of whether each subject had acceptable vision for display screen use (again on a pass/fail basis). This was intended to allow the screeners to be compared to an objective standard (the Optometrist).

Table 4
Overall pass rate comparison between the Optometric and screener data

	Screener					
	City	Vutest	Keystone	Optec	Titmus	Ergovision
Coefficient	.11	.04	.33	.47	.39	.03
Subject Number	196	196	194	23	194	59
p =	.06	.28	<.01	.01	<.01	.41

(Spearman/1-tailed Significance)

A significant correlation was found between the Optometric examination and the overall pass rates of the Optec ($p = .01$), Keystone and Titmus ($p<.01$) systems. The data from the other three screeners were all positively correlated with the Optometric data, but not at a significant level.

4. CONCLUSIONS

The screeners compared well to each other on all the measures of visual function examined. Additionally the newer software vision screeners are generally as accurate as the well established stand alone systems in an overall assessment of whether a display screen users' vision is acceptable for their task. The correlations of the vision screening data to the Optometric data, however, were generally low (with the exception of distance acuity). Although a more thorough discussion of possible factors is outside of the scope of this paper the following need to be considered:

- the accuracy or reliability of the screeners' results
- the accuracy or reliability of the Optometrists' results
- the different functions and use of vision screeners as compared to Optometrists.

Vision screeners for display screen users can have advantages over Optometric examinations in terms of:-
- time- it is quicker to test each individual
- finance- it is generally cheaper to screen subjects
- training- an expert is not usually required to perform the screening
- 'validity'- screening can often be carried out in the users' normal workplace (and for the software systems on their own computer).

In terms of cost / benefits vision screening should be regarded as an efficient option when measuring the vision of display screen users. A well organised regular screening programme can have a positive impact on the occupational health of display screen users.

5. ACKNOWLEDGEMENTS

We gratefully acknowledge the support of Keeler Ltd. in carrying out this study and the following companies for making their equipment available : Warwick -Evans Optical Co. Ltd., City Visual Systems Ltd., Bollé, Essilor (through Central Safety Equipment Ltd.) and Grafton Optical Co. Ltd. In addition we thank R. Thompson from Melson Wingate for conducting the Optometric eye examinations.

REFERENCES

1. McAlister, W.H. and Peters, J.K., 1990, The Validity of Titmus Vision Testing Results, Military Medicine, 155 (9), pp 396-400.
2. Health and Safety Executive, 1992, Display Screen Equipment Work : Guidance on Regulations, Health and Safety (Display Screen Equipment) Regulations 1992, (HMSO, London).
3. Horberry, T.J., Gale, A.G. and Taylor, S.P.,1994, Screeners under Scrutiny, Health and Safety at Work, September 1994, pp 32-34.

Using Visual Acuity to Measure Display Legibility

J. E. Sheedy and I. L. Bailey

University of California, School of Optometry, Berkeley, CA 94720

Abstract

The letters which are used on visual acuity charts must have known legibility in order that meaningful visual acuity measurements can be made. Proper design of visual acuity charts entails measuring the legibility of acuity letters compared to a standard acuity target. The techniques for comparing the legibilities of visual acuity letters have been internationally standardized. These same techniques are used in Experiment 1 to measure the relative legibility of words and letters on 6 different computer displays. In Experiment 2 reading speed and visual comfort measurements obtained in a study of 21 subjects on those same displays. The relative legibility measurements in Experiment 1 correlate closely with reading speed and comfort measurements in Experiment 2 - thereby demonstrating method validity.

1. Background

The legibility of text can be affected by many typographical variables such as font type, type size, letter spacing, line spacing, stroke width, contrast, color, etc. With the advent of video displays we can add other factors such as pixel density, gray scale and monochrome vs. color. The ultimate measure of legibility should be performance on a reading or other task using alphanumeric characters. Reading tasks can be difficult and time consuming to perform and thus it would be useful to have a more easily obtainable measure which bears a good relationship to reading performance - thus providing a surrogate measure of legibility.

The legibility comparison method used in this study is consistent with and significantly derived from the standardized method for measurement of human visual acuity.[1-5] The letters on visual acuity charts must be of a known and consistent level of legibility in order for the clinical measurements to be meaningful and repeatable. To this end, the methods for comparing the legibility of acuity letters (optotypes) have been incorporated into those standards.

The method used in this study is equivalent to using a visual acuity chart composed of characters or words of the particular design (e.g. the font style, stroke width, pixel density, etc.) for which the legibility is to be determined. However, an accurate visual acuity chart of the traditional design (i.e. progressively smaller lines of optotypes) cannot be presented on a video display since the legibility of the letter decreases as it becomes smaller on the screen due to pixelization. Therefore, in this study the characters or words are fixed in size and the angular size is varied by having the subjects view the characters or words at a designed series of distances. Utilizing the same subjects and same method for each of the test conditions enables an accurate determination of the relative legibilities. For lack of a better standard display condition, the legibilities of the test displays are normalized to those obtained with standard visual acuity optotypes.

This legibility measurement method directly tests the ability to perceive letters and words - therefore it would be expected to be related to reading performance. Correlation of the relative legibility measurements to reading speeds and visual comfort measurements using the same display conditions are tested.

2. Experiment 1 - Legibility Comparison

Ten subjects were screened to have 6 meter visual acuity of at least 20/20 (logMAR 0.0) unaided or with spectacle lenses. All testing was performed monocularly and with the same eye of a given subject occluded for all testing.

Test charts were constructed with capital letter optotypes and with lower case word optotypes. The word charts were constructed with the same set of letters used in the Bailey-Lovie[6] visual acuity chart (D,E,F,H,N,P,R,U,V,Z). The word charts were designed with words selected from a set of one hundred 5 letter words that were selected to be commonly recognized and to each contain at least one ascender or descender (in fact, it is difficult to find five letter words that do not have at least one ascender or descender). Three charts each of letters and words were developed to limit memorization effects due to multiple testing.

Letter and word charts were developed using 9 point New Century Schoolbook (NC) font. All charts were printed with a 1200 DPI Linotype printer and were scanned into hard disk storage for display on three Cornerstone Technology monitors (1024, 1280, and 1600) which will henceforth be referred to as A, B, and C respectively. These monitors were selected to provide stepped levels of resolution: B had greater dots/inch than A, and C had the same DPI as B but was monochrome. Charts on each monitor were displayed in both black and white (B&W) mode in which pixels were either black or white and in scale to gray (STG) mode in which gray scale was used to improve letter definition. This provided 6 different display conditions.

Every acuity determination was with 10 optotypes to an acuity line. For each acuity measurement, testing was performed at all distances inclusive of those which enabled at least 90% identification and 10% or less identification. Testing began at the closer viewing distances. The test distances which corresponded with acuity levels of 20/40, 20/32, 20/25, 20/20, 20/16, 20/12.5, 20/10, and 20/8 were 80.22, 100.99, 127.13, 160.06, 201.51, 253.70, 319.35, and 402.11 cm. respectively. At each test viewing distance the subject viewed a different set of 10 letters or characters on the chart while the other sets were screened from view.

Three measurements of each of the test conditions (in randomized order) were averaged to determine a single logMAR value for each subject/test condition. The logMAR results for the lower case words were adjusted upward by log(23/16) in order to equilibrate the lower case letter (without ascenders or descenders) results with those of the capital letters. This essentially adjusted the size of the lower case letters to be the same as the capital letters. The data for each subject were then normalized relative to the average of all conditions tested for that subject. The 10 normalized logMAR values (10 subjects) were then averaged. In order to obtain legibility values relative to standard visual acuity measurements, the logMAR of the test condition was subtracted from the logMAR of the visual acuity measurements with standardized charts. The anti-log of this value is the relative legibility value for the particular condition tested. See the Appendix for additional details regarding the method.

3. Experiment 2 - Reading Speed and Symptom Assessment

In a previous study[7], a group of subjects read text under each of the same six different display conditions in Experiment 1: STG and B&W presented on each of the three different resolution monitors. The text was New Century Schoolbook, so the reading results could be compared to the NC legibility results in experiment 1. The same text scanning and display options were utilized in order to equalize the size of the text under each display condition. Twenty-one subjects participated in the study. During a single test session they performed 6 twenty minute reading trials - one each with the scanned text presented on each display condition. Trial order was randomized, and the number of lines read and were timed and an audible tone signaled the end of a session. At the end of each trial, subjects immediately filled out a symptom questionnaire. Lines read and symptom ratings were the outcome measures of each trial. Experimental details are presented elsewhere[7].

4. Results

Figures 1A and 1B show the relationships between the measured legibilities and the reading performance attained on each of the six display conditions (the three monitors, each configured with B&W and STG). It can be seen that reading performance and relative legibility are positively related to one another. The relationship is stronger for the capital letter legibility measurements.

Figures 2A and 2B show the relationships between the reported symptoms and the legibility measurements for the six display conditions. There is a very strong inverse relationship between the relative legibility measurement and the reported symptoms (better legibility associated with lower symptom ratings) while reading on the display.

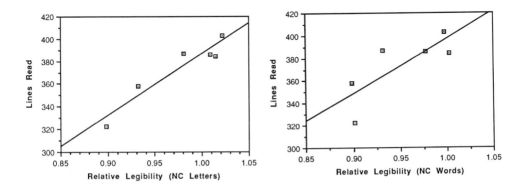

Figure 1A. Relationship of reading performance to letter legibility measurements. 1B. Relationship of reading performance to word legibility measurements. One data point for each of the 6 display conditions for both figures.

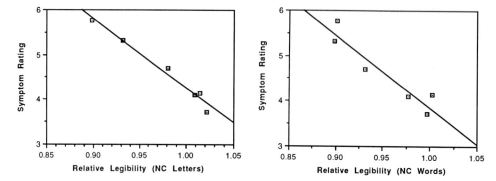

Figure 2A. Relationship of mean symptom rating to <u>letter</u> legibility measurements. 2B. Relationship of mean symptom rating to <u>word</u> legibility measurements. One data point for each of the 6 display conditions for both figures.

5. Discussion

These results demonstrate that the legibility measurements made with a visual acuity method are positively related to reading speed and inversely related to reported symptoms. Since human performance and comfort are the desirable outcomes of display legibility, these results show that this legibility method has validity.

This legibility method is a direct means of using the human visual system to assess relative legibilities. It is likely that relative legibilities measured with this method would integrate all of the aspects of the display which affect the legibility, such as pixel density, gray scale, font design, color, etc. This technique is a viable means of comparing display legibility

6. Acknowledgment

This research was supported by Cornerstone Imaging, Inc.

References

1. Committee on Vision, National Research Council, National Academy of Sciences. Recommended standard procedures for the clinical measurement and specification of visual acuity. Report of Working Group 39, Washington, D.C., 1979. Also in Advances in Ophthalmology 41, 103-148, 1980.
2. Consilium Ophthalmologicum Universale - Visual Functions Committee. Visual acuity measurement standard. Italian J Ophth II/I, 15, 1988 and Arq Bras Oftal 51(5), 203, 1988.
3. American National Standard for Ophthalmics - Instruments - General Purpose Clinical Visual Acuity Charts. Available from Optical Laboratories Association, P.O. Box 2000, Merrifield, VA 22116-2000.

4. International Standards Organization. ISO/DIS 8596, Optics and optical instruments - visual acuity testing - standard optotype and its presentation. Available from American National Standards Institute, NY,NY.
5. International Standards Organization. ISO/DIS 8597, Optics and optical instruments - visual acuity testing - correlation of optotypes. Available from American National Standards Institute, NY,NY.
6. Bailey IL, Lovie JE. New design principles for visual acuity charts. Am J Optom Physiol Optics 53(11), 740-745, 1976.
7. Sheedy JE and McCarthy M. Reading performance and visual comfort with scale to gray compared to black-and-white scanned print. In press, Displays, 1994.

Appendix - Visual acuity method and relative legibility calculations

The recognized standard visual acuity target is a Landolt Ring, which is a circular letter "C" in which the stroke width and the gap in the ring are one-fifth the letter height. The test subject responds by identifying the rotational orientation of the Landolt Ring - usually presented in one of the four cardinal orientations. The gap size or stroke width of the smallest Landolt Ring that can be identified is called the Minimum Angle of Resolution (MAR). A person with "normal" or 20/20 vision is able to resolve an acuity letter when the diameter is 5 minutes of arc and the gap is 1 minute of arc.

On a standard visual acuity chart, several (usually five) different letters of the same size are presented on a single acuity line. The size progression to the next largest line is by a factor of $10^{0.1}$, or 1.2589. The size designation for any line can be given in several different ways as shown in Table 1. The common clinical designations are Snellen fractions in which the numerator indicates the testing distance and the denominator indicates the distance at which the Landolt ring equivalent to the smallest letter that could be identified subtends 5 minutes of arc. The logarithmic progression of letter sizes is shown in Table 1. Another method is to specify the logarithm of the MAR (logMAR). Character charts are more useful clinically than those with Landolt Rings because of easier communication between doctor and patient. The standards require that clinical optotypes be shown to perform equivalently to the Landolt Ring - if necessary they may be size adjusted in order to have the same visibility as the Landolt Ring. Most common visual acuity charts are designed with alphabetic characters that also have stroke widths that are one-fifth the outer dimension of the letter and studies have shown that certain letters have the same visibility as the Landolt Ring (Bennett, Sloan). A minimum of 5 optotypes must be presented at each acuity step.

Each acuity line has a logMAR contribution value of -0.1 (see Table 1), and each optotype on a given acuity line has a logMAR contribution value determined by its proportion of the line. (e.g. If there are 10 optotypes/line, then each has a logMAR contribution value of -0.01, if there are five optotypes/line then each has a logMAR contribution value of -0.02. For calculations it is easier to use 5 or 10 optotypes/line.) The logMAR score is based upon the total number of optotypes properly identified, optotypes properly identified on one line will compensate for optotypes missed on another line. Scoring examples are presented below:

Performance #1:   20/32   10/10 correct
                  20/25   10/10 correct
                  20/20   9/10 correct
                  20/16   4/10 correct
                  20/12.5 0/10 correct

logMAR score is -0.03

This is equivalent to identifying the entire 20/20 line plus 3 additional optotypes on the 20/15 line (not 4, since 1 optotype was missed on the 20/20 line). The logMAR for 20/20 is 0.0, and each additional optotype is valued at -0.01, therefore the logMAR score is -0.03.

Performance #2:   20/32   5/5 correct
                  20/25   4/5 correct
                  20/20   2/5 correct
                  20/16   0/5 correct

logMAR score is 0.08

This is equivalent to identifying the entire 20/25 line plus 1 additional optotypes on the 20/15 line (not 2, since 1 optotype was missed on the 20/25 line). The logMAR for 20/25 is 0.1, and each additional optotype is valued at -0.02, therefore the logMAR score is 0.08.

The relative legibility of two conditions is calculated by subtracting the equivalent logMAR of the test condition from that of the control condition. The anti-log of this value gives the relative legibility factor (RLF). The equation is as follows:

$$RLF = \log^{-1}(logMAR_{control} - logMAR_{test})$$

The RLF is the multiplier factor by which the angular size of the control condition must be multiplied in order to have the same visibility as the test condition.

Table 1.
Angular sizes of optotypes, optotype detail, and visual acuity designations for standard visual acuity measurement systems.

Optotype Height	Optotype Height (Rounded)	Minimum Ang. of Res. (MAR)	logMAR	20 feet Acuity Designation	6 meter Acuity Designation
1.99 min	2.0 min	0.398 min	-0.4	20/8	6/2.4
2.505	2.5	0.501	-0.3	20/10	6/3
3.155	3.2	0.631	-0.2	20/12.5	6/3.8
3.97	4.0	0.794	-0.1	20/16	6/4.8
5.00	5.0	1.000	0.0	20/20	6/6
6.295	6.3	1.259	0.1	20/25	6/7.5
7.925	8.0	1.585	0.2	20/32	6/9.5
9.975	10.0	1.995	0.3	20/40	6/12
12.55	12.5	2.512	0.4	20/50	6/15
15.81	16.0	3.162	0.5	20/63	6/19
19.905	20.0	3.981	0.6	20/80	6/24
25.06	25.0	5.012	0.7	20/100	6/30
31.55	32.0	6.310	0.8	20/125	6/38
39.715	40.0	7.943	0.9	20/160	6/48
50.0	50.0	10.000	1.0	20/200	6/60

Eye strain syndrome, contrast sensitivity and critical flicker fusion frequency : a comparative study.

C. Manganelli, C. M. Locarno, G. Fasolino, A. Capobianco, F. Focosi

Istituto Clinica Oculistica - Universita' Cattolica Sacro Cuore, Roma - Italy -

1. INTRODUCTION

Asthenopic complaints are common in V.D.T. users and several reports underline the importance of different factors on the onset of the eye strain syndrome.
Enviromental agents (1), psycological (2), physical (3, 4) and ocular conditions (5, 6, 7, 8) have been extensively studied. Microclimate, noise, lighting, ergonomic characteristics of the workplace (screen, keyboard, table, chairs) and technical characteristics of the V.D.T.s (contrast, color, size, and shape of characters, flickering) have all been considered as contributing to the genesis of eye fatigue.
Particular attention has also been given to psychological factors linked to stress, misperceptions regarding ocular damage from V.D.T.s as well as personal attitude towards V.D.T. activity.
Physical, especially musculo-skeletal, and ocular conditions have been considered particularly relevant.
In our work we have tested in detail visual function measuring not only visual acuity, but also contrast sensitivity and critical flicker fusion frequency, since we believe that these two additional parameters can be particularly involved in V.D.T. work and hence possibly implicated on the onset of the eye strain.
As a matter of fact, visual dysfunction can be much more complex than described by the Snellen fraction generated in the examination lane. Non acuity parameters can help to complete the visual profile of the patient with eye problems.
Approaching to visual disorders, it is obvious to assess the patient's visual abilities. In principle, a great number of abilities can be tested. In practice, however, the first and often only aspect of vision to be tested is spatial vision in or near the fovea. The most common clinical measures of spatial vision, defined as the ability to see achromatic, two dimensional patterns, are visual acuity tests.
Ways to assess acuity can generally be grouped into three large categories : detection, resolution, recognition.
In tests of detection, the smallest stimulus that the patient can see is determined. Rather than detect a single item, it is possible to measure visual acuity by having patients look for separations between elements in a stimulus such as gratings (resolution). Tests like Snellen letters are examples of recognition : the patient has to name the target (a letter or number) or to name the location of some particular element of the target (direction of an E) : acuity is determined by the size of the

elements of the target. Acuity measures, however, could not contain all the information needed to describe spatial vision since acuity is a one - dimensional answer to a two dimensional problem.

Spatial patterns varying in size and contrast occupy a two - dimensional space (size and contrast) . Acuity test locate the limit of the size dimension (the size below which an item cannot be resolved regardless of its contrast). There is a similar limit in the contrast dimension, a contrast below which an item cannot be detected regardless of its size. Most work in the last twenty years has involved sinusoidal or "sine wave" gratings. A sine wave grating is a pattern of bars whose luminance varies sinusoidally in the direction orthogonal to the orientation of the bars. Such a grating looks like a blurred set of parallel lines. The size of a grating is specified in terms of spatial frequency : the number of sinusoidal cycles for degree of visual space. Contrast sensitivity testing can also be carried on by means of tables with low contrast letters or symbols. (Fig.1).

In conjunction with acuity testing, contrast sensitivity methods provide a more accurate assessment of a patient's spatial vision than does acuity alone.

An other psychophysical method to evaluate visual ability is critical flicker fusion frequency testing. The measurement of central retina critical flicker fusion to light stimuli is one of the few non invasive methods permitting to achieve data on the efficiency of arteriolar retinal as well as cerebral microcirculation and also to assess even the smallest changes of retinal oxygen supply.

Cerebro - retinal hemodynamic conditions are such that the ocular blood flow depends on brain circulation and can be influenced by its changes, which can hence interfere on retinal pigment genesis.

A decrease of critical flicker fusion can be due to blood vessel diseases leading to blood flow reduction or chronic hypoxia, while a strong mental work can induce a marked increase of critical flicker fusion frequency for the well known correlations existing between retinal and cerebral circulation.

Critical flicker fusion frequency can be measured by electronic devices provided with light emitting diodes of different frequencies. The patient is asked to tell the first non flickering LED.

2. SUBJECTS AND METHODS

Among 987 VDU workers 2 groups of emmetropic subjects were identified.
The first group included subjects affected by eye strain syndrome (A group), while the second one was unaffected (B group). VDT work was over 4 hours a day in all cases. The A group consisted of 95 workers (mean age 28.9 years, ranging from 22 to 33, 30 males and 65 females, while the B group covered 50 workers (mean age 29.5 years, ranging from 24 to 40), 30 males and 20 females. All of operators were emmetropic and eye examination, including ocular motility, was normal.
Contrast sensitivity was studied using Regan low contrast letter charts (9), consisting of three tables with letters of decreasing size and contrast (95%, 9% and 3%).
Monocular and binocular tests were carried on at a distance of three meters, with homogeneous lighting of 103 candles / square meter.

Critical flicker fusion frequency was measured using Rispoli-Modugno device (PIL 24/2 Lg RV, 20-60Hz) (10). This device displays 24 red and 24 green LEDs, flickering at 24 different frequencies ranging from 20 to 60 Hz (Fig. 2). A conversion table allows to read the value expressed as Hertz. We examined one eye at a time and the subject was asked to recognize the first non flickering LED.

3. RESULTS

The mean values of A and B groups were compared utilizing Student's test. Contrast sensitivity values (mean +/- 2 SEM) were significantly lower in the symptomatic group than in the asymptomatic one for 9% and 3% contrast charts (t test : Regan 9% 6.000 +/- 0.260 vs 6.462 +/- 0.364, p=0.03; Regan 3% 6.703 +/- 0.242 vs 7.287 +/- 0.428, p=0.01).
Critical flicker fusion frequency values for red colour (20-40Hz) were significantly higher in the symptomatic group (22.420 +/- 1.226 vs 19.900 +/- 2.407, p=0.04) There was no significative difference for the high contrast chart (95%) and green colour.

4. DISCUSSION

The data obtained appear apparently in contrast. The presence of a good contrast sensitivity seems to be related to the lack of eye strain since the subjects achieving higher scores do not complain of ocular symptoms linked to the use of V.D.T..
On the other hand, high values of critical flicker fusion frequency result more frequent in eye strain subjects. To explain these results we hypothesize that a good contrast sensitivity could facilitate the process of visual perception on V.D.T. screen, a condition that could be influenced by the possibility of adjusting contrast, according to personal requirements.
Conversely, the value of critical flicker fusion frequency could influence the degree of subjective sensitivity to screen flickering . As well known, V.D.T. images are electronically generated by stimulating screen phosphorous, which can have several colours, with different refreshing times responsible for screen flickering. The sensitivity to perceive light variations, expressed by critical flicker fusion frequency, could therefore increase the possibility of the eye strain onset for the instability of V.D.T. images (screen flicker cannot be modified and could therefore play an important role in the genesis of eye strain).
In conclusion, it is important to regulate the screen to have an optimized contrast, as well as to advocate the employment of new materials permitting a greater image stability to reduce the onset of the eye strain syndrome in V.D.T. operators. Moreover, contrast sensitivity and critical flicker fusion frequency can be sistematically used in the examination of workers with eye strain, to obtain further information for a better understanding of the mechanism of onset of the eye strain phenomenon.

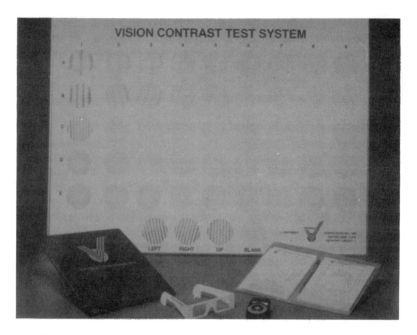

Figure 1. Vision contrast test system.

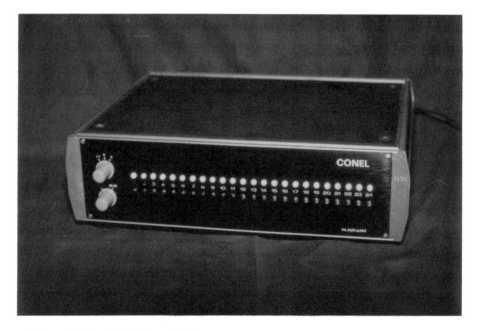

Figure 2. Rispoli-Modugno device.

REFERENCES

1. Gobba F.M., Broglia A., Sarti R., Luberto F., Cavalleri A.: Visual fatigue in video display terminal operators: objective measure and relation to environmental conditions. Arch. Occup. Environ Health 60, 81 - 87, 1988.
2. Smith M.J., Cohen B.G.F., Stammerjohn L.W. : An investigation of health complaints and job stress in video display operations - Human Factors 23, 387 - 400, 1981.
3. De Groot J.P., Kamphins A: Eye strain in V.D.U. users: physical correlates and long-term effects. Human Factors 25, 409 - 13, 1983.
4. Yamamoto S.: Visual muscolar skeletal and neuropsychological health complants of workers using video display terminals and occupational health guideline. Jpn J. Ophthalmol. 31, 171-183, 1987.
5. Boles Carenini B, Di Bari A.: Epidemiological aspects on the ocular pressure and glaucoma in 30000 employees of Italian Telephone Company. Boll. Ocul., 68, 69-84, 1984.
6. Focosi F., Dickmann A., Manganelli C., Tamburrelli C., Buratto E.: Eye problems associated with the use of V.D.U.s: epidemiological study on 1000 cases and a comparison between ophthalmological screening devices and a traditional visit. Proceedings of IV World Congress of Ergophthalmology. Sorrento, May 1985.
7. Ostberg O.: Accomodation and visual fatigue in display work in: Grandjean E., Viglian E. eds. Ergonomic aspects of visual display terminals. London : Taylor & Francis. 41-52, 1980.
8. Rechichi C., Scullica L.: Asthenopie et ecran de visualisation. J. Fr. Ophtalmol. 13, 8/9, 456 - 60, 1990.
9. Regan D., Neima D.: Low contrast letter charts as a test of visual functions. Ophthalmology 90: 1192 - 1200, 1983.
10. Cedrone C., Palmieri N., Stocchi D., Bonfili R.: Frequenza critica di fusione centrale retinica in operatori ai videoterminali. Clin. Ocul., 2, 119 - 123, 1987.

Which is more comfortable for VDT workers, spectacles or contact lenses ?

Toru Suzuki[a], Naofumi Hirose[a], Kenji Ibi[a], Tsuneto Iwasaki[a], Susumu Saito[b] and Shinobu Akiya[a]

[a] Dept. of Ophthalmology, University of Occupational and Environmental Health, Japan
[b] Dept. of Industrial Physiology, National Institute of Industrial Health, Japan

Abstract

We analyzed the intensity of ocular complaints related to eye-strain in 128 VDT workers by means of questionnaires with a self-rating method, and clarified the differences in complaints between VDT workers with spectacles and those with contact lenses, especially in cases of myopia. As a conclusion, we can suggest that although neither spectacles nor contact lenses do not reduce the visual discomfort of myopia totally in VDT work, at least, contact lenses might be helpful to reduce symptoms relating to loss of visual acuity.

1. INTRODUCTION

Clinically, we often see VDT workers whose subjective complaints of eye-strain seem to be strengthened not only by ergonomic factors such as upward gazing direction during VDT work [1] but also by refractive errors without optimal optical lens correction. The power of optical correction is an important problem in discussing optimal correction. Another important problem is which kind of optical device should be used to correct the refractive error of VDT workers, spectacles or contact lenses. Although we often encounter this question clinically, it is hard to find the scientific reports that provide answers.

Recently, we had a chance to examine the occupational health problem of visual complaints of VDT workers, and we tried to analyze the intensity of their complaints. We discuss which device is better for VDT workers in view of their visual comfort.

2. METHOD

2.1. Subjects
This study included 128 VDT workers. They were all female, and their ages ranged from 21

to 41 years old, with an average and standard deviation of 26.0±4.1 years old. They engaged in VDT operation, mainly for data entry, for at least 2 hours a day.

We planned to include only subjects whose near visual acuity was adequate to perform near tasks without particular visual effort. Thus, we excluded VDT workers whose monocular visual acuity at 50 cm was less than 0.7 (approximately 6/9 in Snellen's fractional notation) with their own optical correction if they wore spectacles or contact lenses during VDT work, those with hypermetrope whose refractive value was greater than +1.0D, and those with over-corrected myope, in either the left or right eye.

Visual acuity was measured by the Landolt's ring chart, and the refractive error was measured by an auto-refractometer.

The subjects were categorized in 5 groups as indicated in Table 1.

Table 1. Subject categories

Category	n	visual acuity at 50 cm	visual acuity at 5 m	refractive error (D) mean	S. D.
Control	32	both eye ≧ 0.7	both eye ≧ 0.7	-0.27	0.68
No correction	22	both eye ≧ 0.7	either eye < 0.7	-1.20	0.67
Spectacles	12	both eye ≧ 0.7		-3.14	2.12
HCL	33	both eye ≧ 0.7		-4.39	1.92
SCL	29	both eye ≧ 0.7		-4.51	2.05

The first group (Control) consisted of 32 emmetropic subjects without any optical correction during VDT work. Their monocular visual acuity at 5 m was 0.7 or better in both the left and right eye. This group was regarded as a control group for the other ametrope groups.

The second group (No correction) consisted of 22 myopic subjects without any optical correction during VDT work because of their good near visual acuity. Their monocular visual acuity at 5 m was less than 0.7 in either the left or right eye due to refractive error.

The third group (Spectacles) consisted of 12 myopic subjects with spectacles to correct their refractive errors during VDT work. The fourth group consisted of 33 myopic subjects with hard contact lenses (HCL), and the fifth group consisted of 29 myopic subjects with soft contact lenses (SCL).

There was no statistical difference among the age averages of the 5 groups.

2.2. Analysis of the subjects' complaints

To evaluate the complaints of the subjects, questionnaires with a self-rating scale were used to analyze the intensity of the complaints of 5 symptoms as follows:

1. Feeling of eye fatigue
2. Ocular surface irritation (superficial foreign body sensation, red eye, dry eye, or itchy eye) during VDT work
3. Ocular pain (a deep pain within the eye)
4. Transient blurred vision after VDT work
5. Progression of myopia

The intensity of these complaints was scored as 0 for no complaint and 4 for maximum intensity on a 5 point scale. Then the average score of each complaint was calculated for each subject group, and compared with that of the Control group by t-test.

3. RESULTS

3.1. Feeling of eye fatigue

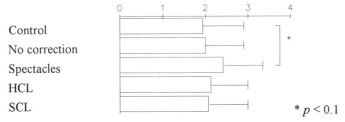

Figure 1 : Average score for feeling of eye fatigue

No clear differences in the feeling of eye fatigue were observed between groups, but the Spectacles group tended to have a higher level of complaint than the Control group as shown in Figure 1 ($p < 0.1$).

3.2. Ocular surface irritation

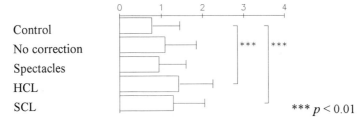

Figure 2 : Average score for ocular surface irritation

The level of ocular surface irritation was found to be significantly more intense among the subjects in both the contact lenses groups than the Control group as illustrated in Figure 2 ($p < 0.01$). Contact lenses are considered to irritate the ocular surface because of the decrease in tear volume during VDT work.

3.3. Ocular pain

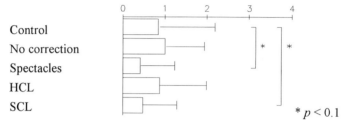

Figure 3 : Average score for ocular pain

The Spectacles group and SCL group tended to have a lower level of complaint than the Control group as illustrated in Figure 3 ($p < 0.1$).

3.4. Transient blurred vision after VDT work and the progression of myopia

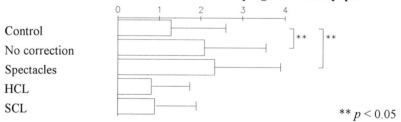

Figure 4 : Average score for transient blurred vision

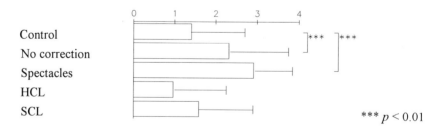

Figure 5 : Average score for progression of myopia

Complaints of transient blurred vision after VDT work and the progression of myopia were found to be higher level among subjects in the No correction and Spectacles groups than in the Control group (Figure 4 and Figure 5). On the other hand, the subjects in both contact lenses groups complained of these two symptoms only at the same level as those in the Control group.

4. DISCUSSION

Table 2. Intensity of the complaints in each group

	feeling of eye fatigue	ocular surface irritation	ocular pain	transient blurred vision	progression of myopia
Control					
No correction				**	***
Spectacles				**	***
HCL		***			
SCL		***			

** : The complaint level of the subjects is higher than that of the Control group at $p < 0.05$.
*** : The complaint level of the subjects is higher than that of the Control group at $p < 0.01$.

The results of this study are summarized in Table 2. There was no clear difference in the feeling of eye fatigue, the most common complaint during VDT work, between groups. However, in analyzing the other complaints related to eye-strain, some differences were found between the subjects with spectacles and those with contact lenses.

The subjects in the No correction group complained of symptoms concerning visual acuity (visual symptom), i.e., transient blurred vision after VDT work and the progression of myopia, much more than those in the Control group. It is suggested from this result that myopia may increase the visual discomfort of VDT workers

The subjects in the Spectacles group complained of these two visual symptoms at the same level as those in the No correction group. On the other hand, although the subjects in the HCL and SCL groups complained of ocular surface irritation much more than the Control group did, they did not complain more of the visual symptoms.

We could not find meaningful relationships between the intensity of the complaints of these visual symptoms and the refractive errors or the visual acuity with correction of the subjects.

Therefore, the subject's condition of their own refraction and the power of optical correction are considered not to be responsible for the difference in visual symptoms between the Spectacles group and Contact lens groups. Some reports suggest that the contact lenses may be effective in controlling myopia progression [2,3]. The stabilizing action of contact lenses on the change in refraction appears to be effective to reduce the visual symptoms of VDT workers. From the aspect of visual comfort, contact lenses are suggested to be superior to spectacles.

Successful contact lens wear is attributed to normal tear volume and stability, but decrease in the tear volume and disturbance of the tear film stability during VDT work are reported [4,5]. Wearing the contact lenses during VDT work is not generally recommended. However, because complaints of transiently or progressively decreased visual acuity with VDT use is a serious problem in occupational health, the findings of this study should be noted.

5. CONCLUSION

Myopia appears to increase the visual discomfort of VDT workers. Although neither spectacles nor contact lenses reduce all the uncomfortable symptoms of myopia during VDT work, they may reduce some of subjective complaints of the operators. Both hard and soft contact lenses might be helpful to reduce the complaints of visual symptoms, but they are irritating to the eye during VDT work.

Myopic VDT workers with enough tear volume to avoid dry eye may be recommended to wear contact lenses to reduce visual discomfort following work with display units.

REFERENCE

[1] Saito S, Sotoyama M, Suzuki T, Saito Sh, Taptagaporn S : Vertical gazing direction and eye movement analysis for a comfortable VDT workstation design. In : Luczak H, Cakir A, Cakir G (eds.) : WORK WITH DISPLAY UNITS '92 : 110-114, Elsevier Sci. Publ., Amusterdm, 1993

[2] Grosvenor T, Prrigin J, Prrigin D, Quintero S : Rigid gas-permeable contact lenses for myopia control. Optom Vis Sci 68 : 385-389, 1991

[3] Shaprio EI, Kivaev AA and Kazakevich : Use of contact lenses in progressive myopia. Vestn Oftalmol 106 : 30-31, 1990

[4] Abe S, Sotoyama M, Taptagaporn S, Saito Sh, Villanueva MBG, Saito S : Relationship between vertical gaze direction and tear volume. In : Work with Display Units '94 (abstract book) : B6-7, Berlin, 1994

[5] Yaginuma Y, Yamada H, Nagai H : Study of the relationship between lacrimation and blink in VDT work. Ergonomics 33 : 799-809, 1990

Dark vergence of the eyes in relation to fixation disparity at different luminances and amounts of blur on a visual display

W. Jaschinski-Kruza

Institut für Arbeitsphysiologie, Ardeystr. 67, D-44139 Dortmund, Germany

1. INTRODUCTION

The conditions of ocular vergence can be related to visual discomfort in extended periods of near-vision, e.g. at VDU work. Different optometric tests and procedures are used for the diagnosis of the vergence state. A clinically common measure is heterophoria, which refers to a resting condition of the extraocular muscles when the fusion stimulus is eliminated or reduced. This is achieved either by a strong cylindrical lens (or "Maddox rod") in front of one eye in the Maddox technique [1], by a monocular vertical prism in von Graefe's technique [1], or by dichoptically separated orthogonal bars in the Polatest [2]. These measures differ in stimulus conditions, test procedures, and some aspects of the physiological concept, and thus may produce similar, but not equivalent results. Their common feature is that the stimulus for fusion is removed or inhibited; however, accommodation is still stimulated and can influence vergence via the coupling of these two oculomotor mechanisms.

If one wishes to study the resting state of vergence free of any fusional, accommodative, and proximal influence one can use a visual field free of any fixation target, e.g. a completely dark surround [3,4] The population mean of dark vergence is about 1 m, but ranges among individuals between infinity and 40 cm (0 - 2.5 meter angle, or about 9 deg). Dark vergence differs very much between subjects (as does heterophoria), but is rather stable within subjects. Research has provided some evidence in support of the hypothesis that subjects with a far dark vergence experience stronger eyestrain in near vision since they have to exert higher convergence effort to fuse a near target, compared to subjects with a near dark vergence who are able to work at distances similar to their resting position [5,6,7,8]. Dark vergence is, on average, more convergent than heterophoria; however both measures are well correlated [9]. Owens and Tyrrell [10] showed that heterophoria can be predicted from the subjects' dark vergence, negative accommodation (from the dark focus to the distant target), and accommodative vergence.

In contrast to dark vergence, fixation disparity is a measure of vergence in viewing conditions that include all cues that occur in normal viewing, e.g. fusion, accommodation, and proximal effects. Fixation disparity is the vergence error (in minutes of arc relative to optimal fixation onto the centers of the foveas of the two eyes) that occurs during binocularly viewing of a near target [11]. The group mean of fixation disparity is about -1' (exophoric), but ranges from about -8' (exo) to 2' (eso) among subjects. Intra-individual variation is smaller. Fixation disparity can also occur in normal binocular vision with good stereopsis. Following Pickwell et al. [12,13] groups of subjects with asthenopic near vision symptoms had a larger exophoric fixation disparity than those without symptoms. According to Sheedy and Saladin [14], esophoric fixation disparity and exophoria larger than 10' tend to be associated with asthenopic complaints.

It is plausible that dark vergence and fixation disparity are not independent concepts. Previous research demonstrated that vergence errors are biased by the individual dark vergence when the fusion stimulus is degraded, e.g. at low luminance or with peripheral retinal stimuli [3]. The present study investigates the relation between dark vergence and fixation disparity with a distinct text target and degraded conditions due to blurring and dimming.

2. METHOD

The stimulus was a paragraph of text with dark letters (18' high) on a bright circular background of 8 deg diameter in a dark surround. A letter "X" in the centre served as a fixation target. The text was produced on a back-projection screen at 50 cm viewing distance by means of a slide projector. Fixation disparity was measured with two dichoptically-presented nonius targets, which were optically superimposed on the fixation target. Luminance was adjusted with neutral density filters to values of 67, 3.8, and 0.1 cd/m^2. Blur was increased by placing lenses in front of the slide projector. To describe the blur levels we determined the power of a convex lens at the eye that produced equivalent blur (after the far point was shifted to 50 cm with a + 2 D lenses). In Condition 1, a plane glass in front of the projector produced a sharp image. When stronger lenses up to -0.75 D were introduced the spectacle lens for equivalent blur increased up to about 6 D and the resulting acuity decreased to 0.1, so that the text almost disappeared and the subject saw a nearly blank blurred circular area.

Twelve subjects took part in Experiment 1, and 18 in Experiment 2. They were drawn from a group of 20 subjects with an age of 28.5 ± 8.5 years (mean and SD). They had good stereopsis and visual acuity of one minute of arc or better. Series of tests of 3 min durations were made. Details are reported elsewhere [15,16].

Table 1
Description of blur conditions in Experiment 1 (mean and SD, n = 6 subjects)

Condition	Lens at objective of slide projector	Spectacle lens for equivalent blur	Resulting visual acuity	Fixation disparity (min arc)
1	plane glass	-	1.94±0.06	-1.27±1.85
2	± 0.00 D	+0.55±0.07 D	1.58±0.12	-1.11±2.21
3	- 0.25 D	+2.09±0.15 D	0.31±0.06	-2.46±3.06
4	- 0.50 D	+2.93±0.10 D	0.20±0.07	-4.48±5.37
5	- 0.75 D	+6.14±0.71 D	0.11±0.03	-6.97±7.93

3.0 RESULTS

3.1 Experiment 1 (Effect of blur)

For the sharpest condition mean fixation disparity was -1.27' (exo), as shown in Table 1. No significant change occurred when the first step of blur was introduced in Condition 2. As blur was further increased, mean fixation disparity became more and more exophoric, reaching -6.97' (exo) when the text in the target had almost disappeared. The effect of blur on fixation disparity was highly significant [$F(4/44) = 8.50$; $P < 0.0001$; analysis of variance with repeated measures].

Figure 1a illustrates the individual fixation disparity in minutes of arc versus dark vergence. Vergence is expressed in meter angle, the inverse of the vergence distance in meters. Thus, 0 meter angle corresponds to vergence at infinity and 2 meter angle to 50 cm. We found a significant correlation of 0.61 [$P < 0.025$] when the target was sharp and an even higher correlation of 0.72 [$P < 0.01$] for the target with the strongest blur. It is mainly subjects who convergence at long distances in darkness, who show larger exophoric fixation disparity. This was expected for blurred targets, but it also appears for the sharp stimulus.

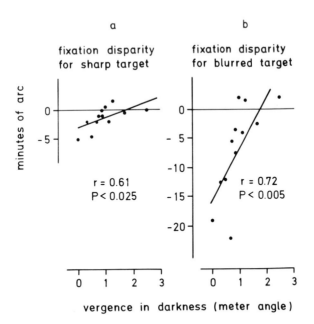

Figure 1. Correlation of dark vergence with fixation disparity for the sharp target (a) and for the strongest blur in Condition 5 (b). P gives one-tailed levels of significance. Regression lines are shown. (From [15]).

3.2 Experiment 2 (Effect of luminance)

Reducing the luminance from 67 to 0.1 cd/m^2 caused fixation disparity to change from - 0.82' ± 2.63' to - 1.41' ± 3.29'. Although small, this exophoric shift of 0.6' reached statistical significance [$F(2/34) = 3.43$; $P = 0.044$]. Figure 2 shows the relation between dark vergence and fixation disparity at two luminance levels. The correlation was significant for the bright ($r = 0.51$; $P < 0.025$) and for the dim target ($r = 0.54$; $P < 0.025$). This pattern of results was very similar to that in the blur experiment.

It appears that blur had a stronger effect on fixation disparity than did luminance. However, the fusion stimulus in the worst condition of the blur experiment was perceptually considerably weaker than it was with the dimmest target in the luminance experiment.

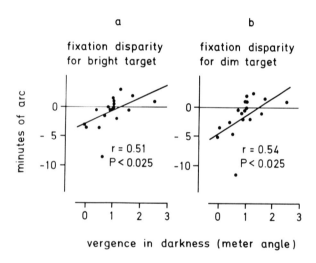

Figure 2. Correlation of dark vergence with fixation disparity for the bright (67 cd/m^2) target (a) and for the dim (0.1 cd/m^2) target (b). P gives one-tailed levels of significance. Regression lines are shown. (From [15])

4. DISCUSSION

Both experiments showed that fixation disparity was more exophoric in subjects with far dark vergence, not only for the degraded targets (which could be expected) but also for sharp, bright stimuli. The correlation coefficient was in the range of 0.5 to 0.6, which was slightly higher that that reported for the correlation between fixation disparity and heterophoria [17].

Thus, previous research on visual near-tasks can be summarized by saying that subjects suffering from near-vision convergence problems tend to be those whose eyes adopt a relatively exophoric position, both in the resting state (measured in darkness) and when fusing a normal stimulus.

This interpretation comes from correlational studies and from comparing groups of subjects; therefore, this scheme of explaining visual fatigue need not be true for a given individual. On the one hand, one finds individuals with a clear exophoric fixation disparity who do not complain of near-vision problems; and on the other hand visual fatigue at the workplace can result from a number of stress factors that are not related to convergence.

In Condition 2 of the blur experiment, fixation disparity was not different from the sharpest condition. (Although the lens used in Condition 2 of the blur experiment was specified as 0.00 D, small irregularities of the power across the lens produced blur similar to a bad CRT-monitor or paper print.) Consequently, the precision of vergence appears not to be impaired by the reduced sharpness that may occur in realistic visual targets. However, this study refers only to short-term periods of observation, corresponding to the three minutes duration of the measurements. It cannot be ruled out that viewing a degraded target over a longer period of time may deteriorate the oculomotor performance. Further, even if oculomotor adjustment is not impaired, the oculomotor effort and strain may have to be stronger in order to maintain a precise adjustment with a degraded stimulus. We all know the feeling of visual discomfort when viewing dim or blurred images. This is reason enough to demand bright and clear visual targets at workplaces, even if short-term measurements do not reveal an effect of slight blur or moderate luminance levels on fixation disparity.

Measuring dark vergence can be difficult in practical application, since it requires a completely dark environment to excude any fixational target. In this respect, heterophoria is an easier measure. In relation to both dark vergence and heterophoria, measuring fixation disparity has the advantage that the state of vergence can be measured in more realistic viewing conditions as accommodation assumes the natural state. The traditional instrument for testing fixation disparity is the *Mallett unit* [11]. However, this clinical test device has nonius bars in a fixed aligned position. This allows testing of whether or not a fixation disparity is present and determining the associated phoria, i.e. the prism correction required to compensate the fixation disparity. For research purposes, Yekta et al. [13] modified a *Mallett unit* to have mechanically adjustable nonius bars. The *Disparometer* [14] also uses adjustable bars, however it does not include a central fusion stimulus, which is present in ordinary visual tasks. The dimensions of these mechanical devices are designed for the conventional reading distance of 40 cm. A more flexible arrangement of the stimulus conditions is possible with a computer-controlled apparatus that was proposed by Bonacker et al. [18]: on a cathode ray tube, both the fusion stimulus and the nonius test bars are presented, the latter can be adjusted with the *Nonius Controller* in steps much smaller than the pixel separation of the visual display unit. With this device it is possible to measure fixation disparity in actual conditions of the workplace, e.g. with respect to viewing distance [19].

REFERENCES

1. Bennett, A.G. & Rabbetts, R.B. (1984) *Clinical Visual Optics*. London: Butterworths, p. 178.
2. Lie, I. & Opheim, A. (1990) Long-term stability of prism correction of heterophorics and heterotropics. *J Am Optom Assoc* 61, 491-498.
3. Owens, D. A. & Leibowitz, H. W. (1983) Perceptual and motor consequences of tonic vergence. In Schor, C. M. & Ciuffreda, K. J. (Eds.) *Vergence Eye Movements: Basic and Clinical Aspects*. Boston: Butterworths, pp. 25-74.
4. Jaschinski-Kruza, W. (1990) Effects of stimulus distance on measurements of dark convergence. *Ophthal Physiol Opt, 10,* 243-251.
5. Owens, D. A. & Wolf-Kelly, K. (1987) Near work, visual fatigue and variations of oculomotor tonus. *Invest Ophthalmol Vis Sci, 28,* 743-749.
6. Tyrrell, R. A & Leibowitz, H. W. (1990) The relation of vergence effort to reports of visual fatigue following prolonged near work. *Hum Factors, 32,* 341-357.
7. Heuer, H. (1993) Bildschirmarbeit und die Ruhelage des Vergenzsystems. *Zeitschrift für experimentelle und angewandte Psychologie, 40,* 72-102.
8. Jaschinski-Kruza, W. (1991) Eyestrain in VDU users: Viewing distance and the resting position of ocular muscles. *Hum Factors, 33,* 69-83.
9. Rosenfield, M. & Ciuffreda, K. J. (1990) Distance heterophoria and tonic vergence. *Optom Vis Sci, 67,* 667-669.
10. Owens, D. A. & Tyrrell, R. A. (1992) Lateral phoria at distance: Contributions of accommodotion. *Invest Ophthalmol Vis Sci, 33,* 2733-2743.
11. Pickwell, D. (1989) *Binocular Vision Anomalies - Investigation and Treatment*. London: Butterworths, p. 37.
12. Pickwell, L. D., Yekta, A. A. & Jenkins, T. C. A. (1987) Effect of reading in low illumination on fixation disparity. *Am J Optom Physiol Optics, 64,* 513-518.
13. Yekta, A. A., Jenkins, T. & Pickwell, D. (1987) The clinical assessment of binocular vision before and after a working day. *Ophthal Physiol Opt, 7,* 349-352.
14. Sheedy, J. E. & Saladin, J. J. (1983) Validity of diagnostic criteria and case analysis in binocular vision disorders. In Schor, C. M. & Ciuffreda K. J. (Eds.) *Vergence Eye Movements: Basic Clinical Aspects*. Boston: Butterworths, pp. 517-540.
15. Jaschinski-Kruza, W. (1994) Dark vergence in relation to fixation disparity at different luminance and blur levels. *Vision Res, 34,* 1197-1204.
16. Jaschinski-Kruza, W. & Schubert-Alshuth, E. (1992) Variability of fixation disparity and accommodation when viewing a CRT visual display unit. *Ophthal Physiol Opt, 12,* 411-419.
17. Pickwell, L.D., Jenkins, T.C.A. & Yekta, A.A. (1987) Fixation disparity in binocular stress. *Ophthal Physiol Opt, 7,* 37-41.
18. Bonacker, M., Schubert-Alshuth, E. & Jaschinski, W. (1994) Precise placement of nonius lines on a personal computer screen for measuring fixation disparity. *Ophthal Physiol Opt, 14,* 317-319.
19. Jaschinski-Kruza, W. (1993) Fixation disparity at different viewing distances of a visual display unit. *Ophthal Physiol Opt, 13,* 27-33.

The vertical horopter and the angle of view

D.R. Ankrum [a], E.E. Hansen [b], K.J. Nemeth [c]

[a] Human Factors Research, Nova Office Furniture, Inc., 949 Lake Street, Suite 3-G, Oak Park IL 60301, USA

[b] Department of Technology, College of Engineering, Northern Illinois University, 203 Still Hall, DeKalb, IL 60155, USA

[c] Center for Ergonomic Research, Department of Psychology, Miami University, 104 Benton Hall, Oxford OH 45056, USA

The existence of a vertical horopter which tilts away from the observer at the top suggests that computer users would experience less visual discomfort with a computer screen tilted back at the top. This study presented the monitor at positive, negative and horopter monitor angles, and at gaze angles corresponding to both eye height and a low position. Postural and visual discomfort were greater with the monitor at a negative angle of view (tilted forward). Subjects expressed a marked dislike for work with negatively tilted monitors. They preferred monitor angles tipped back from the vertical. If glare and reflections are not addressed, the potential benefits of a positive tilting monitor will be lost.

1. INTRODUCTION

The angle of view, also known as the angle of incidence, is the angle formed by the line of sight and the plane of the screen. One reason for adjusting the monitor about the horizontal axis has been to avoid reflected glare [1].

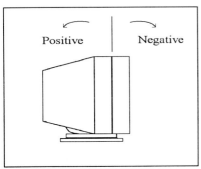

Figure 1. Directions of the angles of view used in this study.

ISO 9241 [2] and ANSI HFS-100 (1988) [3] both allow the angle of view to be from zero to +/- 40 degrees. The top of the monitor may be tilted forward (negative angle of view) or backward (positive angle of view) (Figure 1). Those limits have been intended to reduce the effect of geometric foreshortening. If the only effect of the angle of view is on geometric foreshortening, comfort and preference should vary about equally at both extremes of the allowed limits.

The horopter is the locus of points in space that appear binocularly fused to the observer [4]. Anywhere else in space appears as a double image to the observer. The horopter varies across individuals and with fixation distance and gaze angle.

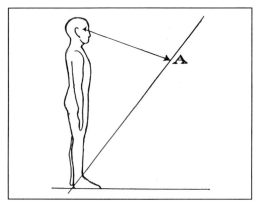

Figure 2. The vertical horopter for fixation at point A.

Horizontally, the horopter is curved with the sides coming closer to the observer [5]. The vertical horopter, however, starts somewhere between the viewer's waist and feet and projects outward, intersecting the point of fixation and continuing in a straight line (Figure 2). If an observer fixates on the center of a vertical wire in the median plane, both ends of the wire will be seen as double until the wire is tilted backward, with its top farther away from the observer [6].

The development of the human visual system is conditioned by its environment during infancy and early childhood [7]. When looking at an intermediate point on the ground, objects below the point of fixation tend to be progressively closer while those above are generally farther away. As a result, the lower visual hemifield is better equipped to see objects nearer than the point of fixation, while the upper visual hemifield is better equipped to see objects that are farther away [8].

For VDT users, a vertical screen orientation results in an angle of view which is inconsistent with the developed abilities of the visual system. In some cases, recommendations have been made to tilt the monitor downward to avoid glare sources [1]. That contradicts the principle of the vertical horopter.

The characteristics of the vertical horopter predict that computer users with a monitor whose top is closer to the eyes than its bottom (negative angle of view) will experience greater discomfort and reduced performance. The present study was conducted to evaluate the effects of monitor height and angle on comfort and performance. The study looks at positive, negative and horopter monitor tilts, and at gaze angles corresponding to both eye height and a low position.

2. METHOD

The subjects were 6 emmetropic students (refractive correction, if needed) with an average age of 21.5 years (range: 20-24) and an average of 6.1 years of computer experience (range: 3-10).

The experimental task involved comparing an accurate list of names, addresses and phone numbers on paper copy to a list on the screen that contained errors. When they found mistakes, subjects corrected the screen image.

There were six experimental conditions involving all combinations of three screen angles and two gaze angles. The three screen angles (measured from the perpendicular to the line of sight) were: "Horopter," tilted back 15 degrees at the high condition and 25 degrees at the low condition, more or less coincident with the horopter [9]; "Positive," tilted back 40 degrees; and "Negative," tilted forward 40 degrees. The gaze angles were: "High," top of screen at eye height; and "Low," top of screen 20 degrees below eye height. The center of the three lines of text on the screen was another 8 degrees lower. The viewing distance was initially set at 66 cm, but subjects were free to alter their postures.

Reflections on the screen were minimized by a combination of indirect lighting and positive screen polarity (dark letters on light background). There was no discernible glare on the screen.

Each session consisted of two 20-minute parts, separated by a 10-minute break. Each subject participated in all six conditions on separate days. The order of conditions was determined by a Balanced Latin Square. At the beginning and end of each condition, subjects rated postural and visual discomfort on a visual analogue scale from 1 to 10 (1 = No, not at all, 10 = Yes, very much). The questions were:

1. I have difficulty seeing.
2. I have a strange feeling around my eyes.
3. My eyes feel tired.
4. My eyes feel numb.
5. I have a headache.
6. I feel discomfort in my neck.
7. I feel discomfort in my upper back.
8. I feel discomfort in my lower back.
9. I feel tired looking at the screen.
10. I feel tired looking back and forth from the screen to the hard copy.

The questionnaire was a modified version of one by Heuer [10] as translated by Jaschinski-Kruza [11]. The last two statements were presented only at the end of the session. At the end of the sixth condition, subjects rated their preferences on a similar visual analogue scale.

3. RESULTS

The change in discomfort was determined by subtracting the initial rating from the rating at the end of the condition. Performance was measured by counting the total number of accurately corrected entries. After participating in all six conditions, subjects rated their preferences. For those scores, higher ratings represent a greater preference for the condition. The data were analyzed initially with a two-way ANOVA. Follow-up tests were performed with a Tukey HSD test. Reported results are significant at the .05 level.

Four measures were found to be significantly different under different viewing conditions: neck discomfort, upper back discomfort, "tired eyes," and "tired looking at the screen."

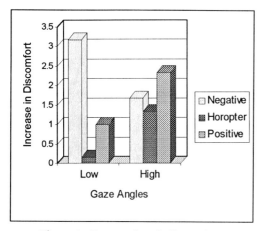

Figure 3. Reported neck discomfort.

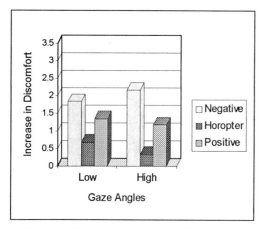

Figure 4. Reported upper back discomfort.

The differences in performance did not achieve significance.

The results for neck discomfort are shown in Figure 3. A significant interaction was found between monitor tilt and gaze angle. At the low gaze angle, the negative monitor angle produced significantly greater increases in discomfort than either of the other angles ($p = .0164$) At the high gaze angle, no significant differences were found.

The same trend was found in the responses to the statement "My eyes feel tired." An interaction was found between the monitor tilt and gaze angle. At the low gaze angle, the negative monitor angle produced significantly greater discomfort than either of the other angles ($p = .0397$).

Changes in upper back discomfort are reported in Figure 4. Subjects reported significantly greater increases in discomfort in the negative monitor angle condition over the other two monitor tilt conditions at both the high and low gaze angles ($p = .0190$). The responses to "I feel tired looking at the screen" followed the same trend with increased discomfort for the negative monitor tilt at both high and low gaze angles ($p = .0488$).

After participating in all six conditions, subjects rated their preferences (Figure 5). Higher scores represent a greater preference for the condition. As in the analysis of several comfort variables, there was a significant interaction effect between gaze and monitor angle ($p = .0110$). In the positive monitor tilt condition the low gaze angle was preferred over the high gaze angle. The two negative monitor tilt conditions were the least preferred of all six conditions.

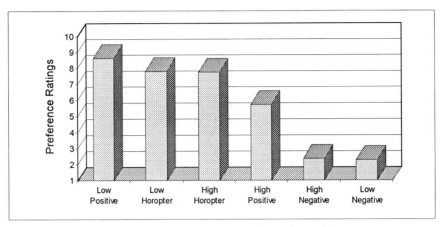

Figure 5. Reported preferences for each condition.

4. DISCUSSION

The results of this study indicate that the vertical horopter may play a role in visual and postural discomfort at computer workstations. A vertical horopter which tilts away from the observer at the top has developed to adapt to a commonly experienced feature of the visual environment. In that environment, objects below a point of visual fixation are usually closer to the observer, while higher objects are usually farther away. In this study, four measures of discomfort, including both postural and visual, showed significant increases when subjects viewed a monitor at an angle of view opposite to the horopter. Subjects clearly disliked the negative monitor tilt condition.

Because the results of this study appear to concur with the physiological mechanism of the vertical horopter, it suggests that monitor tilts opposite to the horopter may contribute to visual and postural discomfort.

In this study, no performance differences were found between any of the conditions. The time period (40 minutes of work) may not have been long enough to reveal effects on performance. Also, because the subjects were working with both hard copy and a screen, the effects of the experimental conditions may have been diluted.

It is inappropriate to consider the angle of view adjustments commonly observed in office environments as reflecting preferred settings due to the constraints of existing lighting systems and equipment. In many offices tilting the monitor back would result in glare from ceiling luminaires. The work environment must be viewed as an integrated whole. If glare and reflections are not satisfactorily addressed, the potential benefits of a positive tilting monitor will be lost.

ACKNOWLEDGMENT

The authors wish to thank Dr. Walter Makous for introducing them to the concept of the vertical horopter.

REFERENCES

1. National Institute for Occupational Safety and Health. (1991). *Publications on Video Display Terminals* (Revised) (p. 78). Cincinnati, OH: U.S. Department of Health and Human Services.

2. International Standards Organization. (1992). *ISO 9241-3: 1992, Ergonomic requirements for office work with visual display terminals* (VDTs) -Part 3: Visual display requirements.

3. Human Factors Society. (1988). *American National Standard for Human Factors Engineering of Visual Display Terminal Workstations.* Santa Monica, CA: Human Factors Society.

4. Tyler, C.W. (1983). Sensory Processing of Binocular Disparity. In Schor, C.M., and Ciuffreda, K.J. (Eds.). *Vergence Eye Movements: Basic and Clinical Aspects.* Boston: Butterworths.

5. Aguilonius, F. (1613). *Opticorum Libri Sex.* Antwerp: Plantin.

6. von Helmholtz, H. (1866/1925). *Treatise on Physiological Optics,* volume 3, translated from the 3rd German edition,. Southall, J.P.C. (Ed.). (p. 429). New York: Optical Society of America.

7. Tychsen, L. (1992). Binocular Vision. In Hart, W.M. (Ed.). *Adler's Physiology of the Eye.* St. Louis: C.V. Mosby.

8. Breitmeyer, B., Battaglia, F., and Bridge, J. (1977). Existence and implications of a tilted binocular disparity space. *Perception,* 6:161-164.

9. Nakayama, K. (1983). Kinematics of Normal and Strabismic Eyes. In Schor, C.M., and Ciuffreda, K.J. (Eds.). *Vergence Eye Movements: Basic and Clinical Aspects.* Boston: Butterworths.

10. Heuer, H., Hollendiek, G., Kroger, H., and Romer, T. (1989). Die Ruhelage der Augen und ihr Einfluss auf Beobachtungsabstand und Visuelle Ermudung bei Bildschirmarbeit (The resting position of the eyes and the influence of observation distance and visual fatigue on VDT work). *Zeitschrift fur experimentelle und angewandte Psychologie,* 36, 538-566.

11. Jaschinski-Kruza, W. (1990). On the preferred viewing distances to screen and document at VDU workplaces. *Ergonomics,* 8, 1055-1063.

VDT-WORK WITH DIFFERENT GAZE INCLINATIONS

I. Lie and K. I. Fostervold

Vision Laboratory, Institute of Psychology University of Oslo
P.O. Box 1094, Blindern, N - 0317 Oslo, Norway
E-mail: K.I.Fostervold@psykologi.uio.no

1. INTRODUCTION

Visual and oculomotor consequences of sustained excessive near-work have been research topics in visual perception and optometry for almost 50 years (1,2,3). These issues have received renewed interest in recent years with the massive introduction of VDTs into almost every sector of employment, indicating subjective complaints to be aggravated under prolonged interactive VDT work (c.f., 4,5,6,7)

From the point of view of visual ecology our eyes are primarily developed for prolonged scanning and fixation operations at longer distances and for intermittent focusing activity at near distances (8,9). Under natural scanning conditions of every-day life, eye movements are closely integrated with head and body movements. With small visual fields at close distances, like a VDT screen, this eye-head-body scanning programme is "arrested" and the natural dynamic vergence and accommodation performance is changed into mainly static muscle activity (10).

When working at short distances, vision is usually engaged in eye-head co-ordination activities requiring a downward gaze. This is normally found to be the case in reading, sewing, handicraft work, etc. The recommended position of the VDT screen, making a gaze angle of 5° to 20° degrees below the Frankfurter plane, represents, therefore, a very rare exception from what may be considered natural working conditions at near.

Investigations of the resting states of the oculomotor systems in different gaze directions suggest that work with downward gaze could serve to reduce visual fatigue (11,12,13). Corresponding results in favour of downward gaze are reported for accommodation (14) and for eyelid position, showing eye irritation to be reduced when the eye lid covers an increased part of the eye ball with downward gazing (15).

These results on visual fatiguing are supported by a recent study from our laboratory, showing a smaller increase of subjective symptoms during a period of proof-reading when the screen was lowered from 15° to 45° (16). Two follow-up studies are reported in the present paper.

These studies were supported financially by:
Tandberg Data A/S and The Norwegian Research Council

2. METHOD

In both studies the VDT-task required visual search for meaningful words in an array of letter strings. The ratio of meaningful to meaningless words was 1 to 5. Different measures of visual fatigue were compared under two conditions of gaze inclination; 15° and 45° under the Frankfurter plane.

2.1 Study 1

In Study 1, 12 female subjects were recruited from the office staff at the University of Oslo. Their mean age was 30,8 years, and the age span was from 21 to 38 years. All subjects were experienced VDT-users and had VDT-work, mostly data entry and routine data dialogue, as a major part of their working day. All of them had a history of problems related to VDT-work. Their symptoms varied, but could be summarised as astenopic symptoms and visual fatigue. The study was set up as a within-subject, repeated measures design, with subjects run in a counterbalanced way (ABBA) (17). Under both conditions the VDT-task was presented as a single-spaced, WordPerfect 5.1, document on a 14-inch monochrome monitor (HR monitor 31.11, Ericsson Information systems AB, Sweden), with light (amber) characters on dark background. The monitor had a refresh rate of 50 Hz and the resolution was 720 x 350 pixels. The subjects were comfortably seated on a multi-adjustable chair and were given time and individual instructions on how to do necessary adjustments in order to prevent postural discomfort. The table and chair were then adjusted to obtain a viewing distance of 57 cm.

Each work session lasted for 1 hour, with an inter-session period of at least 1 day. The subjects were instructed to work as quickly and accurately as possible, without pauses. Work-related symptoms were measured after 5 minutes of work and immediately after each work session, using a paper and pencil test, the 14 item - 7-step Cantril scale, developed by the authors. Modifications of this symptom scale have been used in other studies (10,18). A measure of productivity was also computed. The number of meaningful words identified during each work session was registered and the percentage of words identified from the total number of meaningful words in the document calculated.

2.2 Study 2

In Study 2, 60 unselected female subjects participated from an introductory class in Psychology. The mean age was 22,9 years, and the age span was from 19 to 33 years. 35 of the subjects had some form of optical correction and nearly half of them (19 subjects) wore this correction daily. The subjects were randomly divided into two groups in a traditional parallel group design. The work session was increased from one to two hours and pre - post measures of contrast sensitivity and refraction were included together with a follow-up symptom questionnaire. Both reduced contrast sensitivity and myopization have been shown to indicate oculomotor fatigue (18,19, 20) and the follow-up questionnaire was included because subjects in the first study often reported an increase in subjective symptoms *after* the work session was completed. Apart from the above mentioned differences this study follows the same procedures as Study 1. It also includes the same productivity measure and symptom scale, with the addition of one item (Do you experience a general feeling of tiredness?).

Measures of contrast sensitivity were done, at a distance of 6 metres, with a VCTS 6500 chart. (Vistech Consultants Inc., Dayton, Ohio, USA). Work related changes in contrast sensitivity may be a combined effect of spatial frequency adaptation and myopization. To maximise the effect of myopization, the ordinary testing distance (3,3 m - 10 feet) was extended to 6 m. The VCTS 6500 measurements were done in a room with stable artificial light conditions (30-70 ft.-L). Measurements of refraction were done with an autorefractometer (RM-A3000B, Topcon Corporation, Tokyo, Japan). The measurements were repeated ten times on each eye, to ensure representative values.

The monitor used in this study was a 14-inch low radiation colour monitor (TDV 5330, Tandberg Data A/S, Oslo, Norway) and the VDT-task were, under both conditions, presented as a single-spaced, Word for Windows, 2.0, document with dark characters on light background. The monitor had a refresh rate of 72 Hz., non-interlaced, with a resolution of 800 x 600 pixels. The font used was 12 point, Times Roman.

3. RESULTS

In Study 1, we observed an increase in subjective symptom strength, pre - post VDT work, in both conditions of gaze inclination. As shown in figure 1 this increase was larger under the 15° condition than under the 45° condition.

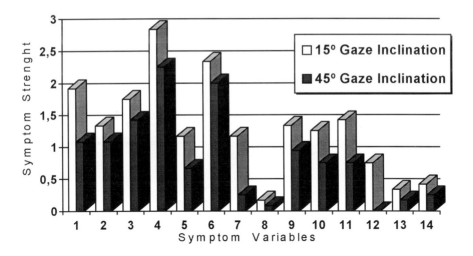

1.Pain, tension behind/around the eyes; 2.Pain, tired/dryness of eyes; 3.Focusing difficulties; 4.Pain, tension in the neck/shoulders; 5.Headache; 6.Pain, tension in the back; 7.Dizziness; 8.Nausea; 9.Problems with linetracking; 10.Concentration problems; 11."Foggy" letters, words or numbers; 12."Doubling" letters, words or numbers; 13."Jumping" letters, words or numbers; 14.Shivering text.

Figure 1. Study 1, Subjective Symptom Scores. Difference, Pre - Post, VDT - Work.

When computed as an aggregated symptom score this difference was statistically significant (t= 2.48, df=11, p < .050).

In Study 2, when unselected subjects were used, pre - post work measurements of subjective symptoms still showed a significant increase in subjective symptoms. However, the results did not show any significant difference between the two experimental conditions. Interestingly enough, this picture is slightly different when we consider the subjects who wore optical corrections daily. Assuming these subjects to be more symptomatic than the other subjects, it is interesting to find that the aggregated symptom score for this subsample approaches statistical significance (t= 1.97, df=16, p = .066). Analyses of single variables in this subsample showed two significant results, "pain, tension in the neck/shoulders" (t= 2.58, df=16, p < .050) and "Pain, tired/dryness of eyes" (t= 2.30, df=16, p < .050). These variables showed the largest increase in symptom strength under the 15° gaze inclination.

Analyses of the follow up questionnaire showed that as many as 93% of the sample experienced increased symptoms in the hours after the work session was completed. Nevertheless, only one symptom variable showed significant differences between the two gaze inclinations. This variable indicates that subjects working with the 15° gaze inclination have more "concentration problems" in the hours after the work session was completed than subjects working with the 45° gaze inclination (t=2.67, df=45, p= .011).

Figure 2, show the pre-post measurements in contrast sensitivity for the two experimental groups of Study 2. Both groups show reduction of contrast sensitivity, the reduction being significantly smaller for 45° gaze inclination compared to 15° gaze inclination. (F=4.28, df=57, p<0.05).

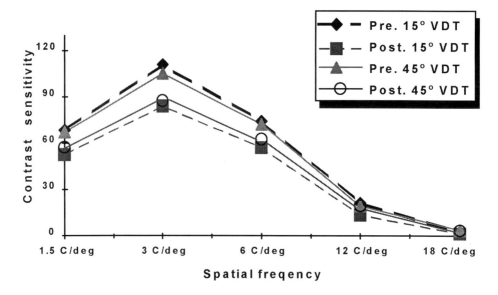

Figure 2. Changes in contrast sensitivity. Pre/post VDT work, 15°and 45° gaze Inclination.

Figure 3, present the results from the pre-post refraction's done in Study 2. As this figure indicates, subjects working with the 15° gaze inclination experienced a change in the direction of myopa during the 2 hour VDT-work session. This is contrary to the group working with the downward gaze angle, whose change was in a hypermetropic direction. The difference of refraction change between the groups is statistically significant (t= -2.03, df=57, p < .050).

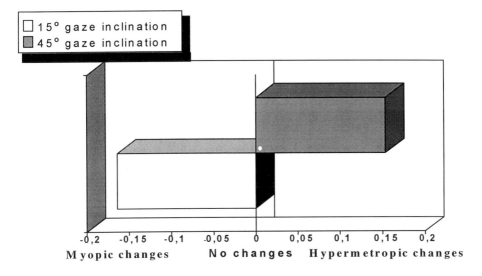

Figure 3. SPH - refraction: Pre/post-test difference. 15° gaze inclination vs. 45° gaze inclination.

Measurements of productivity did not show any statistical significant results. However, there was a tendency toward higher productivity under the 45° gaze inclination in both studies.

4. CONCLUSIONS

The results from these studies are consistent with the common finding that even short periods of VDT-work have a detrimental influence upon both visual functions and subjective symptoms. The negative effects are, however reduced when gaze angle inclination is shifted from 15° to 45° below the Frankfurter plane, suggesting that the VDT-screen should be positioned according to a downward gaze of about 45°. This suggestion is currently being tested in a 2-year field study in Norway.

REFERENCES

1. C. Behrens and S. B. Sells, Experimental studies of fatigue of accomodation. In, Plan of research and observation on recession of near point of accomodation following a period of interpolated work on the ophthalmic ergograph. Archives of Ophthalmology, 31 (1944) 148.
2. K. Brozek, E. Simons and A. Keys, Changes in performance and in ocular functions resulting from strenuous visual inspection. American Journal of Psychology, 63, (1950) 51.

3. W. J. Smith, A review of literature relating to visual fatigue. In, Proceedings of the Human Factors Society, 23rd Annual Meeting, (1979) 362.
4. O. Østerberg, Accomodation and Visual fatigue in display work. In, E. Grandjean and E. Vigliani (eds.), Ergonomic Aspects of Visual Display Terminals, , Taylor & Francis, UK, London 1980.
5. P. Padmos, Visual Fatigue with work on visual display units: The current state of knowledge. In, Van der Ver and G. Mulder (eds), Human Computer Aspects: Psychonomic Aspects. Springer Verlag, Germany, Berlin, 1988.
6. E. Grandjean, Ergonomics and Health in modern Offices, Taylor & Francis, UK, London,1984.
7. F. W. Campell and K. Durden, The Visual Display Terminal Issue: A consideration of it's Physiological, Psychological and clinical background. Ophthalmic and Physiological Optics, 3, (1983) 175.
8. J. J. Gibson, The Ecological Approach in Visual Perception, Houghton Mifflin Company, USA, Boston, 1979.
9. L. Manas, Visual Analysis. The Professional Press Inc., USA, Chicago, 1968.
10. I. Lie and R. Watten, VDT work, oculomotor strain and subjective complaints. An experimental and clinical study. Ergonomics, 37(8), (1994) 1419.
11. H. Heuer and D. A. Owens, Vertical gaze direction and the resting posture of the eyes. Perception, 18, (1989) 363.
12. H. Heuer, Visual Work With Different Gaze Inclination. In, H. Luczak, A. E. Çakir and G. Çakir, (eds), Work With Display Units '92. Technische Universität Berlin. Institut für Arbeitswissenschaft. Germany, Berlin, (1992) B-16.
13. S. Saito, S. Taptagaporn, S. Saito, M. Sotoyama and T. Suzuki, Eye Movement Analysis of Vertical Gazing Position and Dark Vergence for Comfortable VDT Workstation Design. In, H. Luczak, A. E. Çakir and G. Çakir, (eds), Work With Display Units '92. Technische Universität Berlin. Institut für Arbeitswissenschaft. Germany, Berlin, (1992) B-12.
14. T. Takeda, K. Hashimoto, K. Ikeda and N. Hiruma, Accomodation Induced by Line of Sight. In, H. Luczak, A. E. Çakir and G. Çakir, (eds), Work With Display Units '92. Technische Universität Berlin. Institut für Arbeitswissenschaft. Germany, Berlin, (1992) B-10.
15. T. Suzuki, S. Taptagaporn, M. Sotoyama, S. Saito and S. Saito, Application of the Ophthalmological Aspects of Ocular Position to VDT Workstation Design. In, H. Luczak, A. E. Çakir and G. Çakir, (eds), Work With Display Units '92. Technische Universität Berlin. Institut für Arbeitswissenschaft. Germany, Berlin, (1992) B-14.
16. T. Paulsen, Proof-Reading from VDU: The Effect of Vertical Gaze Direction on Speed, Acuity, Subjective Discomfort and Preference. Institute of Psychology. University of Oslo, Norway, OSLO, 1990.
17. J. M. Neale and R. M. Liebert, Science and Behavior An introduction to methods of research Prentice - Hall, Inc. USA, Englewood Cliffs, N. J. 1980.
18. R. Watten, I. Lie and S. Magnussen, VDU work, contrast adaptation, and visual fatigue. Behavior & information technology, 11(5), (1992) 262.
19. R. Lunn and W. P. Banks, Visual fatigue and spatial frequency adaptation to video displays of text. Human factors, 28, (1986) 457.
20. R. Watten, & I. Lie, Time Factors in VDT-Induced Myopia and Visual Fatigue: An Experimental Study, Journal of Human Ergology, 21, (1992) 13.

Stress and health problems due to alteration of binocular vision at visual display units

K. Fassbender[a], M. Georgi[a], J. Wahl[a], H. Mayer[b], E. Kraus-Mackiw[a], D.-B. Braun[a], C. Danckwardt[a] and J. Dürr[a].

[a]Ergophthalmological Research Unit, Ruprecht Karl University,
P.O.Box 102369, D-69013 Heidelberg, Germany

[b]Stress Research Unit, Ruprecht Karl University,
P.O.Box 102369, D-69013 Heidelberg, Germany

1. INTRODUCTION

Asthenopia at visual display units (VDUs) has been found to correlate with the quality of binocular vision (1). The German trade association norm G37 takes this into account by setting a screening test which, in addition to its main objective of testing vision, selects subjects with phoria or deficiencies in fusion and stereoscopic vision.

These selected persons undergo a supplementary investigation by the ophthalmologist, who then has to evaluate if, or under what conditions, the subject could work at VDUs without any risk to health.

The aim of this study is to establish whether these tests are sufficient to assess the prevalence of binocular deficiencies and to verify their correlation with asthenopia and other health complaints, which has already been demonstrated for the close work performed by seamstresses (2, 3, 4).

2. METHODS

740 persons working on VDUs in two different companies (A,B) were investigated in accordance with the German trade association norm G37. The study also included 152 members of university staff, working on VDUs who had shown abnormalities of vision in routine examinations by the works doctor. A group of 847 workers from four garment factories (seamstresses) with tasks requiring near vision served for comparison.

The investigations were performed with different vision test instruments in use for this purpose, namely Binoptometer (Oculus) (company A), R7 and R12 (Rodenstock) (company B and garment industry) and Ergovision (Essilor) (university). Binocular deficiencies were diagnosed if phoria, stereoscopic vision or fusion did not fulfill the criteria for every vision test instrument and its respective test disc (according to the instructions for use).

2.1. Phoria

R7, R12 and Ergovision select subjects if exophoria exceeds 2cm/m or if esophoria, hypophoria or hyperphoria exceed 1cm/m. The Binoptometer selects eso- and exophorias of more than 3 cm/m and hypo- and hyperphorias of more than 1cm/m.

2.2. Stereoscopic vision

R7 and R12 select subjects with a stereoacuity worse than 60 seconds of arc, Ergovision and Binoptometer worse than 120 seconds of arc.

2.3. Fusion

All vision test instruments select subjects who show suppression or double vision. All vision tests were carried out at near distance (55cm) with the subjects' corrective lenses. Based on this data, the prevalence of binocular deficiencies was determined.

2.4. Subjective well-being and health status

In Company B subjective well-being and the health status of the employees were additionally assessed using the Freiburg Symptom Inventory (Freiburger Beschwerdenliste, FBL) (5,6) and questionnaires concerning visual symptoms and current work place. The correlation between health complaints and binocular deficiencies was investigated. For statistical analysis the chi square-test was used.

3. RESULTS

The prevalence of binocular deficiencies found with the screening methods ranged between 5% and 35% (see Table 1).

Table 1
Investigated employees

	N*	Mean age (years)	Employees wearing spectacles	Binocular vision disturbed**
VDU work:				
Company A	612	35	60 %	5 %
Company B	128	35	58 %	35 %
University	152	39	31 %	22 %
Reference group:				
Garment industry (seamstresses)	847	31	30 %	26 %

* Numbers of employees tested
** Relates to phoria, fusion and stereoscopic vision.

In company B, in the subgroup with binocular deficiencies, a higher percentage of employees suffered from other health complaints than in the subgroup without binocular deficiencies (see Table 2).

Table 2
Subjective well-being and general health in relation to binocular deficiencies in 128 subjects working on VDUs (Company B).

Health complaints	Binocular vision disturbed (%)	Binocular vision not disturbed (%)
Shoulder and back pain**	67	30
Blurred vision at VDU**	45	19
Autonomic symptoms**	58	29
Psychosomatic symptoms**	64	33
Visual stress index:		
- ocular fatigue	73	58
- burning eyes	45	32
- watering eyes	45	45
- sensitivity to light*	51	28
Subjective stress feeling*	70	45
Neuromuscular complaints*	73	45

* $p < 0.05$ ** $p < 0.005$

4. DISCUSSION

Screening tests revealed prevalences of binocular deficiencies of 5%, 22%, 26% and 35%. These results are determined not only by the different cut-off values applied by the different vision test instruments, but also, even more, by the scope for interpretation of the testers. The 5 % value came from company A, whose works doctor is insensitive to the problems being investigated, and naturally passes this attitude on to his staff.

According to the trade association norm G37, one of the minimum requirements to "pass" the screening test is normal phoria and stereoscopic vision. Since there is no further definition of what "normal" is, this decision is left to the constructor of the vision test instrument or the test disc.

An investigation in which the same parameters (phoria, fusion and stereoscopic vision) were studied with different methods (cover test, Worth test, prism test, Titmus stereo test and synoptophore) came to similar results (1): 20.6 % of the employees showed impairment of binocular vision.

The lower percentage may be due to the classification of well-compensated heterophoria (24.7 %) as normal. However, if binocular vision is assessed with supplementary methods, binocular vision deficiencies amount to 60% of cases (7).

The most important information about wether the function of the physiological double eye is generally exact, only intermittently exact or non-existent, is gained by the experienced observer when the test subject is required to perform persuit movements. If fixation in the two eyes is accompanied by symmetrical corneal light reflexes and if the two eyes can follow the object of interest with smooth persuit movements, this is proof of normal fusion. If, on the other hand, jerky eye movements are observed, either unilaterally or in alternation, depending on the direction or distance of gaze, this indicates the need to regain, by way of compensation, the common horopter (8).

When the test subject holds Bagolini striated glasses (at 45° and 135°) he can subjectively experience the potencial instability of his sensory-motor behavior as an explanation of his visual complaints (9).

The positive correlation observed in this study between binocular vision deficiencies and health complaints suggest that even small deviations from exact binocular vision should be selected by a screening test in routine occupational health tests, even if they represent a "normal" condition. The main task of the ophthalmologist is then to investigate refraction and the flexibility of accommodation in regard to extent and promptness. If differences are found here between the two eyes, even small refractive errors should be corrected in jobs with high visual demands in order to facilitate binocular cooperation.

In binocular deficiencies, the loss of time and the uncertainty caused by recurrent interruptions of bifoveal fixation, explain the higher prevalence of stress sensations, psychosomatic symptoms and shoulder and back pain in this group. The latter represents a major problem in VDU work (10).

The finding that a higher percentage of employees at VDUs than employees doing other types of close work wear spectacles is consistent with the result of an Allensbach survey in Germany (commissioned by the "Kuratorium Gutes Sehen" in 1993), which additionally found these differences to be most pronounced in the age group between 30 and 44. Concerning the low percentage of the university sample (31%), it must be taken into consideration that it is based on a selected sample of problem cases.

5. CONCLUSION

Since small deviations from exact binocular vision are widespread and since subjects with such deviations, if working at VDUs, bear a higher risk of complaints, it is important especially for software ergonomists to aim at "clear design that will reduce binocular stress". The most important requirement arising from the results of this study is that works doctors need to be better educated about problems of binocular vision.

ACKNOWLEDGEMENTS

We are gratful to Kersti Wagstaff, M.A., John Webster, B.A., and Dieter Windfuhr, University of Heidelberg, for their careful preparation of the manuscript.

REFERENCES

1. Piccoli B, Gratton I, Pierini F, Catenacci G, Raimondi E, Farulla A. Asthenopia and objective ophthalmological findings in a population of 2058 VDT operators in region Lombardia. G Ital Med Lav 1989; 11:267-71.

2. Mayer H. Stress durch Probleme des Sehens bei der Arbeit. In: Wissenschaftliche Vereinigung für Augenoptik und Optometrie e.V. (ed) Die Brille für den Bildschirmarbeitsplatz. WVAO, Mainz, 1991; 2:13-16.

3. Mayer H. Gesundheitliche Beschwerden und Stress durch Probleme des Sehens bei der Arbeit. Optometrie 1991; 38:125-28.

4. Mayer H, Kraus-Mackiw E. Streß bei visueller Arbeit. NOJ 1992; 34:18-23.

5. Fahrenberg J. Die Freiburger Beschwerdenliste FBL. Z Klin Psychol Psychother 1975; 4: 79-100.

6. Hampel R, Fahrenberg J. Die Freiburger Beschwerdenliste. Gruppenvergleiche und andere Studien zur Validität. Forschungsbericht des Psychologischen Instituts der Albert Ludwig-Universität, Freiburg/Breisgau,1982; 7.

7. Wahl J, Fassbender K. Basic parameters and empirical constructs of binocular processes. In: Grieco A, Molteni G, Occhipinti E, Piccoli B (eds) Work With Display Units '94. University of Milan, Institute of Occupational Health, Milan, 1994; 1:P20-21.

8. Kraus-Mackiw E. Heterophories and work at near point. In: Grieco A, Molteni G, Occhipinti E, Piccoli B (eds) Work With Display Units '94. University of Milan, Institute of Occupational Health, Milan, 1994; 3:B25-26.

9. Bagolini B. Tecnica per l'esame della visione binoculare senza introduzione di elementi dissocianti (Test del vetro striato). Boll Ocul 1958; 37:195-209.

10. Smith MJ, Carayon P, Sanders KJ, Lim SY, LeGrande D. Employee stress and health in jobs with and without electronic performance monitoring. Applied ergonomics 1992; 23: 17-28.

Results of an ergophthalmologic and oculistic survey on a sample of video display unit workers and non-exposed subjects.

F. De Marco, D. Colombini, M. Meroni, E. Occhipinti, A. Petri, A. Soccio, E. Tosatto, C. Vimercati

CEMOC - AZIENDA USSL 41, via Riva Villasanta, 11, 20145 Milano, Italy

1. INTRODUCTION

A sample of 863 VDU workers underwent an ergophthalmic and oculistic survey aimed at evaluating the prevalence of ocular pathologies and symptoms and the correlation with various visual overloading factors linked to the work environment and the characteristics of VDU use, in according to some studies available in field literature (1,2,3,4,5,6,7).
All the subjects were given a questionnaire aimed at highlighting the characteristics of the work environment and ocular anamnestic data.
Analysis was made of one hundred and sixty voices on the questionnaire covering:
Age; Length of employment on VDUs; daily hours at VDUs; type of work; their evaluation of indoor air quality, lighting and noise; VDU work station lay-out, with particular reference to the natural and artificial light sources; the characteristics of VDTs, furniture and accessories; work satisfaction assessment, stress and constructive atmosphere at work; ocular anamnesis; type and frequency of impairments to the eyes, the breathing passages, the osteoarticular system and general symptoms occurring due to work.
The ocular symptoms were evaluated both analytically and using a points system which gave a value to each symptom in relation to how frequently it occurred (0=never, 6=every day). The points were then added together to give a value which has been used in some statistical analyses.
The subjects examined underwent various tests: all the subjects underwent ophthalmometry testing, the anterior segment and accessory organs of the eye were also tested and their lenses were tested with a lens meter; 24 subjects underwent VISIOTEST; 55 subjects had VISIOTEST and orthoptic tests to evaluate the main binocular functions for close distances; 786 subjects had dynamic refraction and orthoptic tests.
Based on the symptoms reported, impairments found and existing ocular pathologies, 328 subjects were sent to a specialised oculist.

A sample of 134 nursery school teachers (all female) was used as a control group for evaluating the prevalence of ocular symptoms.
The data were analysed using Chi-square test, analysis of variance and logistic regression analysis.
Only the main results concerning ocular problems will be presented.

2. RESULTS

The control group had an average age of 36.7 (SD=7.5).
Of the VDU users, 37% are male (average age 38.7; SD=9.3) and 63% female (average age 35.3; SD=7.7).
Both sexes show similar average of length of employment with VDUs (M=6.2 years, SD=4.2; F=5.2 years, SD=3.6) and a similar average of daily hours of VDU use (M=3.6 hours, SD=1.8; F=3.3 hours, SD=1.7), even though the males always have slightly higher values.
Most of the people worked on data loading, data acquisition and word processing tasks.
The prevalence of refractive defects are similar in the control group and in the VDU users and only a greater prevalence of emmetropic subjects showed up in the control group over 40 years old.
The daily hours of VDU use were grouped into three classes: 0 to 1 hours (101 subjects, or 11.6%), from 2 to 4 hours (540 subjects, or 62.3%) and over 4 hours (226 subjects, or 26.1%).
Table 1 displays the percentages of subjects manifesting ocular disturbances with a frequency of at least a few times a month, divided by hours of daily VDU use and the last column shows the results of the Chi-square test.

Table 1.
Prevalence (in percentage) of subjects reporting asthenopic symptoms, divided by hours of VDU use. (*1 : at distance -*2 : close up).

SYMPTOMS	CONTROL	HOURS OF VDU USE			p
		< 2	2 - 4	> 4	
Dry eyes	2.2	2	2.4	5.7	0.076
Burning eyes	12.0	13.9	19.6	24.8	0.012
Lacrimation	5.9	7.9	7	10.6	0.315
Photophobia	1.4	7.9	8.5	6.2	0.036
Eye-strain	25.3	28.7	38.5	46	0.0003
Foggy vision *1	9.1	5.9	7.8	12.3	0.15
Foggy vision *2	6.7	8	6.1	7.5	0.85
Double vision	0	1	0.8	0.8	0.75
Frontal headaches	9.7	12.9	10.8	11.5	0.88

Burning eyes, photophobia and eye-strain were found in significantly higher numbers in the VDU operators than in the control group.

Foggy vision at a distance and close up, double vision and headaches occurred in both the VDU and the control groups in similar numbers.

It should be noted that the subjects considered as the control group still manifest visual disturbances of which the tired eyes symptom reaches 25%.

Five symptoms, dryness, burning, lacrimation, photophobia and ocular fatigue were considered related, even if in varying degrees, to the daily number of hours of VDU use.

The averages obtained by adding the frequency scores for those five symptoms were evaluated using variance analysis (max value=30).

VDU users have significantly higher averages than the control group (control group=1.7; 0-1 hours of daily VDU use=3.1; 2-4 hrs=3.5; >4 hrs=4.3; p=0.00).

It should be noted that it is the scores of the VDU users with more than four hours of daily use that determine the significance of the statistical analysis.

Subjects that manifested at least one of the cited five asthenopic symptoms with a frequency equal or greater than a few times a month were considered affected by asthenopic impairments.

The data that follows relates to subjects classified with this criteria.

The prevalence of subjects with symptoms in the control group was significantly lower than among the VDU users (control group=34.3%; 0-1 hours of daily VDU use=42.6%; 2-4 hrs=48.1%; >4 hrs=56.6%; p=0.0005).

The frequency of disturbances increases with greater use among the operators in a statistically significant way, even though a third of the control group show asthenopic symptoms.

In the groups examined, no correlation was found between the frequency of asthenopic symptoms and the gender of the subjects.

In the sample analysed, the position of the VDU with respect to the window, the screening of the windows and lights, the type of work surface and the colour of the walls did not demonstrate a correlation to the asthenopic symptoms.

Screen reflections did reveal itself as an important factor in determining ocular symptoms.

The greater percentage of subjects with asthenopic impairments occurs among these reporting screen reflections (screen reflections=symptomatics 63%, non screen reflections=45%; p=0.000).

The greatest frequencies being among subjects that use VDUs for more than 4 hours a day (symptomatics=71%).

The general lighting assessment was also seen to be an important element associated with ocular disturbances.

The prevalence of subjects manifesting asthenopic symptoms among those that reported that the lighting was poor (58%) or excessive (68%) was significantly higher (p=0.0002) than among those that reported comfortable lighting (46%).

Those who reported excessive lighting showed a significantly higher average of symptom score (excessive lighting=symptom average 5, poor lighting=4.2, comfortable lighting=3.2; p=0.000).

The presence of air-conditioning, stale air, unpleasant smells, airborne dust and tobacco smoke within the work place, did not show a correlation to asthenopic symptoms.

However, the subjects that reported that the air was too dry (dry air= symptomatics 61% vs normal air=48%; p=0.0001) or who were unsatisfied by the air quality (unsatisfied= symptomatics 56% vs satisfied=44%; p=0.0006) manifested a significant increase in asthenopic symptoms.

Subjects with refractive defects reported a greater number of asthenopic disturbances, with the exception of purely presbyopic or myopic subjects. For brevity's sake, only emmetropia and refractive defects with the major occurrence of ocular symptoms are presented: emmetropia= symptomatics 42%, hypermetropic astig. + hypermetropia=62%, myopic astig. + myopia + presbyopia=65%, myopic astig.=67%, myopia + presbyopia= 68%, hypermetropia + presbyopia=73%, hypermetropic astig.=79%, hypermetropic astig.+ prebyopia=87%.

Subjects that do not have the right correction manifest a greater percentage of asthenopic disturbances in comparison with emmetropic or appropriately corrected subjects but the difference is only significant for subjects not corrected for distance (not corrected =68% vs corrected =47%; p=0.0002).

Subjects with impairments of the *fundus oculi* or the anterior segment did not report asthenopic symptoms in any significantly greater percentages than the subjects without impairments.

Subjects showed impairments in close up and distant divergence; distant convergence; subjective and objective ocular deviation angle (measured with the synoptophore) did not manifest asthenopic symptoms in significantly greater numbers than the subjects without impairments.

Near point of convergence impairments showed a significant correlation with asthenopic symptoms (symptomatics with good NPC =48%, fair =60%, poor=64%, absent=50%; p=0.05).

Impairments in fusional convergence for un-corrected near sight were also revealed to be associated with the asthenopic symptoms (symptomatics with normal fusional convergence=47%, at lower limit=46%, insufficient=63%; p=0.02).

Subjects with ocular deviation revealed by the close cover-uncover test showed a significantly greater prevalence towards asthenopic symptoms than those with orthophoria or mild exophoria , who made up 48% of the sample (symptomatics with normal CT=45%, with impairments=53%; p=0.02)).

Exotropia and intermittent exotropia were revealed as being the impairments found in the highest percentage of subjects with ocular disturbances (around 60%).

The sample examined did not show significant differences in the prevalence of refractive and ocular motility defects due to the number of daily hours of VDU use or the number of years of VDU use.

The average scores for the constructive atmosphere at work (0=very poor, 10=very good), stress (0=no, 10=extremely stressful) and work satisfaction (0=completely unsatisfied, 10=completely satisfied) were analysed in relation to the hours of VDU use, asthenopic symptoms, screen reflections, overall assessments of lighting and air quality.

Subjects who used VDU's for a period of over 4 hours a day had average scores for stress that were significantly higher than those who used VDUs for 2 to 4 hours (0-1 hours =7, 2-4 hours = 6.4, >4 hours =7.2; p=0.003).
There were no differences in the stress scores due to other parameters.
Average scores for the constructive atmosphere at work were significantly lower in subjects reporting asthenopic disturbances (asymptomatic=7.4, symptomatic=6.4, p=0.008) and in those who said they were unsatisfied with the air quality (satisfied=7.6, unsatisfied =6.6; p=0.002).
There were no differences in the constructive atmosphere at work scores due to other parameters.
With reference to work satisfaction, a significant number of subjects claiming to be less satisfied were among those who reported asthenopic disturbances (asymptomatic=7, symptomatic=6.2; p=0.002) and those who said they were unsatisfied with the air quality (satisfied =6.2, unsatisfied =7.6; p=0.000).
There were no differences in the work satisfaction scores due to other parameters.

3. CONCLUSIONS

The results of this survey confirm that numerous factors are correlated to asthenopic symptoms in VDU workers.
The factors emerging from the survey can be summed up as follows:
daily hours of VDU use; the presence of screen reflections; air quality; individual factors like: refractive defects, optical correction, binocular function impairments.
The opinion that the asthenopic syndrome has multi-factorial origins is widely shared in the field literature.
However, in the VDU work environment these factors do not act in isolation but rather run together to a variable degree to determine ocular symptoms.
Certain questions remain: Are some factors of greater relevance? How much weight do the single factors carry when they act together? Towards which elements should preventive or corrective interventions be primarily addressed?
A solution was tried that applied the logistic regression analysis, constructing a model with which to predict the asthenopic syndrome on the basis of data from the survey.
Obviously, in defining the model simplifications had to be made, such as trying to reduce the greatest possible number of variables to just the dichotic ones.
The presence of at least one of the following ocular disturbances were considered as a dependent variable: dry eyes, burning eyes, lacrimation, photophobia and eye-strain with a frequency of at least a few times a month and, as covariate ones, all the factors cited that had demonstrated a statistically significant association with the asthenopic symptoms.
Each single factor was eliminated in successive steps on the basis of the level of significance when compared with all the others.
In this way a model was obtained which allowed us to correctly classify 62% of the subjects.

On the basis of the data available, 4 factors played a significant role in determining ocular symptoms, in the conditions in which all the cited factors act together:
1. The daily hours of VDU use (in particular, the use of VDUs for over 4 hours a day)
2. Screen reflections (that came out as the factor with greatest weight)
3. Near point convergence impairments
4. Refractive defects (particularly, close vision defects), whether vision was corrected adequately or not.

This data seems to highlight the nucleus of factors that determine the asthenopic syndrome and can indicate the priority objectives of an evaluation and prevention system that considers work organisation, working environment and individual characteristics.

It is not possible to establish whether the model obtained can be generalised, but the size of the sample studied allowed us to establish that it can reasonably represent aspects of other working situations.

In conclusion, we hope that there will be an increasing number of surveys that evaluate the joint role of the various factors associated with the ocular symptoms of VDU users. This would help make better use of preventive and corrective interventions on the environment and work organisation and the preventive and therapeutic ones for the workers.

REFERENCES

1. A. Belisario, D. Nini, E. Gennari, A. Modiano, G. Olivetti, L. Bassein "Sintomatologia oculare in un gruppo di operatori videoterminalisti." In Monduzzi (ed.): Atti del 53° Congresso della Soc. It. di Medicina del Lavoro e Igiene Industriale - Stresa 10-13 Ottobre 1990, 433.
2. L. Scullica, C. Rechichi "Influenza dei vizi di refrazione sulla insorgenza della astenopia in lavoratori addetti a videoterminali (inchiesta epidemiologica su 29614 soggetti)." Boll. Ocul: 69, suppl. 5, 41 (1990).
3. A. Di Bari, F.M. Grignolo, G. Maina, A. Sonnino "Risultati di una indagine ergoftalmologica in operatori al VDT." Boll. Ocul.: 69, suppl. 5, 93 (1990).
4. A. Di Bari, F.M. Grignolo, B. Boles Carenini, G. Maina "Analisi fattoriale dei disturbi lamentati dagli addetti a terminali video." Boll:Ocul.: 69, suppl. 5, 129 (1990).
5. World Health Organization "Visual display terminals and workers' health." WHO Offset Publication 99, 85 (1987).
6. G. Hermans "Office work and eyestrain." Abstracts, IXth International Congress of Soc. Ophthal. Europea, Brussels, May 23-28 1992, 95.
7. L. Rose "Workplace video display terminals and visual fatigue." J. Occup. Med., 29, 231 (1987).

Testing a proposed ergophthalmic protocol for monitoring the health of video display unit workers.

A Petri., D. Colombini, F. De Marco, M. Meroni, E. Occhipinti, A. Soccio, E. Tosatto, C. Vimercati

CEMOC - AZIENDA USSL 41 via Riva Villasanta, 11 - 20145 Milano, Italy

1. INTRODUCTION

From the very first signs of the asthenopic syndrome in VDU workers (1,2,3,4,5,6,7), specialised medical surveillance was studied, the structure of which is still the subject of much debate in Occupational Medicine.

EEC directive 270/90 aims at providing medical surveillance for VDU workers but it does not provide practical indications as to which protocols should be adopted, particularly in the case of ocular-visual problems.

This regulation leaves room for extreme situations: rapidly carried out visual screening on the orthoanalyser (by people that are not necessarily qualified) on the one hand, and complex diagnostic protocols (8,9,10) on the other which require a lot of time, high costs and the constant presence of an oculist.

The aim of this work is to establish a standard protocol that would provide adequate ergophthalmic monitoring for VDU users.

2. MATERIALS AND METHODS

Three different medical-check protocols were evaluated, using a sample of VDU users, with the aim of obtaining practical indications about which type of test to carry out.

Four hundred and ninety two subjects were investigated: 122 men, with an average age of 39.7 (SD 8.5) and average length of employment on VDUs of 6.3 years (SD 4.3) and 370 women - av. age 35.4 (SD 7.4) and av. length of employment of 4.5 years (SD 3.4).

The subjects of the survey were VDU users with a daily VDU use that varied between 1 and 7 hours; 66% used VDUs for a period between 2 and 4 hours.

In order to establish which ergophthalmic tests represent the minimum requirements for the VDU workers'medical surveillance, an ample ergophthalmic protocol was used in this study as a reference. This will be described as protocol C.

Later it was decided that the sample group be subjected to two protocols called A and B, made up of a lesser number of ergophthalmic tests. The idea was to evaluate which and how many ocular impairments would not have been diagnosed by applying protocols A or B in place of protocol C.

The first table shows protocol A, the simplest, which consists of a test using the Essilor company's VISIOTEST orthoanalyser; ophthalmometry; examination of the anterior segment and accessory organs with a slit lamp; lensmeter test.

Table 1
Protocol A

- visiotest
- ophthalmometry
- examination of the anterior segment and accessory organs with a slit lamp
- lensmeter test

The second table shows protocol B which consists of protocol A, as well as voluntary extra-ocular motility testing; objective and subjective near point of convergence tests; distant and near cover-uncover tests for both natural (un-corrected) and corrected vision (with subject's own lenses); near fusional divergence and convergence prism tests for both natural and corrected vision.

Table 2
Protocol B

PROTOCOL A +
- voluntary extra-ocular motility testing
- objective and subjective near point of convergence tests
- distant and near cover - uncover tests for both natural an usual corrected vision
- near fusional divergence and convergence prism test for both natural and usual corrected vision

The third table shows protocol C, which consists of protocol B without the "VISIOTEST" but with near and distant visual acuity testing for natural, corrected and optimally corrected vision with optotype; colour vision, using Ishihara tables; stereopsis, with the Titmus and Lang Stereo tests.

Protocol C also included: near and distant cover-uncover tests with optimum correction; Worth's four dot test over a short distance; synoptophore testing of binocular functions; near fusional divergence and convergence prism tests with optimally corrected vision.

This study did not take fundus oculi impairments and intraocular pressure into consideration. These pathologies can only be picked up by a test carried out by an oculist and this is not considered necessary for a basic ergophthalmic protocol.

Obviously, any subjects manifesting particular symptoms or impairments were referred to an oculist.

The results of the tests of protocols A and B were then compared with those of protocol C which was considered the reference protocol.

An evaluation was made of the prevalence of impairments found during protocol C testing in subjects that did not manifest impairments in protocols A and B.

Table 3
Protocol C

- ophthalmometry
- examination of the anterior segment and accessory organs with a slit lamp
- distant and near visual acuity testing for natural, usual corrected and optimally corrected vision with optotype
- colour vision, using Ishihara tables
- stereopsis with the Titmus and Lang stereotests
- voluntary extra-ocular motility testing
- distant and near cover-uncover tests for both natural, usual corrected and optimally corrected vision
- objective and subjective near point of convergence test
- Worth's four dot test over a short distance (natural, usual corrected and optimally corrected vision)
- synoptophore testing of binocular functions
- near fusional divergence and convergence prism tests for both natural, usual corrected and optimally corrected vision

3. RESULTS

The fourth table shows the overall frequencies and percentages of the impairments found in the protocol C testing, in subjects that were cleared in protocol A testing.

In order to keep brief, the table does not include the results of the tests that had the same results in protocols A and C.

Certain ocular functions, such as near point convergence and ocular motility, are not shown up by the orthoanalyser. However, the table does show the occurrence of subjects with impairments to the near point of convergence and ocular motility, shown up in the protocol C tests among those who were classified normal by all the protocol A tests.

As the table shows, protocol A was considered inadequate for screening impairments in ocular deviations. In fact, the cover-uncover test showed impairment percentages between 15% and 27% in subjects that would have been considered normal had only the results of protocol A been used.

Another limitation of protocol A is that it does not give an evaluation of fusional divergence and convergence. Impairments in these functions go to make up ocular symptoms and, as this table shows, they are manifested in between 32% and 43% of the subjects classified as normal in the tests of protocol A. Moreover, the use of just protocol A would not recognise subjects that need convergence exercises at home or clinic, who in this study represent 6.6% and 5.3% respectively.

Table 4
Overall frequencies and percentages of impairments found in subjects cleared in protocol A

TEST	IMPAIRMENTS	
	N.	%
– distant visual acuity	33	7.1
– near visual acuity	16	3.7
– voluntary extra-ocular motility	3	1.0
– obj. & subj. near point of convergence	42	13.1
– cover test natural-near	69	26.7
– cover test usual correction- near	16	14.8
– cover test optimal correction-near	3	26.7
– Worth test natural-near	3	1.7
– fusional divergence synoptophore test	5	3.9
– fusional convergence synoptophore test	45	35.4
– fusional divergence prism natural-near	25	10.9
– fusional convergence prism natural-near	100	43.1
– fusional divergence prism usual correction-near	8	8.2
– fusional convergence prism usual correction-near	32	32.0
– fusional convergence prism optimally correction-near	2	22.2
– home convergence exercises	20	6.6
– clinic convergence exercises	16	5.3

It is relevant to point out that among the subjects who showed normal visual acuity in the VISIOTEST (in both protocols A and B), 3.7 % did not have correct close visual acuity and 7.1% did not have correct distant visual acuity.

In comparing protocols B and C, a complete match was found. The impairments found in protocol C were in fact the same as those identified by protocol B but in greater depth. Only four subjects did not manifest any impairments under protocol B and the same four did not show any impairments under protocol C.

Obviously, many of the impairments found were not of clinical relevance (for example, light close exophoria, initial presbyopia, etc.).

Thus protocol B was seen to be adequate for screening impairments revealed by protocol C.

5. CONCLUSIONS

Based on the data obtained, protocol B can be used as a basic protocol for the ergophthalmic monitoring of VDU workers if the VISIOTEST is substituted.
In fact, the visual acuity test is replaced by optotype, the stereopsis tests by Titmus or Lang stereo tests and the colour vision test by Ishihara tables (table 5).

Table 5
Proposal for an ergophtalmic protocol

- ophthalmometry
- examination of the anterior segment and accessory organs with a slit lamp
- lensmeter test
- distant and near visual acuity testing for natural, usual corrected and optimally corrected vision with optotype
- voluntary extra-ocular motility testing
- objective and subjective near point of convergence test
- distant and near cover-uncover tests for both natural and usual corrected vision
- near fusional divergence and convergence prism tests for both natural and usual corrected vision
- stereopsis with the Lang or Titmus stereotest
- colour vision, using Ishihara tables

In this way the visual conditions created are less artificial.
This provides an easier and more precise study of visual acuity and any resulting correction.
Protocol A, on the contrary, even though it is easier to administer, allows impairments to be overlooked.
Knowledge of this impairments is important, particularly for the preventive medicine that the ergophthalmic screening is aimed at.
There is the question of how long it takes to carry out the tests of each of the three protocols proposed. Carrying out protocol B does not increase the time needed, given that 20 minutes are needed on average, as opposed to the 15 minutes needed for protocol A. Moreover, there is a saving over the 40 minutes needed for protocol C.
It would appear therefore that the time taken to carry out the tests would not limit the adoption of protocol B for mass testing.
These times do not include the collection of data concerning the working environment, visual and ocular anamnesis and anamnesis of general pathologies of oculistic interest.
The added tests from protocol C can be included to provide a more detailed diagnosis for subjects that manifest impairments in protocol B, while leaving any further testing to a visit to an oculist.

To sum up, the tests of protocol B are given to staff trained in Orthoptics, Orthoptists - Ophthalmic Assistants, leaving the coordination and the decision whether to refer the patient to an oculistic examination to the Occupational Health Doctor.

REFERENCES

1. F.Gobba, F. Ruberto, F. Bergamini, A. Broglia "Variazioni del potere refrattivo ed astenopia quali indici di affaticamento visivo nei lavoratori a VDT." In Monduzzi (ed.): Atti del 53° Congresso della Soc. It. di Medicina del Lavoro e Igiene Industriale - Stresa 10-13 ottobre 1990, 421.
2. A. Belisario, D. Nini, E. Gennari, A. Modiano, G. Olivetti, L. Bassein "Sintomatologia oculare in un gruppo di operatori videoterminalisti." In Monduzzi (ed.): Atti del 53° Congresso della Soc. It. di Medicina del Lavoro e Igiene Industriale - Stresa 10-13 ottobre 1990, 433.
3. C. Rechichi, A. Rizzotti, C.G.M. Tringali, L. Scullica "Influenza nella durata di applicazione al videoterminale sulla insorgenza della astenopia." Boll. Ocul.: 69, suppl. 1, 101 (1990).
4. A. Di Bari, F. M. Grignolo, G. Maina, A. Sonnino "Risultati di una indagine ergoftalmologica in operatori addetti al VDT." Boll. Ocul.: 69, suppl. 5, 93 (1990).
5. G. Hermans "Office work and eyestrain." Abstracts, IXth International Congress of Soc. Ophthal. Europea - Brussels, May 23-28, 1992, 95.
6. M. De Concini, M. Gabrielli, A. Betta "Astenopia e funzionalità oculare nel lavoro al videoterminale." Atti del Corso di Aggiornamento dell' Ass. It. Ortottisti-Assistenti di Oftalmologia - Trento, 13 novembre 1993.
7. World Health Organization Geneva "Visual display terminals and workers' health." Who Offset Publication 99,85 (1987).
8. P. Apostoli, F. Vigasio, F. Semeraro, B. Quadri, L. Alessio, C.A. Quaranta "Utilità e significatività delle visite oculistiche preventive per l'avvio al lavoro degli operatori ai VDT." In Monduzzi (ed.): Atti del 53° Congresso della Soc. It. di Medicina del Lavoro e Igiene Industriale - Stresa 10-13 ottobre 1990, 515.
9. P. Cenni, F. Farnè, V. Guerrieri, G. Valdè "Videoterminali: criteri ergonomici e funzionalità visiva. Studio di un campione di utenti ENEA dell' area di Bologna." In Monduzzi (ed.): Atti del 53° Congresso della Soc. It. di Medicina del Lavoro e Igiene Industriale - Stresa 10-13 ottobre 1990, 531.
10. Gruppo Italiano per lo studio dei rapporti tra Lavoro e Visione "Il rapporto tra lavoro e visione sotto il profilo medico preventivo: primi orientamenti per un corretto approccio ergoftalmologico secondo il Gruppo Italiano per lo studio dei rapporti tra Lavoro e Visione (G.I.L.V.). Parte seconda: metodo."
Med. Lav.: 84, 4, 324 (1993).

EYE DISORDERS IN EMPLOYEES WORKING AT VDU: LONGITUDINAL STUDY.

ASSILS (Voluntary Mutual Assistence Association of Telecomunication Workers): B. Bagolini, R. Bellucci, B. Boles Carenini, S. Borra, C. Ceccarelli, G. Coccia, A. Di Bari, F.M. Grignolo, D. Lepore, G. Maina, M. Miglior, F. Molle, E. Monaco, R. Morbio, C. Rechichi, B. Ricci, G.F. Rubino, L. Scullica, G. Sibour, P. Troiano, M. Turbati.

This study was designed to include two successive surveys on more then 70,000 employees of the Italian Telecommunication Company. The organization and scientific coordinations were entrusted to a national interdisciplinary scientific committee including: University of Turin Eye Clinic, University of Verona Eye Clinic, University of Messina Eye Clinic, University of Milan Eye Clinic, University of Milan Eye Clinic, University of Turin Institute of Industrial Medicine. To date 23,621 subjects have already undergone two complete ophthalmological examinations including ophthalmometry, biomicroscopy, autorefractometry, ophthalmoscopy, orthoptic examination and tonometry. The group under study includes 8,125 females (34.4%) and 15,496 males (65.6%); the mean age of the females was 40.7 ($\pm$ 8.7) and that of males 38.6 ($\pm$ 8.2) years. The control group include the subjects who do not use VDT or work at VDT less than two hours/day and who represent forty per cent of population. Differences found over 3.96 years elapsed between the two visits with regard to refractive status, ocular motility, ocular pressure and ocular pathology were evaluated. Data were collected from May 1986 to December 1993. During the visit a questionnaire was administered in order to evaluate the subjective level of discomfort, somatic complaints and workplace conditions. Subjective symptoms of eye strain (asthenopia) were defined according to the presence of the following nine symptoms: headache, tearing, eye smarting, eye heaviness, photophobia, ocular itching, blurred vision, double vision, reduced vision. Each symptom was graded from 0 to 2 on the basis of both its frequency and its appearance during work shift: this produced a global asthenopia score from 0 to 18. The mean asthenopia score (Table 1) increases from 2,2 to 2,4 and was found to be different in males and females respectively, in that mean values of females were higher than those of males in both examinations; however, for females they turned out to be decreased in the second examination (from 3,3 to 3,2), whereas for males there was a statistically significant ($p < 0.001$) increase of asthenopia (from 1,7 to 2).

Table 1
Asthenopia mean score: comparison between two opthalmological examination

	MALES			FEMALES			TOT		
	n°	mean	±σ	n°	mean	±σ	n°	mean	±σ
FIRST EXAMINATION	15498	1.7	2.2	8128	3.3	3.2	23626	2.2	2.7
SECOND EXAMINATION	15320	2.0	2.4	8085	3.2	3.0	23405	2.4	2.7

Asthenopia mean score increases in controls (from 1,6 to 1,9); whereas in VDT users is unmodified.
Asthenopia mean score variation according to use-no use VDT variation, is presented in Table 2. The highest increase in asthenopia mean score (+ 0.60) was observed among the 3.426 subjects who where classified as controls at first examination and as VDT users at the second examination, having increased the daily hours spent at VDU. In the 12.402 subjects classified as VDT users in both examinations asthenopia mean score was unmodified.

Table 2
Delta asthenopia mean score

		SECOND EXAMINATION (03/89-11/93)	
		CONTROLS	VDT USERS
FIRST EXAMINATION (1/86-7/88)	CONTROLS	+0.28 (n.5798)	+0.60 (N. 3426)
	VDT USERS	-0.12 (N. 1556)	+0.06 (N. 12402)

Those classified as VDT users at first examination who became controls at the second showed a slight decrease of the asthenopia mean score (+ 0.12). It should be emphatized the increase (+ 0.28) recorded in the 5.798 subjects classified as controls at both examinations.
In both examinations (Fig. 1) there was also a statistically significant relationship ($p < 0.001$) between asthenopia mean score and hours spent at VDU for both males and females.

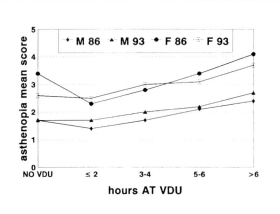

Fig. 1: Asthenopia mean score at vdu: comparison between two opthalmological examination

The hours spent daily at VDU by females were basically the same at the time of the first and second examination, whereas for males there was a slight increase in 1993.
In the second examination refractive status variations were observed in 26.3% of males and 33.5% of females (changes of more than 0.25 diopters were considered as significant): in particular changes toward myopia were found in 11.1% of males and 10.7% of females and toward hyperopia in 15.2% of males and 22.8% of females.
No correlations were found between VDT use and refractive modifications.

In both sexes changes toward myopia were significantly associated with changes in the mean asthenopia score (0.5 in males and 0.3 in females) (Table 3).

Table 3
Asthenopia mean score variation and refractive variation

	MALES			FEMALES			TOT		
REFRACTIVE VARIATION (86/93)	n°	mean	±σ	n°	mean	±σ	n°	mean	±σ
MYOPIC CHANGE	15498	17	2.2	8128	3.3	3.2	23626	2.2	2.7
UNMODIFIED	10461	0.3	2.9	5087	-0.02	3.8	15448	0.2	3.2
HYPEROPIC CHANGE	15320	2.0	2.4	8085	3.2	3.0	23405	2.4	2.7

The oculomotor and lachrymal status are essential for visual comfort and, if altered, can cause tearing, eye burning, eye heaviness and blurred vision. Evaluation of ocular motility was made using the cover test in near and distant vision; ocular deviations have been measured by prisms. We use also the Maddox-Wing test phorias to allow comparisons with the data collected during 1869-93 investigation, when the prismatic measurement was not performed. Seven classes of ocular motility have been identified: ortophoria, esophoria, exophoria, other types of phoria, esotropia, exotropia, other types of tropia. Stereopsis has been evaluated by Lang stereo-test, and considered good, sufficient or poor. We also investigated lachrymal film functions using the Scirmer I for quantitative analysis, the Jones test for quantitative analysis of basal secretion, and Break-Up Time, for qualitative analysis. We identified four symptoms related to visual fatigue, oculomotor and lachrymal film disturbances: tearing, blurred vision, eye burning and eye heaviness. The results show a great significance between each symptoms and lachrymal film evaluation tests. This statistical evidence is also found with the Mantel-Haenszel test for linear association. The same statistical analysis show a good general association between all symptoms and near Cover-test results, confirmed by Mantel-Haenszel test for linear association only for eye burning, eye heaviness and tearing. All symptoms are related with age and sex. All this data have been than related with VDU work parameters. To summarise the results of our statistical analysis it would seems that ocular motility and lachrymal film alterations play an important role in producing some asthenopic symptoms. Particularly, exophoria and esophoria seem to be most capable of induce VDU stress. In the second examination phoric status variations were observed in 20% of cases (changes of more than 5 prismatic diopters were considered as significant). No correlations were found between VDT use and phoric modification (Table 4).

Table 4: Asthenopia mean score variation and phoria variation

	MALES			FEMALES			TOT		
PHORIA VARIATION (86/93)	n°	mean	±σ	n°	mean	±σ	n°	mean	±σ
EXOPHORISATION	1881	0.5	3.0	1060	0.2	3.8	2941	0.4	3.3
UNMODIFIED	7265	0.4	2.9	4395	-0.01	3.8	11660	0.2	3.2
ESOPHORISATION	2475	0.4	3.0	1094	-0.08	4.0	3569	0.3	3.3

During the ophthalmic examination the intraocular pressure was measured by means of a Goldmann tonometer in all patiens over 40 years old and in those younger where there were symptoms, signes or case histories of glaucomatous risk. The mean values of intraocular pressure at first and second checks were not significant different. In both checks the increase and prevalence of ocular hypertension were significantly correlated with the age of subjects. No statistical significance was found between intraocular pressure values and VDU use, years of VDU use and daily hours at the VDU (Table 5).

No substantial variations were observed in the prevalence of ocular pathology between 1986 and 1993. External eye disease, sometimes suspected related to VDTs, did nto increase. The increase in the diagnoses of optic nerve head abnormalities and the decrease in the diagnoses of discromatopsias reflects the more stringent criteria of classification adopted in the second visit. The increase in the number of subject found affected by age related macular degeneration is probably due to the growing age of the operators examined. These pathologies do affect only a minimal percentage of workers. The conclusion is that VDT work did not lead to more impairments in the ophthalmic health of the operator studied over four years as compared to the impairments expected because of age.

Table 5: Prevalence of ocular hyperthension

	VDU USE			
	NO VDU (%)		VDU (%)	
FIRST EXAMINATION	9		1.1	
SECOND EXAMINATION	1.0		0.9	
	VDU USE (%)			
	NO VDU	<1	1-4	>4
FIRST EXAMINATION	1.4	0.9	0.9	1.1
SECOND EXAMINATION	1.3	0.9	0.9	0.9
	DAILY HOURS AT VDU (%)			
	< 1h	1-2 h	3-4 h	>4 h
FIRST EXAMINATION	1.0	0.7	0.9	1.2
SECOND EXAMINATION	0.9	1.1	1.0	0.8

No relation was found between the time spent at VDU and prevalence of ocular pathologies (Tab 6). For pinguecolas there is a higher prevalence in the group of workers with no or low VDU workload. No difference was found as for the time spent of VDU.

Our results point to the conclusion that VDU use is neither a cause, even after several years, of permanent organic ocular damages nor tends to worsen them. As far as refraction, motility and ophthalmic pathology are concerned, no VDU effect is found. In our population VDU use was shown to involve an adaptation of the operators over time, that asthenopia increase possibly according to task, age, hours, spent at VDU and environment.

The number of working hours at the VDU, four or more, the worker personality, sex, age, educational level and work organization, appear to be as important as the work place, the environmental condition and status of the ocular apparatus.

Table 6
External ocular pathology considered as for time spent at VDTs

	VDT ≤2H/DAY (n.=11,165)		VDT ≥4H/DAY (n.=7,329)		P
	N.	%	N.	%	
CONJUNCTIVITIS:					
- ALLERGIC TYPE	54	0.48	40	0.55	NS
- CHRONIC TYPE	16	0.14	20	0.27	NS
PTERYGIUM	42	0.38	17	0.23	NS
PINGUECOLA	411	3.68	205	2.98	0.012
BLEPHARITIS	96	0.86	65	0.89	NS
CHALAZION	37	0.33	28	0.38	NS
CATARACT CONGENITAL	10	0.09	10	0.14	NS
LENS OPACITIES, MINOR	336	3.01	199	2.70	NS

REFERENCE

1. Epidemiologic Survey of Ocular Disorders among VDT Operators: an italian multicentric research on 31,570 subject. Boll. Ocul. 1989; 68 (Suppl. 7): 3-123.

2. Rubino G.F. Work With Display Units '89. Elsevier N. Holland 1990.

3. Rubino G.F. "Longitudinal Survey of Ocular Disorders and General Compliants in VDU operators". HCI; 1:768-773, Orlando, 1993.

ASSESSMENT OF MECHANICAL EXPOSURES IN ERGONOMIC EPIDEMIOLOGY: a research program and some preliminary data

Winkel J[1,2,3], Balogh I[2], Hansson G-Å[2], Asterland P[2], Kellerman M[2], Byström J[2], Ohlsson K[2]

[1] Natl. Inst. of Occup. Health, Div. of Appl. Work Physiol., S-171 84 Solna, Sweden
[2] Dept. Occup. & Environ. Med., Div. of Ergonomics, Univ. Hospital, Lund, Sweden
[3] Dept. Community Health Sciences, University of Lund, Sweden

1. INTRODUCTION

Several investigations of musculoskeletal disorders suggest that the workrelated fraction is 30-40% (5), and for some occupations it may amount to 50-90% (4). The workrelated fraction is the fraction of observed cases that would not have occurred if no one in the population were exposed. Improved ergonomics may therefore offer a considerable potential for improved musculoskeletal health. Consequently, the emphasis of ergonomic epidemiology is now gradually shifting from qualitative risk identification to quantitative assessments of exposure-effect relationships, which is needed for practical ergonomic interventions. Quantitative exposure assessments require more precise and accurate exposure methods than those generally applied in ergonomic epidemiology.

The workrelated fraction of musculoskeletal disorders may be due to physical work load and psychosocial factors. The relative significance of these two kinds of exposures is frequently discussed but difficult to assess (cf. 14). This is partly due to poorly defined mechanical exposures as well as insufficient exposure methods.

Imprecise estimates of mechanical exposures (due to poor assessment and/or poor definition) may imply that the calculated relative risks are *underestimated* compared to the psychosocial risk factors, if the latter are assessed with higher precision in the same study and are correlated to the physical work load factors (10).

In considering the above mentioned issues, the present paper discusses strategies for assessment of physical work load. A research program for valid and reliable job exposure assessment in large populations is described and some preliminary data will be presented. The program is run by an "Exposure group" at the University of Lund, Sweden. It is an integral part of the "Malmö Shoulder-Neck study" investigating mechanical and psychosocial risk factors for shoulder-neck disorders in a nested case-control study comprising 15.000 individuals (16). This, in turn, is part of the SOUND network comprising 10 departments in the Sound region (Copenhagen/Denmark and Lund+Malmö/Sweden), all focusing on occupational musculoskeletal research issues.

2. EXPOSURE DEFINITION

"Physical work load" is often assessed in terms which are difficult to discriminate from psychosocial exposures (e.g. 1). It has been suggested therefore that "physical work load" should be confined to mechanical forces arising in the human body due to *mechanical* demands in the work environment (14). Conceptually, mechanical exposure may be expressed as an unlimited number of force vectors, one for each point in the body, each varying in length and direction according to time (14). A sufficient operational quantification of mechanical exposure may therefore comprise three main dimensions: amplitude (e.g. posture), repetitiveness (e.g. lifting frequency) and duration (e.g. hours of VDU work) (15).

3. EXPOSURE ASSESSMENT STRATEGIES

An overview of the literature shows that the most common way of classifying mechanical exposure in ergonomic epidemiology is by job title (2,15). Burdorf (2) reviewed 72 studies on low back pain and 38 of these assessed exposure by job title only. Questionnaire was used in 27 studies, observational methods in 7 and direct measurement techniques in 6.

3.1 Exposure assessment by job title

According to our preliminary results the exposure of workers having the same job title may vary within a wide range (figure 1). This is in agreement with several previous studies (e.g. 7). Risk estimates in terms of job titles, therefore, do not offer a practicable basis for ergonomic interventions.

3.2 Exposure assessment by self-report

Self-report (questionnaire or diary) provides the possibility of studying a large number of individuals at a modest cost. Furthermore, by this single instrument you may collect information concerning a variety of different exposure variables. In addition, the questions may be designed to aim at exposure in general while direct methods may only convey exposure information about the particular recording period. Therefore, self-report seems to be the more appropriate instrument in epidemiologic studies. However, the reliability and validity may be questioned.

Quantification of exposure by scales comprising more than 2-3 points reduces the reliability and validity considerably as estimated by kappa statistics (13, Wiktorin et al., manuscript). Consequently, only a 3-point rating scale has been used in the present questionnaire study of mechanical exposures (figure 1). Some preliminary self-reported exposure data are presented in this figure for two of the investigated occupational groups: cleaners and office workers. The data show large variances within as well as between the occupational groups.

Office workers and cleaners are two commonly occurring jobs in our study group and they were selected for the field investigation in the development of the job exposure assessment strategy (see below in chap. 4).

When exposure is assessed by self-report, dependent misclassification is a crucial issue which needs to be addressed (cf. 12,13). In the "Malmö Shoulder-neck study" this issue is carefully investigated. In figure 2 we present some preliminary data on rated perceived exertion (RPE) during a working day in relation to average relative heart rate increase recorded by a Sport Tester PE 3000®. The figure illustrates that for these subjects no correlation between the two investigated parameters could be demonstrated. This is in agreement with a previous study by Wigaeus Hjelm et al. (12). Furthermore, there may be a tendency towards a higher perception of exertion among the cleaners indicating complaints compared to the healthy ones. Any conclusions must, however, wait until all 100 subjects have been investigated (see chapt. 4.1).

3.3 Exposure assessment by systematic expert observations

A recent review by Kilbom (8) concluded that postures of trunk and arm may be difficult to classify into more than two to three categories by systematic expert observations. Furthermore, it was concluded that postures of neck and head as well as repetitive movements may be difficult to assess and manual handling can only be assessed crudely by this kind of method. These conclusions correspond to our experience from previous studies (3).

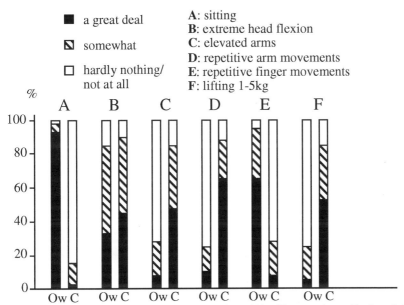

Figure 1. Some selfreported exposure data for 663 office workers (Ow) and 159 cleaners (C). Each staple indicates the percentage of the individuals indicating "a great deal", "somewhat" and "hardly nothing/not at all".

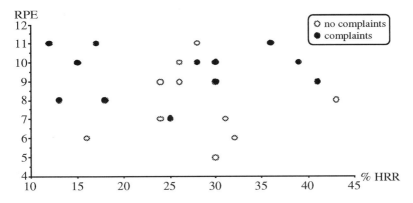

Figure 2: Some preliminary data on rated perceived exertion (RPE) obtained by the questionnaire in relation to average heart rate increase during one working day in percent of the heart rate range (%HRR). Each dot represents a subject.

3.4 Exposure assessment by direct measurements

Based on the above review of exposure assessment strategies, direct measurement techniques appear to be needed to obtain exposure data offering a sufficient accuracy for practical interventions. Furthermore, data obtained by technical measurements are not confounded by psychosocial exposures, which may occur when using self-reports. However, direct technical methods are rarely used due to high resource demands. Furthermore, it may be questionned if direct recordings during a few hours are generalisable across time. Thus, new cost-effective strategies including direct technical methods and proper weighting of these across time need to be developed to obtain a breakthrough for ergonomic epidemiology in relation to risk assessment and workplace interventions.

4. PRESENT JOB EXPOSURE ASSESSMENT STRATEGY

It has been suggested that a thorough description of job exposure should comprise quantitative assessment of 'task exposure', i.e. exposure of the different body parts due to each task, weighted according to 'task distribution', i.e. occurrence and duration of the different tasks included in the job (14). 'Task distribution' is assessed by self-reports which are evaluated. Furthermore, special emphasis is put on development of sensors, data collecting and analysis systems as well as software for assessment of 'task exposure' (see Table 1). The aim is to optimize exposure accuracy with particular consideration to manpower when using the above mentioned Job exposure assessment strategy. Apart from these research issues, the group also investigates exposure/outcome relationships based on the questionnaire data (see 16) and types of diagnoses among the cleaners and office workers.

TABLE 1: Main research issues. Notice the relationship to the presented Job exposure assessment strategy.

Task distribution (Self-reported):
• definition of task
• validity of diary and interview in assessment of task distribution
• test-retest reliability of diary: between-day, between-week
• between individuals within job variability of task distribution
• between days within individuals within job variability of task distribution
Direct technical methods
• transducers
• loggers
• software
Task exposure (assessed by Direct technical measurements):
Test-retest reliability: significance of *duration* and *repetition* of measurements, variation according to *task* and *job*
Job exposure:
• Assessment based on task exposure weighted according to task distribution
• comparison of job exposure assessed by questionnaire and the above strategy
• misclassification of self-reported exposure due to: *disorder, age, gender, occupation*
Other issues:
• occurrence of mechanical exposures in tasks and jobs
• discrimination between mechanical and psychosocial exposures

4.1 Study design
'Task distribution' of 100 workers (50 cleaners and 50 office workers) is assessed during 2 weeks by a diary. Task exposures of the same workers are recorded by direct technical methods during 1-3 ordinary working days depending on method. Job exposure is calculated and compared to the job exposures assessed by using an ordinary questionnaire. The significance of disorders, gender, age and occupation for the classification of exposure by self-report is investigated.

4.2 'Task distribution'
Wiktorin et al (manuscript) has pointed out that exposures pertaining to the whole body (e.g. tasks duration) compared to part of it (e.g. duration of neck flexion) may be quantified in more detail than indicated above (chapt. 3.2). We are therefore testing different self-

reporting procedures for assessment of task distribution. So far a systematic interview has been validated in relation to continuous whole-day expert observations of task duration. As illustrated in figure 3, the agreement seems to vary considerably according to occupation. One crucial issue is how to define a task in some occupations and thus to define the thru task duration (figure 3B). Due to this, we are also developing and evaluating a diary as an alternative tool in the assessment of task duration.

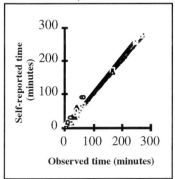
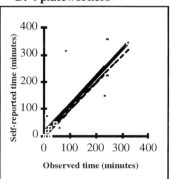

FIGURE 3. Agreement between self-reported and observed duration of tasks. Each subject rated 1-7 tasks.. Line of identity: thin; regression line: thick. Left: 29 observations (symbols) of 6 subjects. Right: 17 observations (symbols) of 4 subjects.

4.3 Direct technical methods

Our needs for direct technical methods are only partly fulfilled by available equipment and software. Therefore, we have developed transducers, data loggers and computer programs for analysis.

Transducers: A triaxial accelerometer has been developed. It is used as an advanced inclinometer (6). The main advantages of this sensor are, that it may be mounted in a arbitrary orientation on the body segment, and has not any limitation in the range of movements that can be recorded. As the total acceleration can be calculated, it is possible to determine if the interpretation of the measurements as inclination is relevant, a feature not possible with ordinary inclinometers. Sampling rate is 20 Hz, which is sufficient to determine, not only the angular distributions, but also dynamic properties, e.g. the angular velocity distribution for the forward/backward movements of the head.

Logger: A data logger has been constructed (Hansson et al., to be published). The logger is small (140 x 80 x 30 mm), has a low weight (350 g), and is battery operated. The sampled data are stored on credit card sized (86 x 54 x 3.3 mm) PCMCIA flash memory card, which, so far, has a maximum capacity of 20 Mbytes. The logger contains a real time clock, that stamps each recording with date and time. A push button may be pressed to mark different events, e.g. the beginning and end of different work tasks, during the recording. Three different loggers have been built; (1) recording of wrist angles for both hands simultaneously, max recording duration: 34 h's; (2) for simultaneous recordings from 4 triaxial accelerometers, max recording duration: 11 h's; (3) for simultaneous recording of two channels of raw EMG, max recording duration: 1 h 20 min. The recording durations can in practise be extended unlimited by removing the full memory card and inserting a new, erased one; a procedure which only takes a few seconds. The memory cards are read on an IBM compatible personal computer (PC) equipped with a PCMCIA interface. The computer programs for the different analyses are run off line on a PC. Since no data reduction is performed in the logger, both extensive quality control, and detailed analysis of dynamic properties are possible. The use of automated quality control, especially of EMG, is of great importance, in order to avoid exposure misclassification in the epidemiological analyses.

Software: The direct technical recordings give rise to a huge amount of data. The raw data need to be checked for noise and artifacts, reduced and weighted according to task distribution to obtain an estimate of job exposure. All these steps require development of appropriate software. Algorithms for analysis and description of task exposure as well as graphical user-friendly interfaces for inspection of signal quality and marking the beginning and end of the different tasks are now being implemented. At present, further development of the software is planned in order to minimize the required time for handling the data.

4.4 Task exposures

These are estimated by posture recordings using the above mentioned triaxial accelerometer for recording head, upper arm and trunk postures. Right and left wrist postures are recorded by Penny & Giles biaxial goniometers (Hansson et al., manuscript). Load on upper right and left upper trapezius is assessed by surface EMG normalized according to Mathiassen et al (9). Duration of sitting is assessed by a posimeter (11), number of foot steps by a pedometer (11) and heart rate by a Sport Tester PE 3000$^©$.

5. CONCLUSION

So far the presented Job exposure assessment strategy seems to be promising as an effective tool offering reliable exposure data at a modest cost in ergonomic epidemiology.

REFERENCES

1. Armstrong T.J., Buckle P., Fine L.J., Hagberg M., Jonsson B., Kilbom Å., Kuorinka I.A.A., Silverstein B.A., Sjøgaard G., Viikari-Juntura E.R.A. Scand. J. Work Environ. & Health 19 (1993), 73-84.
2. Burdorf A. Scand J Work Environ Health 18 (1992), 1-9.
3. Fransson-Hall C., Gloria R., Karlqvist L., Wiktorin C., Winkel J., Kilbom Å., Stockholm MUSIC 1 Study Group. Appl Erg (In press).
4. Hagberg M., Wegman D.H. British Journal of Industrial Medicine 44 (1987), 602-610.
5. Hansen S.M. Nordic Counsil of ministers, Copenhagen, Denmark 1993.
6. Hansson G.-Å., Björn F., Carlsson P.: A new triaxial accelerometer and its application as an advanced inclinometer. In: Proceedings of The 9th International Congress of ISEK. Ed by Florence, Italy, June 28 - July 2 1992, Abstracts 207.
7. Karlqvist L., Winkel J., Wiktorin C., Stockholm MUSIC 1 Study Group. Appl Erg 25 (1994), 319-326.
8. Kilbom Å. Scand J Work Environ Health 20 (1994), 30-45.
9. Mathiassen S.E., Winkel J., Hägg G. J Electromyogr Kinesiol (In press).
10. Phillips A.N., Smith G.D. J Clin Epidemiol 44 (1991), 1223-1231.
11. Selin K., Winkel J., Stockholm MUSIC 1 Study Group. Appl Erg 25 (1994), 41-46.
12. Wigaeus Hjelm E., Winkel J., Nygård C.-H., Wiktorin C., Karlqvist L., Stockholm MUSIC I Study Group. J Occup Med (In press).
13. Wiktorin C., Karlqvist L., Winkel J. Scand J Work Environ Health 19 (1993), 208-214.
14. Winkel J., Mathiassen S.E. Ergonomics 37 (1994), 979-988.
15. Winkel J., Westgaard R. Int J Ind Ergon 10 (1992), 85-104.
16. Östergren P.-O., Balogh I., Ektor-Andersen J., Hanson B.S., Isacsson A., Isacsson S.-O., Lindbladh E., Ranstam J., Winkel J., Ørbæk P.: The "Malmö Shoulder-neck study" - design and preliminary results from the baseline investigation. In: Proceedings of PREMUS. Ed by Montreal, Canada (In press).

ELF Magnetic Field Exposures in an Office Environment

P. N. Breysse[a]

[a] Johns Hopkins University, Center for VDT and Health Research, 615 N. Wolfe Street, Baltimore, Maryland 21205, USA

1. Introduction

The use of video display terminals (VDTs) and other sources of extremely low frequency (ELF) magnetic fields have been investigated as a potential cause of adverse reproductive outcomes among women (1-2). Recent reviews, however, generally conclude that there is no association between VDT use and adverse reproductive outcomes (3,4). Schnorr et al. and Lindbohm et al. characterized exposure based on spot field measurements in front of VDTS, while all other studies defined exposure based on time spent using VDTS. These surrogates of actual exposure may not adequately classify individuals as exposed and nonexposed. Since methodological issues associated with investigating reproduction outcomes and defining appropriate exposure variables are very complex, additional investigation of VDT use and ELF field exposures in office environments is therefore warranted to conclusively address this question. Little information on personal exposure estimates for VDT workers can be found in the published literature.

Any electrical equipment or electric wire which draws electrical current will emit ELF fields. Many types of equipment including electric typewriters, photocopiers, and VDTs are therefore potential sources of ELF exposure in an office environment. Previous investigations of ELF field strengths in front of VDTs indicate exposures in the range of 1 to 7 mG (5).

The purpose of this paper is to review published information on ELF magnetic field exposures to office workers and to review recently published guidelines for conducting office related electric and magnetic field exposure assessments.

2. Background

The unit of magnetic field flux density used in this paper is the milligauss, mG. Magnetic field flux densities are typically measured using either hand held survey meters or data-logging personal exposure meters (PEMs). Hand-held survey meters are typically used to evaluated field sources and to identify areas of high exposure. PEMs, such as the Emdex, are used to determine time integrated personal exposures over periods such as a complete work shift. Data-logging software for PEMs can be programmed to measure the three orthogonal components of the magnetic field at predetermined intervals. An example of an office worker full-shift exposure record produced by an Emdex PEM is contained in Figure 1.

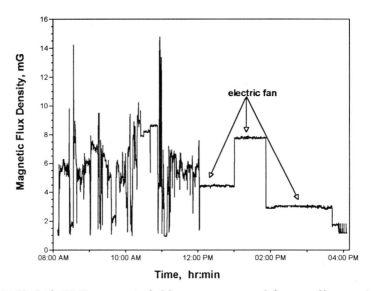

Figure 1. Full-shift ELF magnetic field exposure record for an office worker.

There are many sources of ELF fields in a office environment. As depicted in Figure 1, ELF magnetic field exposure patterns are therefore complex. In most cases it is not possible, or very difficult, to apportion exposure to specific sources such as a VDT. In the case of Figure 1, the dominant exposure source in the afternoon was traced to the use of a small desk-top electric fan while the contribution of the VDT is uncertain.

3. Office Environment ELF Magnetic Field Exposure

In a recent study Breysse et al. (6) evaluated the ELF exposure of fifteen females working in a U.S. government office environment, all of whom used VDTs. The workers were monitored for a full shift, 5.8 to 8 hr, using Emdex PEMs. Emdex dosimeters were placed in belted hip pouches and the clerical workers were instructed to wear the hip pouch during as much of their shift as possible. Results of this study are summarized in Table 1.

In this study typical magnetic flux densities in the office environment ranged from 1.3 to 27.4 mG and were associated with office equipment (e.g., VDTs and photocopiers) and with current flowing through the electrical distribution network in the building. The highest flux density measured, 27.4 mG, was associated with an electric utility chase. Time-weighted average (TWA) magnetic flux density exposures over the full-shift ranged from 1.0 to 6.5 mG with a mean of 3.2 ±1.5 mG.

Table 1
Summary of Time-Weighted Average Resultant Magnetic Flux Density Exposures for Female Clerical Workers

Worker	Sample Time, Hrs.	Magnetic Flux Density, mG (S.D.).*	Worker	Sample Time, Hrs.	Magnetic Flux Density, mG (S.D.).*
1	8.0	4.9 (2.2)	9	7.8	2.2 (1.3)
2	6.6	2.3 (2.0)	10	5.8	2.5 (1.1)
3	7.9	1.9 (1.1)	11	6.5	1.3 (0.5)
4	7.0	6.5 (2.6)	12	7	1.9 (0.7)
5	7.9	1.0 (1.0)	13	7	1.7 (0.8)
6	7.3	1.2 (0.6)	14	7.6	1.7 (2.1)
7	7.3	1.3 (0.7)	15	7.8	1.5 (1.5)
8	7.5	2.0 (1.2)	-	-	-

* Resultant full-shift TWA

The higher fields associated with worker 1 were likely due to her extensive use of an electric typewriter and the presence of a small tabletop fan. The electric typewriter was found to produce a variable exposure pattern that fluctuated between 1 and 5 mG, with the size of the peaks depending on the typewriter functions used. None of the other sampled clerical workers reported extensive electric typewriter use. The small tabletop fan, located on worker 1's desk, produced fields ranging from 4 to 7 mG.

Sources which may produce the higher fields associated with sample worker 4 were investigated using the Emdex dosimeter, which was used to record the field changes at the worker's desk when different types of office electrical equipment were successively turned on. With everything turned off except the overhead lights, the background magnetic flux density was found to be approximately 5 mG, 2-3 times higher than those measured in other areas. Upon further investigation, the source of this elevated background was found to be an electric wire conduit running underneath the floor (i.e., along the ceiling deck of the floor below). Fields as high as 25 mG were found at floor level in worker 4's area, and when the false floor deck was removed, levels as high as 70 mG were measured at the true floor deck. The flux density increased to between 6 and 7 mG when a small desktop fan was turned on. Turning on a nearby photocopier, a printer, and all nearby computers did not significantly increase the magnetic flux density in the area.

The results of this investigation are compared to other studies in Table 2. These studies include assessments for a group of office working non-craft telephone company workers evaluated as a part of a large epidemiologic investigation of leukemia in telephone lineworkers, and two different sets of office workers employed in the electric utility industry.

Table 2
Summary of published literature on magnetic flux density exposures to office workers.

Author	Population	Sample Size, N	Mean Magnetic Flux Density, mG
Breysse, et al. (6)	government workers	15	3.2
Breysse, et al. (7)	telephone company	55	1.5
Sahl et al. (8)	electric utility workers	55	1.8
Theriault et al. (9)	electric utility workers	102[a]	1.3

[a] number of work weeks measured

In general, the time-weighted average magnetic field exposures presented in the above table are less than 2 mG. The average for the 15 government workers is skewed by the two elevated estimates discussed above. If these two values are removed from the calculation, the mean becomes 1.7 mG which is more in line with the other published results.

4. Summary of Workshop on VDT and Office Environment Exposure Assessment

A report of a VDT Exposure Assessment Workshop, sponsored by the Johns Hopkins University Center for VDT and Health Research, was recently published. (10) Workshop participants included investigators involved in previous and ongoing studies of VDTs. The purpose of the workshop was to develop a standardized exposure assessment approach to be used to investigate the potential health effects associated with the types of fields produced by VDTs.

The workshop concluded that an assessment approach should contain three levels or components:

- an evaluation of the VDT as a source of exposure,
- personal monitoring (including non-occupational), where feasible, and
- a characterization of the spatial distribution of field levels within the office or work area.

It was recommended that a test method for Visual Display Units (11) developed by the Swedish National Board for Measurement and Testing (MPR), now known as Swedish Board for Technical Accreditation (SWEDAC), be used to standardize all laboratory and field based exposure assessments. This test method, commonly referred to as the MPR2 Test Method for Visual Display Units, lists the type of test equipment to be used, equipment calibration, measurement geometry, and measurement uncertainty. Whenever possible, at least one representative terminal from each VDT model encountered in a given study should be submitted for a complete or partial MPR2 evaluation. As a minimum, health effects investigations should, report the VDT manufacturer, model and serial number.

It was also recommended that an *in situ* MPR2 evaluation be conducted. This assessment would mimic the MPR2 measurement protocol as closely as possible without removing the VDT from its normal use environment. It was recognized, however, that the presence of other office equipment or high background field levels in an office area can make interpretation of these results problematic and lead to unknown measurement errors.

In addition to characterizing the VDT as a source of exposure, it is important to evaluate a person's total field exposure using PEMs as described above. To date, only personal exposure meters for ELF magnetic fields are available. The workshop recommended that, wherever possible, the study subjects be asked to wear the PEM for a 24-hour period. Twenty-four hour exposure records allow the investigator to evaluate non-occupational sources of exposure which may be relevant to a health effects investigation. Based on the exposure record from a PEM, a number of indices or metrics of exposure, such as time-weighted average, the daily peak, and time above some field level may be calculated.

Due to the wide variety of potential field sources in an office environment, a comprehensive exposure assessment should also include an evaluation of background field levels in each office area. It was recommended that this assessment evaluate background field levels in an office as the average of five field measurements spaced throughout the office area.

Following the above assessment approach, exposure definitions can be developed which are based on the fields from the VDT (determined in a laboratory and/or *in situ*), office background field levels, and personal exposure. More traditional exposure surrogates based on hours of VDT use and distance from VDT can also be used.

5. Conclusions

The health effects, including adverse reproductive outcomes, associated with exposure to ELF magnetic fields are currently the focus of a great deal of public and scientific debate. Although recent reviews generally conclude that VDT use does not represent a reproductive hazard, sufficient concern still exists to warrant investigation. In this context, it is important to evaluate sources of potential ELF magnetic field exposures and attempt to place them in perspective with other potentially exposed groups.

References

1. Lindbohm M, Hietanen M, Kyyrönen P, Sallmén M, von Nandelstadh P, Taskinen H, Pekkarinen M, and Hemminiki K (1992): Magnetic fields of video display terminals and spontaneous abortion. *Am. J. Epidemiol.*, 136(9):1041-1051.
2. Schnorr TM, Grajewski BA, Hornung RW, Thun MJ, Egeland GM, Murray WE, Conover DL, Halperin WE (1991): Video display terminals and the risk of spontaneous abortions. *N. Engl. J. Med.*, 324: 727-733.
3. American Medical Association Council on Scientific Affairs (1987): Health effects of video display terminals. *JAMA*, 257(11):1508-1512.
4. Mariott IA, Stuchly MA (1986): Health aspects of work with visual display terminals. *J. Occup. Med.*, 28:833-848.
5. Stuchly MA, Lecuyer DW, Mann RD (1983): Extremely low frequency electromagnetic emissions from video display terminals and other devices. *Health Phys.*, 45:713-722.
6. Breysse PN, Lees PSJ, McDiarmid MA, and Curbow B (1994): ELF magnetic field exposures in an office environment. *Am. J. Ind. Med.*, 25:177-185.
7. Breysse PN, Matanoski GM, Elliott EE, Francis M, Kaune W, and Thomas K (1994): 60 Hz magnetic field exposure assessment for an investigation of leukemia in telephone linemen. *Am. J. Ind. Med.*, 26, 68-691.
8. Sahl JD, Kelsh MA, and Greeenland S (1993): Cohort and nested case-control studies of hematopoietic cancers and brain cancer among electric utility workers. *Epidemiol.*, 4(2)104-113.
9. Theriault G, Goldberg M, Miller AB, and et al. (1993): Cancer risks associated with occupational exposure to magnetic fields among electric utility workers in Ontario and Quebec, Canada, and France: 1970-1989. *Am. J. Epidemiol.*, 139(6):550-572.
10. Breysse PN, Gray R (1994): Video Display Terminal (VDT) Exposure Assessment: Workshop Report. *Appl. Occup. Environ. Hyg.*, 9(10):671-677.
11. National Board for Measurement and Testing: Test method for visual display units: visual ergonomics and emission characteristics (MPR2), Report No: MPR 1990:8 1990-12-01 (1990).

The definition and assessment of quality of images on VDUs
Part I: Relationships with asthenopia

B. Piccoli

Istitute of Occupational Health - University of Milan

1. INTRODUCTION

The work of a VDU operator normally requires an intense visual effort which consists in continuous observation of: i) key-board, ii) screen, iii) documents.
This type of near visual work (<1 m) mantained often for many consecutive hours, requires an intense activation of accommodation and convergence mechanisms. Besides this, in cases where the illumination is not ergonomically designed (i.e. high luminance ratio), overloading of the structures which control the pupil diameter and the retinal sensitivity, can occur.
At present, among the various medical problems linked with VDU work, particular interest and attention is being given [13,14] to the high prevalence of ocular and visual disturbances ("VDU operators asthenopic syndrome" or "VDU asthenopia") that researchers have high-lighted during many investigations in populations of intensively exposed workers.
The epidemiological research done in the 80's in this field also supports quiet clearly the existance of a positive correlation between the intensity and the prevalence of asthenopic disturbances and the "characteristics" of the display [1,2,3,4].
The hypotheis that the "quality" of the image can have, both in subjective and objective terms, an important role in asthenopia pathogenesis can definitely be sustained.

2. A NEW APPROACH

The asthenopic symptomathology which VDU operators suffer from is a rather complex phenomenon and has a multifactorial etiology. The researches done at the end of the 80's have permitted a much more diverse and probably even more realistic picture to be drawn up, compared to the one of the past. From the literature [5,6,7,8,9,10,11,12,15,16,17], it emerges that the possible causes of this particular symptomatology are essentially connected to three types of variables:
a) ophthalmological pattern of the subject;

b) environmental characteristics of the work place (both chemical and physical);
c) intensity of the "visual work load".

In work-places with VDUs (mostly offices) many, if not all of these types of variables generally co-exists and work synergistically, giving rise to asthenopic disturbances (Table 1).

Table 1
Possible causes of asthenopia in VDU operators

Variable	Asthenopic factors
Subject	Ophthalmological alterations incompatible with the comfortable performance during near visual tasks (ametropia not well corrected, ocular motility impairments, etc.)
Environment	Presence of agents irritative to the ocular surface (I.A.Q problems, inadeguate microclimate, etc.) or those disturbing the visual processes (high luminance ratios, excessive flickering, shadow casting problems, etc.)
Visual work-load	Short observation distance, prolonged duration, frequent "scrolling", bad screen-image quality, etc.

It is important to note that the first two types of variable are present independently from the VDU use and the third one is only partially associated to it.

This assumes greater importance if one considers that, normally, these operators spend only a part of their work day at the VDU while the rest is passed, sometimes in other offices, performing tasks not requiring the use of any computer-based equipment.

The hypothesis that in these kind of operators the screen-image quality could be the element most responsible for asthenopic disturbances is certainly acceptable, particularly for those intensively exposed with a predominance of screen-observation. However, the subjective evaluations and the ophthalmological symptomatology reported in relation to the "quality" of the image on their VDT or PC, may be strongly conditioned by variables not directly connected to the use of this equipment.

Such variables must then be adequately considered and checked during investigations that wish to make a realistic evaluation of cause/effect relationships between "screen-image quality" and possible related asthenopic effects.

Another aspect that appears to be important in this area of research, which is evident from an analysis of the literature (see part 3 of this paper) and that we have already had to deal with in some of our experimental investigations [18], is that the subjective evaluation and the ophthalmological symptomatology reported by operators in connection with the "screen-image quality", seems to be associated to two distinct groups of factors.

One is of a strictly optical/physical nature (character sharpness, contrast, jitter, etc.) and the other of a visual-cognitive nature (method of image presentation, effect of the context on image organization, level of interpretability of text and symbols, etc.).

It could therefore be possible, especially in VDU operators performing sophisticated tasks such as CAD, CAM, CAE, CG, DTP, etc, that some of the asthenopic disturbances normally attributed to a strictly visual overload are instead associated, mainly or partially, also to perceptive-cognitive processes linked with the recognition and interpretation of the pictorial representation on the VDU screen. In this regard it should be noted that among the most frequent complaints reported by VDU operators are disturbances like difficulty in concentration, reading fatigue, headache, which could certainly be connected to overloading of superior cortical functions.

3. CONCLUSIONS

The optical-physical and perceptual-cognitive aspects regarding VDU image-quality are usually studied separately but their effects, whether positive or negative (sensation of visual comfort versus asthenopia), are the result of a rather complex psycho-physiopathological process. To date the role and the interaction of the different variables involved have not been clearly established. In this context the visual capacity of the subject together with the environmental characteristics of the work place could play per se a major role. For these reasons, a correct assessment of a VDU image quality and of its relation with visual comfort has to provide, for the collective sequence of images produced during the different tasks, an adequate evaluation of "physical" and "psychological" aspects.

This kind of approach should allow, besides a more precise quantification of the different factors involved, also a more effective indication of the necessary improvements and rationalization to be made.

A research group on this topic was formed for the WWDU '94 Conference at the Institute of Occupational Health of the Univeristy of Milan. Besides occupational health doctors, the group is composed of physicist and experts in cognitive psychology.

The aim of the group is to set up, through interdisciplinary studies, an integrated approach for the analysis and evaluation of "image quality" in the occupational use of VDUs.

This work, together with the second and third parts which follow, represent an initial contribution on this matter.

REFERENCES

1. E. Grandjean, Ergonomics in computerized offices, p. 63, Taylor & Francis, London, 1987.
2. U. Bergqvist, Video display terminals and health, Scand. J. of Work Env. and Health, suppl. 2 vol 10, p. 48, 1984.
3. J. Roufs, The man-machine interface, p. 57, The Macmillan Press, London, 1991.
4. J. Meyer et al., Discomfort and disability glare in VDT operators, WWDU 89, Elsevier, Amsterdam, 1990.
5. L. Scullica, C. Rechichi, The influence of refractive defects on the appearance of asthenopia in subjects employed at videoterminals, Bollettino di Oculistica, anno 68, suppl. 7, 1989.
6. L. Bonomi, R. Bellucci, Consideration on the ocular pathology in 30000 personnel of the Italian Telephone Company, Bollettino di Oculistica, anno 68, suppl. 7, 1989.
7. B. Bagolini et al., Study on ocular motility in Telephone Company employees working with VDT: preliminary conclusions, Bollettino di Oculistica, anno 68, suppl. 7, 1989.
8. B. Piccoli et al., Astenopia ed obiettivita' oftalmologiche in una popolazione di 2058 operatori VDT in Lombardia, G. Ital. Med. Lav., 267-271, 1989.
9. D. Norback, C. Edling, Environmental occupational and personal factors related to prevalence of sick building syndrome in the general population, Brit. J. of Ind. Med., 451- 462, 1991.
10. D. Norback et al., Indoor air quality and personal factors related to the sick building syndrome, Scand. J. of Env. Health, 121-128, 1990.
11. P. Wolkoff et al., A study of human reactions to office machines in a climate chamber, J. of Exp. Analysis and Env. Epid., Suppl. 1, 1992
12. L. Molhave et al, Integration and adaptation in eye irritation, Proceedings of Indoor Air Congress, pp. 35-40, 1993.
13. S. Kjaergaard et al., Objective eye efforts and their relation to sensory irritation in a sick building, Proceedings of Indoor Air Congress, pp. 117-122, 1993.
14. W.H.O.,Visual display terminals and workers' health, Offset Publication 99,Geneva,1987.
15. W.H.O., Update on visual display terminals and workers' health, Geneva, 1990.
16. W. Jaschinski-Kruza, On the preferred viewing distance to screen and document at VDU workplaces, Ergonomics, 1055-1063, 1990.
17. W. Jaschinski-Kruza, Is the resting state of your eyes a favorable viewing distance for VDU-work?, Proceedings of WWDU Congress 1986 Stockholm, pp. 526-538, Elsevier, Amsterdam, 1987.
18. I. Gratton, B. Piccoli et al, Change in visual function and viewing distance during work with VDTs, Ergonomics, 1433-1441, 1990.
19. B. Piccoli et al., Studio sulle caratteristiche e sull'efficacia degli schermi per unita' video con tubo a raggi catodici, Arc. Sc. Lav., 35-43, 1991.

The definition and assessment of quality of images on VDUs
Part II: Physical aspects

S. Orsini[a], L. Milanesi[b]

[a]Health Physics Department of I.C.P. - Milan
[b]Advanced Biomedical Technology Institute of C.N.R. - Milan

1. INTRODUCTION

From the early advent of photographic reproduction up to the advent of electronic images, the evaluation of quality has been performed "visually".
This technique is still considered nowadays as a particular case of the so-called "perceptual assessment of image quality".
In the framework of medical images, for instance, much attention is paid to the comparison of the judgements of medical experts and of lay-people. Indeed, the assessment and appreciation is highly dependent on the degree of skill of the observer, and the images are said to be "appreciation oriented" [5,7].
Many studies have highlighted the importance of increasing the human-computer interface and it is now generally accepted that such interface can affect work efficiency, increasing individual stress and in the long term also job performance. In this context the Video Display Unit (VDU) is very important because it can remarkably compromise the man-computer interaction. In several applications a very large number of different VDUs ranging from workstation with 21" CRT colour screen, LCD (Liquid Crystal Display) up to screen for video for VR (Virtual Reality) applications [2,3,4,6,8].
The problem associated with the various types of VDUs are related to physical and psychophysiological issues [1,5,7].

2. IMAGE QUALITY FACTORS

Physical factors rely upon:
a) instrumental techniques based on radiometric assessment ;
b) instrumental techniques referring to a standard human observer.

The human observer is not yet wholly represented by a "filter" weighing the input of measure instruments. The evaluation still relies upon pshychophysical techniques, thus passing from physical to observer-related factors.

After standard calibration procedures (temporal calibration included) according to various guidelines or specialized literature sources the relevant characteristic to be taken into account are in table 1.

Table 1.
Relevant characteristics

Hardware & software	Colour properties	Motion and perception
- nature of the display	- contrast	- flicker
- spatial resolution (pixel per inch and pixel shape)	- sharpness or pictorial quality	- jitter
	- colour values	- continuity of motion
- PSF, LSF, MTF, TMTF (*)	- dominant wavelength	- viewing conditions
- shape of photometric emission lobe(s)	- purity	- phychometric functions
	- chromaticity coordinates	- phycological constraints
- colour rendering	- gamma	- subjective judgments (of brightness, presentation time, etc.)
- coding algorithms	- threshold	

(*) Point Spread, Line Spread, Modulation Transfer and Temporal Modulation Transfer Funtions

3. CONCLUDING REMARKS

- Photometry and colorimetry refer, in principle, to steady state situations.
- The assessment they allow are well codified, even if some problems still deserve further consideration.
- Traditionally, non-steady state situations are referred to continuity of motion and to the so-called stability in time (flicker avoidance) and in space (jitter minimization).
- The advanced research is now faced with the assessment of the characteristics of transient situations.
- Physiologically, these imply the responses of post-receptoral structures in the visual chain, which, being neural, respond only transiently.
- At the mathematic site, coding algorithms are to be transferred from the spatial to the temporal domain.
- In a specific field like the virtual reality and multimedia applications, new display technology have been developed. In the stereo display a new kind of problem will arise(i.e. in using an immersing display the difference in term of visual acuity and of interpupillary distance in relation to intense occupational activities must be taken into account).

- With the recent progress of Flat Panel Display technology the quality of the image will soon be as good as the CRT-VDU image, and more in general, the integration of the multimedia applications, television, networking will enable us to organize new ways of working and communicating.

REFERENCES

1. R.S. Berns, R.J. Motta, M.E.Gorzynski: CRT Colorimetry. Part I and II:Theory and Practice. Color reseach and application, Volume 18, Number 5, 299-314, 315-325; October 1993.
2. M.T. Bolas: Human factors in the design of an immersive display. IEEE Computer Graphics & Applications. pp. 55-59, 1994
3. Commission of European Communities and European Parliamnet Visual display units. Ergonomics hints for users. July 1987.
4. S.R. Ellis: What are Virtual Environments?. IEEE Computer Graphics & Applications. pp 17-22, 1994.
5. S. Ericksson: Perceptual threshold for jitter in VDUs Displays, Vol 13, N.4, 187-192; 1992.
6. Fisher et al.: Virtual Interface Environment Workstations. Proc. Human Factors RSoc. 32nd Ann. Meeting, Human Factors Society, Santa Monica, Calif. pp 91-95, 1988.
7. R.L. Ronchi: Il concetto di qualità nella riproduzione a colori. Luce n. 6, 43-47; 1991.
8. J.A. Waterworth:Multimedia technology and Applications. 1991 - Ellis Horwood L.ed.

The definition and assessment of quality of images on VDUs
Part III: Visual-cognitive factors

N. Bruno, A. De Angeli, W. Gerbino

Department of Psychology, University of Trieste

1. INTRODUCTION

The advent and widespread commercial success of Graphical User Interfaces (GUI) require increased attention to visual cognitive processes governing the recognition and interpretation of pictorial representations on visual display units. Typical GUI's are object-oriented interfaces that allow direct manipulation from the user in a window-based system. They are based on (a) continuous visual representation of dialogue objects, (b) simplified sets of rapid, reversible, and incremental actions on such objects, and (c) immediate feedback. Simultaneously presented windows (screen portions wich display one set of output) can represent independent processes. Icons allow to display task operations and concepts as pictorial of objects. Ideally, communication is achieved by unambiguous and immediate manipulation of objects by input devices such as a mouse, light pen or touch-screen. Interacting whith a GUI system, users can perform a number of tasks such as navigating between windows in a simulated layout, searching for objects, and acting on these objects. Actions include explicit activation of functions or operations, and restructuring of the layout for instance by dragging icons.

2. FRAMEWORK

We present a conceptual framework for evaluating the quality of graphic information on visual displays. The framework is based on two concepts.
1) Usability.
"The effectiveness, efficiency, and satisfaction with which specified users achieve specified goals in particular environments" [1]. A graphic system is usable to the extent that users can achieve specific goals accurately, without undue attentional effort, and in a comfortable manner. The operationalization of these three attributes and of the context of use therefore provides a natural benchmark for the assessment of quality of graphic information in a system [2].
2) Perception-action cycle.

Cognitive processes unfold in time. While acting on the environment, we obtain information; these information affect our set of expectations about the environment, which then guides new actions [3]. The cyclic nature of cognition provides a powerful framework for understanding the interaction of human users with a computer interface. From the point of view of cognitive engineering, Norman [4], among others, developed a version of the perception-action cycle for the analysis of interfaces. Within this framework, users incrementally develop and maintain active representations of the system by acting on it and by observing the consequences of these actions. Thus, perception, cognition, and action are interlcaved according to a principle of mutuality.

3. GUIDELINES

Constraints posed by visual-cognitive processes are critical for optimizing graphic displays from the point of view of system usability. They depend not only on low-level visual functions, but also on higher-level factors affecting the perception and the interpretation of the simulated layout, the understanding of possibilities for action, and the correct attribution of causes and effects in the chain of events that occur during the interaction with the system . We have summarized these constraints in seven classes of guidelines to be used in the evaluation of graphic displays. Guideline 1 reflects a fundamental limitation of the human information processing system. Guidelines 2 to 4 summarize constraints on the choosing, organizing, and displaying items in meaningful ways. Guidelines 5 to 7 summarize constraints on eliciting and controlling user actions.

Guideline 1: Magical number seven.

In a variety of domains, the channel capacity of the human information processing system is limited to 7±2 units of information, or "chunks" [5]. Chunks can be single items or groupings of items (see Guideline 4).

Guideline 2: Sensitivity.

The ability to detect and discriminate items such as letters and figures mainly depends on the sensitivity of the visual system to contrast , flicker , and color [6, 7].

Guideline 3: Visibility.

During the course of many visual activities such as reading or scanning a set of graphical objects, observers attempt to identify or localize an item. The visibilty of a given item within a group of distractors typically depends on factors such as form, size, color, and orientation [8]. In most domains, visibility is limited by the channel capacity of the human information processing, system (see Guideline 1). In some specific domains, however, it is not: and specific items can be localized and identified effortlessly even in fields that greatly exceed the channel capacity. This phenomenon is known as preattentive *pop-out* and should be exploited in the design of interfaces whenever specific items must be retrieved for a given task.

Guideline 4: Grouping.

Human observers spontaneously group items into coherent wholes. Factors affecting grouping include item proximity, similarity, and motion; good continuation, closure, symmetry, and simplicity of forms; observer habits [9]. Grouping principles provide important guidelines for organizing information spatially and temporally whithin a graphical display.

Guideline 5: Sequencing.

In typical window-based interfaces, items such as letters, words, digits, and pictures are presented serially at temporal rates that can depend on user actions or be specific to a given process. Items in the stream of information can be involuntarily suppressed if the temporal characteristics of the sequence are not appropriate to a given task and to the nature of the displayed items [10].

Guideline 6: Causality.

Human observers spontaneously experience causal relationships when specific constraints, such as velocity, timing in the onset of events, and temporal phase, are satisfied [11].

Guideline 7: Affordance.

Within the framework of the perception-action cycle, potential uses, or *affordances, of* an object emerge in the mutuality of available information and the observer's repertoire of actions and representations [12]. The notion of affordance is closely related to that of *articulatory directness*, the relationship between the physical form of an item and its meaning [4]. Within the theory of affordances, meanings are action afforded by an item, and graphical objects provided in a display have specific meanings depending on relationships between their form, size, and movement, on one hand, and potential actions from a user on the other. This implies that ways to elicit appropriate actions from users may differ depending on the characteristics of an interface, and the representation of the user within the interface itself.

REFERENCES

1. International Standards Organization (1993). Ergonomic requirement for office work with visual display terminals (VDTs): Part 11 giudance on specifying and measuring usability. ISO CD 9241- 1.3
2. Nielsen, J. (1993). Usability Engineering. NJ: Academic Press.
3. Neisser, U. (1976). Cognition and reality. San Francisco, CA: Freeeman.
4. Norman, D. A. (1986). Cognitive engineering. In D. A. Norman & S. W. Draper (Eds.). User centered systems design: New perspectives on human-computer interaction. Hillsdale, NJ: Erlbaum, 31-61
5. Miller, G.A. The magical number seven, plus or minus two: some limits on our capacity for processing information. Psychological Review, 63, 81-97.
6. Robson, J.G. (1966). Spatial and temporal contrast-sensitivity functions of the visual system. Journal of the Optical Society of America, 56, 1141- 42.
7. Smith, V., & Pokorny, J. (1975). Spectral sensitivity of the foveal cone

photopigments between 400 and 500 nm. Vision Research, 15, 161-171.
8. Treisman, A., & Gelade, G. (1980). A feature itegration theory of attention. Cognitive Psychology, 12, 97-136.
9. Wertheimer, M. (1923) Untersuchungen zur Lehre von der Gestalt. Psychologische Forschnung. 4, 301-350
10. Raymond, J.E., Shapiro, K. L., & Arnell, K M. (1992). Temporary suppression of visual processing in a RSVP task: An attentional blink? Journal of Experimental Psychology: Human Perception & Performance, 18, 849-86
11. Michotte, A. (1954). La perception de la causalité. Louvain: publications universitaires.
12. Gibson, J. J. (1979). The Ecological Approach to visual perception. San Francisco, CA:Freeman.

VDTs: problems arising when the physical ergonomics are perfect

L. A. Le Leu

Staff Health and Occupational Medical Unit, Woden Valley Hospital, Yamba Drive, Garran A.C.T. 2605, Australia

1. INTRODUCTION

I wish to deal with aspects of the workplace which, perhaps not visible, may play a major role in work injuries. I'll cover obvious matters like work structure and the work area, and less-often-described matters such as ease of software use. I am assuming most VDT work is word processing and that, the more 'natural'/ intuitive the software is to use, the fewer the problems. I will not cover particular injuries, but the problems are broadly describable as 'musculoligamentous' and 'stress-based'

2. Work structure

2.1.1. Division of work and supervision

An obvious area of concern, yet some companies ignore it. In a single work area there may be a gross disparity between the work performed by individuals due to many factors e.g. a VDT operator being, historically, assigned to a particular executive, and the practice continuing when facilities are 'shared'. A worker's load is then entirely dependent upon the assigned executive's activity. Sometimes certain individuals have no work while others are overwhelmed; not a recipe for office harmony.

Solution: dispense - but carefully - with the operator-executive link and have a supervisor divide the work up uniformly. The operator-executive link may be jealously guarded out of pride or even low work-load. Other jealousies may be unearthed by making one operator in the area supervisor. Consider importing the supervisor. But appointing an outsider to institute change has its good and bad points. The final result, once the difficulties have been overcome, may be increased productivity, industrial peace, and decreased injury rates.

An alternative view: the above strategy, may cause more problems and friction. Changes in work practices and/or the distribution of work may fail to consider the psychological and social issues that relate to work tasks/skills and territories. Having a supervisor divide up the work as opposed to being a 'facilitator' of necessary change is somewhat paternalistic. The situation can be seen as an opportunity to redesign the physical (including workloads) and social conditions of the work area to provide greater autonomy and responsibility within a work unit. To thus involve the worker in the process of change is in keeping with the principles of industrial democracy. This may achieve an easier transition.

2.1.2. Supervisors themselves

The supervisor must be informed of the hazards associated with VDT work. Despite massive publicity in Australia about overuse injuries, some supervisors still ignore these conditions or abuse those said to have them.

Some very authoritarian and driving supervisors push their workers to the limits, resulting in injury. For example, a VDT operator in a hospital Psychology department, whose workplace was 'ergonomic', had to work continuously at the keyboard to cope with the load imposed by her supervisor. She complained about arm and neck pain to the supervisor and was virtually laughed out of the office. The problem became worse and finally she could not continue in that area. When she put in a compensation claim, the supervisor tried to have it disallowed. Fortunately other workers in the office were so horrified by this that they independently submitted a report, which led to the claim being accepted.

Another example: a VDT operator in a hospital Social Work department who was driven by an apparently mild-mannered supervisor and developed arm pain.

In both cases the supervisors were professional health-care workers who, one might naively expect, would display a similar degree of concern for their workers as they do for their patients.

2.1.3. Provision of rest breaks and their observance

Rest breaks reduce musculoligamentous problems but I know no good double blind trial demonstrating that. In most interventions in the workplace, including rest breaks, one must be aware of the Hawthorne effect; indeed, that effect might be very useful.

Rest breaks are only as good as the extent to which they are observed. Software which provides automated rest breaks - including taking the operator through a series of exercises - make the person feel more of an automaton than before.

2.1.4. Length of Shift

An equivocal area. In other fields - such as the hospital setting - longer shifts result in increased fatigue and risk of injury. Certainly that seems to be so in hospital work, with which I am most familiar. There is evidence for this effect in the VDT literature as well, but some recent research conducted by Worksafe in Australia gave the paradoxical result that computer operators moving from 8 hour to 12 hour shifts had decreased injury.

2.1.5. Variation of tasks

Historically the office worker - at least, early this century - was performing a range of tasks from filing to copying using a variety of techniques. More recently, with the development of the VDT, the range of tasks for many has contracted. Perhaps, for those who remain, the range will once again broaden as the word processor finally assumes its function as a glorified pen - in the hands of the people writing the material.

With further development of voice translator programs and their spread throughout industry, the word processing pool will finally fade out. This does not mean that medical problems with the use of the VDT will fade out but they will become less common.

As the size of the word processor pool diminishes the socialisation, which may have prevented some injury will reduce with eventual social isolation. Job insecurity will be another rising factor.

Another parallel development: the subsuming of simple tasks by automation and technology e.g. personal dictation, document scanning, means increased productivity with increased job complexity of the human operator. This will require increased level of training and better adaptability to change.

The definition of 'office' is shifting from dedicated roles and functions to incorporate many job titles. For example some work undertaken by nurses can be described as office work. They maintain data bases for pathology results, quality assurance, patient notes, triage, and treatment protocols, while also retaining an "office" with a VDT. This comes under the broad heading of multi-skilling and "job enrichment".

Rest breaks and task variety are quite similar in that they break monotony and provide opportunity for alternate activity. For employers to adopt them such work practices must be seen as productive and health enhancing rather than as lost time or inefficiency.

2.1.6. Social isolation

We shall see more of this with the increase in 'telecommuting'. Cases of 'stress' have been observed in people working at their VDTs at home; the underlying cause seems to be social isolation. These may be people whose self-esteem arises from their job and from the people they work with.

There are potential benefits of telecommuting but some 'downsides' as workers must accept more responsibility, less supervision for their work and also manage the competing interests within this 'new' environment. Ergonomic standards at the office are, these days, usually good. How can the employer provide the same good conditions of lighting, work breaks, and so on, and how can he provide support for the isolated worker? Some workers will have a positive benefit; other will have the reverse.

Most of those who do telecommute do well as reflected in workers compensation costs. There is an absence of journey accidents (accidents occurring to and from work). A Sydney consultant, Anne Moffat, says that less compensation claims are made by teleworkers despite the general belief that most accidents occur in the home.

This does not necessarily mean that they have fewer accidents, but they might not report them for fear of losing the privilege of home-based work. Teleworkers are more likely to blame themselves for accidents in their own homes.

3. Software structure

Most of the word-processing software available today comes from the United States. Word processing software has become easier to use and quite complex manoeuvres have been reduced to simple actions such as clicking a pointer on a button. Such techniques are 'intuitive' or, at least, become almost 'natural' for us in the same way that the initially alien environment of the motor car becomes an extension of ourselves with time. But there are still many conventions that have to be learned and our ease of adaptation may depend upon the extent to which we share the software developer's background.

3.1.1. Language

Language is said to be one of the things which makes us human. It may also be one of the things which divides us. But we take pride in our languages and the works that have been created in them. While we understand our languages are dynamic things - they develop with time - we like to think that we will be doing the developing and not some foreign agency.

As the authors of documents become increasingly those who enter them into the word processor it may be the language problems that jar, that irritate, and result - in combination with other factors - in 'injury'.

Software developers are paying far more attention to different language requirements than before. Earlier software operations retained many U.S. expressions; even the date format was invariable. We have made some progress since then but much more is needed.

There are many spelling differences between Australian and U.S. English. It would be easy for us to adopt U.S. spelling but, in doing so, we would be destroying a large part of our heritage - so there are many who jealously guard our spelling, our pronunciation, and that part of our vocabulary which we can call our own. Such differences, which may seem trivial to some, are intrusive; a constant impediment to the tool we are using being virtually assimilated into ourselves.

3.1.1.1. Spell checkers

The early spell checkers in English were almost all of U.S. origin. For many Australians they were largely useless. More recently software companies have attempted to provide spell checkers closer to the Australian version of English. This trend will continue as their manufacture becomes simpler and add-on user dictionaries can be produced in Australia itself. Hence an influence that was subverting Australian English should now assist in its preservation. And those who care about our language will write more effortlessly in it using the word processor.

3.1.1.2. Workload monitoring

The computer can do many things at once - including monitoring of output and productivity. This may be a hazard to workers. We have seen the musculoligamentous scourge caused in industry by so-called piece work the more you finish, the more you get paid. The same thing would be expected with VDT operators. Overuse injuries are often associated with some form of psychic stress, either arising from the workplace or without, attempts to monitor levels of work through the VDT could only add to that stress - with resultant injury.

3.1.2. Instruction manuals

Unfortunately there has not been the same sort of improvement in instruction manuals. They now occupy many more pages than before - apparently to improve readability but, more likely, making them more difficult to photocopy. They make lots of assumptions about prior knowledge, make long leaps of logic, and are often ungrammatical. Poorly written manuals read by persons with inadequate grounding in software operation, may cause health problems from frustration, uncertainty, and unnecessary repetition of work.

3.1.3. Over-engineering

Many software packages have every possibility continually available and, sometimes, one can end up doing something unplanned. A journalist colleague who spends 90% of his time at the keyboard says of word-processors:

"They tend to be over designed for what I want. Try to do something simple and you often find you're locked into some bizarre function which counts every second full-stop and turns it into a tabulated, indexed dot point with a border and three footnotes. Getting out of such functions can be a lot harder than getting into them."

To avoid such frustration there needs to be a mechanism, at installation, to remove functions you are never going to use. This requires good documentation so that you know precisely what you are losing. Even now that is beyond some software manufacturers.

4. Management expectations

I shall try to deal with these in a little detail in my presentation but, in my experience, the attitudes of some managers towards VDT operators are summed up in the following list:

4.1.1. That everyone is created equal with equal capacity

This is not just the attitude of some managers, but also of many fellow workers. "We are all doing the same work; how come you are having problems?" We are prepared to accept human variability in a range of other activities yet, when it comes to operating machinery - and the keyboard is no exception - supervisors expect everyone to be able to perform at the same high rate.

4.1.2. That perfect physical ergonomics are enough

We've had an ergonomist in; we've spent a few hundred dollars on furniture; and still you complain!

4.1.3. That all worker fears are groundless

The scientific evidence is, indeed, pointing in this direction so perhaps the managers may be right. Alas, some unscrupulous salesmen are exploiting the fears of VDT operators to sell their equipment just as, in earlier times, amulets would have been sold to ward off evil spirits. There is, for example, a brisk trade in 'radiation' screens for VDTs. If an operator sees others with these accoutrements, it is natural that he will worry that he lacks such a screen.

Similarly with the low-radiation monitors: it is difficult to explain to an operator that they were made 'low-radiation' merely because that was achievable, not because there were any detectable health effects with the existing monitors. While the purveyors of the low-radiation monitors might say the label is just an expression of technical sophistication, the purchaser will see it as a positive health point and buy it, incorrectly, on those grounds.

Nevertheless, worker fears that are based on reality or deliberately purveyed myths, should be dealt with sympathetically and positively. To do otherwise is to create unnecessary new administrative and health problems.

4.1.4. That injuries resulting while using a VDT are unrelated to the VDT

This occurs, most often, in relation to musculoligamentous injuries arising from excessive work pressure. The supervisor may deny that there is a relationship and may try to resist compensation. This is more likely to happen in Australia where there has been a highly polarised debate about VDT-related injuries - especially overuse injury.

On the one side you have those who view the VDT as a work of the devil responsible for a range of worker health effects ranging from miscarriages to visual deterioration. Perhaps some of these people go home to use their own PCs without a second thought, consistent with the unexpressed view that only events at work result in injury.

5. Worker expectations
5.1.1. To be treated as an individual
5.1.2. Fears to be taken seriously

Even if there is, after all, no basis for some of the reported scares at least provide us with up to date information and, where necessary, discussions with those who know.

5.1.3. Adequate explanation and reassurance where appropriate

As above.

5.1.4. Correct optics

5.1.5. Medical examinations

These should be limited to visual assessment. Provide the ergonomics are good, and the monitor and software are recent, the visual task of operating a VDT should be little different from that of reading paper-based material. We do not examine people who are to do a lot of reading in their work, or provide them with purpose-designed spectacles, or arrange for regular examinations. Why should we do this with VDT operators? Since the size of print on a VDT screen can be adjusted over a very wide range as can its contrast with the background, a good VDT should present a less challenging visual task than having, for example, to plough through hundreds of journal articles for research or presentation.

5.1.6. Workplace participation and consultation
5.1.7. Participation in OHS
5.1.8. Free flow of OHS information
5.1.9. Workplace assessments and monitoring

6. Conclusions

Undue concentration on physical hazards can lead to neglect of social and psychological aspects of the work environment which, though less well understood, are likely to provide a basis for much of the distress and concern about workplace hazards. This is important in three ways: (1) when assessing the workplace; (2) when communicating information about the work environment; and (3) when planning a work environment.

Behavioral Cybernetics, Quality of Working Life and Work Organization in Computer Automated Offices

M. J. Smith

Dept. of Industrial Engineering, University of Wisconsin
1513 University Avenue, Madison, WI 53706, USA
email MJSMITH@macc.wisc.edu

Abstract

Computer automation has emerged as a predominant work process in the 1980's, and it appears this technology will remain dominant through the 1990's. Work organization structures and processes originally designed for non-computerized work have not been very successful in dealing with the transition to computerized work. While economic benefits of computerization have been achieved, the extent of the benefits has been much less than expected due to transition problems. In addition there have been substantial human resource problems concerning work design, ergonomics, and stress. New ways of organizing computerized work are needed, especially approaches which can capitalize on the technological flexibility of computers and associated communications systems. One potential organizational approach builds on theory taken from behavioral cybernetics, which defines the control aspects of human behavior in work processes. Behavioral cybernetics emphasizes the need for real-time feedback of performance, self determination in decision making, and self regulation of the work process. This theory defines human behavior in terms of dynamic systems undergoing change. These same concepts can be applied to organizations undergoing computerized automation to provide real-time direction for the work process design to achieve an appropriate system balance. This paper will explore the application of behavioral cybernetics to the organization of computerized work processes for enhancing the quality of working life.

1. BACKGROUND

In the highly competitive global economy computer technology can be an economic advantage. As Smith & Carayon (1995) have indicated new technology can have several economic benefits: (1) lowered production costs through the use of more efficient machines, (2) reduced workforce, (3) a cheaper, less skilled workforce, (4) improved product quality and conformity, (5) increased "up-time" or productive time, (6) enhanced flexibility of the production system to meet market needs, and (7) lowered insurance costs by reducing worker risks. Evidence from case study research indicates that some benefits are realized, while others are not (OTA, 1984, 1985, 1987; Lindstrom,

1993). There is also emerging evidence that the introduction of new technology can be detrimental to the production process and to the employees (Majchrzak, 1988; Smith & Carayon, 1995). Cyert and Mowery (1988) have discussed how the competitiveness of a global economy has led to applications of technology primarily for efficiency purposes with few benefits for the quality of working life. Advanced technology leads to more products per employee, increased product quality and a reduction in the workforce to achieve efficiency. The results have often been a smaller workforce, doing jobs for less pay that have decreased cognitive content and control (Cyert and Mowery, 1988). Such conditions have been associated with employee stress and ill health (Smith, 1987; Smith and Carayon, 1995).

One of the major influences that new technology has on the workplace is the way in which the work is organized (Bradley, 1989; Westlander, 1993; Smith and Carayon, 1995). The inherent flexibility in advanced automation can be capitalized on by moving away from linear production flow and moving toward flexible distribution of production flow. This means that smaller groups of employees at separate or remote locations or in small groups can be coordinated to produce final products. Such remote integration requires sophisticated scheduling control and substantial monitoring of current status in real-time to have an efficient and integrated process. The process of data collection and processing, the way in which such tasks are continuously monitored, the nature of supervision of the process and the design of the tasks have been linked to lower quality of working life (Smith et al, 1981, 1992; Majchrzak, 1988).

Many workplaces with traditional organizational structures that have been designed for non-computerized work systems have encountered problems when implementing computerized automation (OTA, 1985; Bradley, 1989; Cohen, 1984). However, some research indicates that computer implementation can successfully improve several aspects of the work process including production and the quality of working life (Huuhtanen, et al 1993; Lindstrom, 1993). Some theoretical development and research has been carried out to determine the most effective work organizational design strategies for companies moving to or increasing the extent of computer automation.

2. ORGANIZATIONAL PROCESSES AND COMPUTER AUTOMATION:

Several major theoretical approaches have emerged for addressing the automation of workplaces such as sociotechical systems, participative management, action research, macroergonomics, knowledge based systems, and balance theory. These approaches are discussed in more detail in Smith and Sainfort (1989) and Smith and Carayon (1995). The worker involvement and participative approaches have been very successful in improving productivity and quality in manufacturing and assembly work (Lawler, 1986). These rely on a shift from alienation and confrontation to cooperation and co-determination (Gardell, 1971). Cooperation usually develops from joint concern for the success of a work process. Continued success and cooperation come after a track record of mutual benefit is demonstrated. Compromise and concession to the other side's needs are hallmarks of participative processes.

Bradley (1993) has described the organizational and psychosocial context of the introduction and use of knowledge based computer systems which can be used for work organization benefits. The central features are: (1) influence/power and education, (2) communication and work content, (3) leadership and management roles, and (4) key dimensions of life quality. She further discusses the effects and changes at work which the design of knowledge based systems will influence. These include: (1) the perception of having less time and being closer to each other, (2) the quality and structure of contacts and collaboration at work and in private life will be different with computers, (3) the qualitative aspects of communications which carry emotions such as trust, confidence and security will be more essential, (4) private life will be emphasized over work, (5) the traditional division on gender aspects of society, the individual's self perception and identity will be strengthened, (6) the distinction between work and leisure will diminish, and (7) basic education and training will define the nature of computerized communications.

Westlander (1993) describes an ambitious organizational redesign project at Swedish Telecom Services which used a multi-disciplinary team approach to provide redesign of organizational structure, task distribution, managerial and supervisory focus, and models of control. Over a period of three years an action research paradigm was used to eliminate work environment problems for telephonists. The approach included a collaborative effort with the telephonists and the research team to redesign the work environment. This was put in the context of a "village" comprised of groups of employees with emphasis on intra-group harmony as well as across group harmony (Soderberg, 1993). The intra-group organization led to greater community and cooperation within a group, but led to a weaker sense of community across groups and a low sense of global organizational belonging (Soderberg, 1993). Changes in global organizational structure independent of the local plant changes may have contributed to these results.

Venda and Hendrick (1993) have defined the importance of taking a broader perspective of organizational design using a top down process incorporating various levels of human decision making. This approach examines the integration of technical and personnel subsystems which are seen as interdependent. "Mutual" adaptation of each subsystem provides more flexibility than either approach singularly. Smith and Sainfort (1989) indicated that any redesign process produces "trade-offs" among specific improvements and obtaining the best "overall" work process. Bohnhoff, Brandt and Henning (1992) have called for a balance between people and technology. According to Smith and Carayon (1995) there are two aspects of "balance" when addressing job and organizational design. These are (1) system balance and (2) compensatory balance. System balance is based on the idea that a workplace or process or job is more than the sum of the individual components of the system. The interplay among the various components of the system produces results that are greater (or lesser) than the additive aspects of the individual parts. It is the way in which the system components relate to each other that determines the potential for the system to produce results. Thus, proper balance must consider the effects of a single change on all of the elements of the system.

The second type of balance is "compensatory" in nature. It is seldom possible to optimize all aspects of a work system simultaneously. This may be due to financial considerations, or it may be because it is impossible to improve all job characteristics due to inherent aspects of job tasks. Compensatory balance uses one or more positive elements of the system to balance the negative elements in the system. This produces an overall positive balance in the system.

3. BEHAVIORAL CYBERNETICS AND ORGANIZATIONAL PROCESS:

Smith and Smith (1966) and Smith, Henning and Smith (1994) have defined characteristics of behavioral cybernetics which are central to the human performance control process. The foremost of these are self determination, self regulation and real-time feedback control. Self determination indicates the need for persons to exercise judgment over their own actions. This assumes that the person has the ability to take action without direction. At an organizational level this principle requires a sharing of "power" with the employees to provide autonomy of action. As with individual behavior and performance, this principle also recognizes that the sharing of power shifts not only authority, but also responsibility for actions to the employees and work groups. In a work organization this power sharing often occurs at the group level such that work groups or departments are given the opportunity for self determination in meeting the objectives of the organization. This principle is in conformity with sociotechnical theory (Gardell, 1971) and participative management theory (Lawler, 1986).

Self regulation is related to self determination, but defines the action at the level of individual employees. This principle recognizes the need for individual "control" of the action at the personal level. Thus, there is the requirement for providing instrumental control and decision latitude to each individual employee at the task level. Various theorists have shown the relationship of such control for individual stress responses to technology (Sainfort, 1991). In this control process, real-time feedback is essential for individual employees to be able to make good decisions and to direct their responses for effective performance. A large body of literature has established that feedback is crucial for the very best performance and learning (Smith and Smith, 1966). Such feedback provides the guidance mechanism for achieving proper responses for high level performance.

Behavioral cybernetics has defined essential characteristics of human performance systems, and these characteristics have special relevance for dynamic systems. The application of real-time feedback and personal decision making enable quick responses to changes in the environment. With dynamic feedback and the authority to respond there is no delay between the system's needs and the employees' responses. However, a potential weakness of this approach is the emphasis on the group and individual levels of the organization. This neglects the need to coordinate the responses of various individuals and groups to achieve larger organizational goals. To meet such needs Ting, Smith and Smith (1971) and Smith, Henning and Smith (1994) have defined system level feedback parameters which integrate the responses of many individuals and groups to provide direction for concerted organizational efforts.

This process is termed "social tracking" (Ting, Smith and Smith, 1971) which establishes feedback and tracking mechanisms for jointly meeting the objectives of the organization. Such systems require coordination of these processes which may be best mediated through knowledge based systems as discussed by Bradley (1993) and the macroergonomic approach of Hendrick (1986). In addition this process of social tracking within a group and among groups using dynamic feedback may produce more positive results in organizational cohesion and cooperation than observed by Westlander (1993) and Soderberg (1993). This cybernetic process changes the role of the computer technology from that of a "task processing" machine to a synchronized network of information and knowledge that can assist employees in meeting organizational demands. Thus, the employees are "in control" of their own tasks, have tasks rich in cognitive content and decision making, have social and organizational context to their work activities, and can dynamically balance their demands to meet the work system's needs at any given time. This cybernetic system approach meets many of the positive work organization characteristics described by sociotechnical systems, participative management, action research and macroergonomics. By using a dynamic feedback process it provides a mechanism to coordinate sub-systems, to enhance job task characteristics and to provide dynamic response flexibility as technological characteristics of the work process change.

In summary, the rapid changes in the office workplace due to computerization have produced many ill effects for workers, particularly the deskilling of jobs and less stability in employment. These negative effects have limited the economic benefits of computer automation while also causing health problems for workers. Behavioral cybernetic theory proposes an approach to workplace design where dynamic change in the workplace can be capitalized on to promote improved job design, better productivity and enhanced health. Most computer systems strive for standardization of methods and procedures, computer control over the process and limited inter worker communication. Behavioral cybernetic theory demonstrates that the real power of computers and related communications systems is that they can enable individuals to do tasks using individual work methods and style, provide greater capability for individual task control, and promote participation through ease of communication with coworkers. Properly designed computing systems have the capability to give workers a unique identity, and such capability promotes worker satisfaction, performance and health.

This paper provides only a brief snapshot of how behavioral cybernetic theory can assist in the design of work organizations undergoing technological change. Specific details of action are missing.

REFERENCES

Bohnhoff, A., Brandt, D. and Henning, K., 1992, The dual design approach as a tool for the interdisciplinary design of human-centered systems. Intern. J. of Human Factors in Manufacturing, 2(3), 289-301.

Bradley, G. (1989). Computers and the Psychosocial Work Environment. London: Taylor & Francis.

Bradley, G. (1993). Towards a knowledge sharing organization, In M.J. Smith and G. Salvendy (Eds.) Human Computer Interaction: Applications and Case Studies, Amsterdam: Elsevier, 869-873.

Cohen, B. (1984). Human Aspects in Office Automation. Amsterdam: Elsevier.

Cyert, R.M. and Mowery, D.C. (1988). The Impact of Technological Change on Employment and Economic Growth. Cambridge: Ballinger Publishing Company.

Gardell, B. (1971). Alienation and mental health in the modern industrial environment, In L. Levi (ed.) Society, Stress and Disease Vol. 1. London: Oxford University Press, 148-180.

Huuhtanen, P., Leino, T., Niemela, T. and Ahola, K. (1993). Mastering the changes in information technology: a follow-up study of insurance tasks, In M.J. Smith and G. Salvendy (Eds.) Human Computer Interaction: Applications and Case Studies, Amsterdam: Elsevier, 703-708.

Lawler, E. (1986). High Involvement Management. San Francisco: Jossey Bass.

Lindstrom, K. (1993). Finnish longitudinal studies of job design and VDT work, In M.J. Smith and G. Salvendy (Eds.) Human Computer Interaction: Applications and Case Studies, Amsterdam: Elsevier, 697-702.

Majchrzak, A. (1988). The Human Side of Factory Automation. San Francisco: Jossey Bass.

OTA. (1985). Automation of America's Offices. Washington, DC: Office of Technology Assessment, U.S. Congress.

OTA. (1987). The Electronic Supervisor. Washington, DC: Office of Technology Assessment, U.S. Congress.

Sainfort, P.C. (1991). Stress, control and other job elements: a study of office workers. Inter. J. of Industrial Ergonomics, 7, 11-23.

Smith, K.U. and Smith, M.F. (1966). Cybernetic Principles of Learning and Educational Design. New York: Holt, Rinehart & Winston.

Smith, M.J., Cohen, B.G.F., Stammerjohn, L. and Happ, A. (1981). An investigation of health complaints and job stress in video display operations. Human Factors, 23, 387-400.

Smith, M.J., Carayon, P., Sanders, K., Lim, S. and LeGrande, D. (1992). Employee stress and health complaints in jobs with and without electronic performance monitoring. Applied Ergonomics, 23, 17-27.

Smith, M.J. (1987). Occupational stress, In G. Salvendy (Ed.) Handbook of Human Factors. New York: John Wiley, 844-860.

Smith, M.J. and Sainfort, P.C. (1989). A balance theory of job design for stress reduction. Inter. J. of Industrial Ergonomics, 4, 67-79.

Smith, M.J. and Carayon, P. (1995). New technology, automation and work organization: stress problems and improved technology implementation strategies. Inter. J. of Human Factors in Manufacturing, 5, 99-116.

Smith, T.J., Henning, R.A. and Smith, K.U. (1994). Sources of performance variability, In G. Salvendy and W. Karwowski (Eds.) Design of Work and Development of Personnel in Advanced Manufacturing. New York: John Wiley & Sons, 273-330.

Soderberg, I. (1993). How the design of premises supports a new organizational structure as viewed by full-time operators in large-scale teleservices, In M.J. Smith and G. Salvendy (Eds.) Human Computer Interaction: Applications and Case Studies, Amsterdam: Elsevier, 839-844.

Ting, T., Smith, M.J., and Smith, K.U., "Social Feedback Factors in Rehabilitative Processes and Learning. American Journal of Physical Medicine, 51, 1971.

Venda, V, and Hendrick, H. (1993). Qualitative and quantitative analysis of human decision-making complexity, In M.J. Smith and G. Salvendy (Eds.) Human Computer Interaction: Applications and Case Studies, Amsterdam: Elsevier, 636-641.

Design of Usability Laboratories for Computer Networking Products

C. Bracci[a] and M. Taylor[b]

[a]IBM, Human Factors and Usability Dept., p.le Giulio Pastore 6, 00144 Rome, Italy. Email: bracci at vnet.ibm.com

[b]Human Factors and Usability Consultant, Via Aventina 20, 00153 Rome, Italy Email: mc2985 at mclink.it

1. Background

The Rome Networking Software Laboratory (RNSL) designs and produces software for use in computer telecommunications networks. An integral part of this development process is the Human Factors Department. Human Factors or Ergonomics has been applied to the development of usable software since the early '80s. The Human Factors & Usability group is an integral part of a development process that recognizes that "Ease-of-Use" is a key quality factor. This process is multidisciplinary and requires the active participation of the end user. A key tool in this development process is the usability test is a purpose built usability laboratory.

The laboratory consists of an observation area and a subject area. The subject area is designed to make the user feel at ease and to simulate a modern workplace. The observation area must provide an efficient workplace were the observation team can observe and record what the user is doing.

2. Our Objectives

The design of tests for the evaluation of networking systems requires the simultaneous observation of more than one user. The tests typically simulate the interaction between two independent users in two different locations.

The objectives of the usability test are to:
- Test the software, not the user
- Ensure that the design fits the user, not the programmer
- Simulate realistic work situations with real users
- Allows tests to be repeated and refined throughout the development cycle
- Measure completion of tasks and not functions and features
- Verify overall user satisfaction with the product

Based on experience gained by IBM since the early 80's in the planning and use of usability laboratories we designed a lab that physically placed the observation area between the 2 users.

The objectives of the usability laboratory are to provide a:
- Modern workplace for the users that allows them to work with the product as naturally as possible and puts them at ease.
- An efficient workplace for the observation team which typically consists of the Designer, Information Developer, Human Factors Specialist, System Test and the Customer

3. The Problem

Human-Computer interaction is an interaction between people with the computer system acting as a representative of one or several humans. The networking systems that are developed at the laboratory are macro systems where there are numerous users with a variety of roles. These users tend to be working cooperatively where their decisions affect the system and the other users interactions. This interactivity is compounded as the systems are used in real-time. The flow of information between these users is illustrated in Figure 1. The information that is being exchanged is of two types: network information and human communications. By placing the observers in between the two users it is possible to better analyze and understand the broad picture and the details.

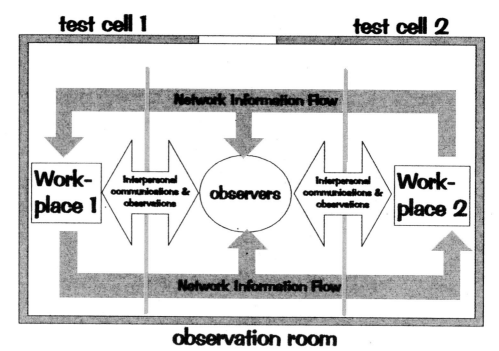

Figure 1. Flows of Information in a Networking System

4. The Solution

The laboratory was designed using three large offices as a starting point. Our requirement for being able to observe two users simultaneously was met by placing the observation area between the two subject areas. Metaphorically speaking, we placed ourselves in the interface between the two users. This analogy was particularly powerful for new observers who could immediately relate to the interaction between the two users. The observers view the users directly through the one-way mirror as well as using computers, audio and video equipment to log as much of the data as possible. It is worth noting that the secret in conducting usability tests is not so much the collection, collation and analysis of data, but rather that the team decide as a group which problems need to solve and how. It is this consensus of opinion that makes this such a powerful tool in terms of speeding up the development of usable software.

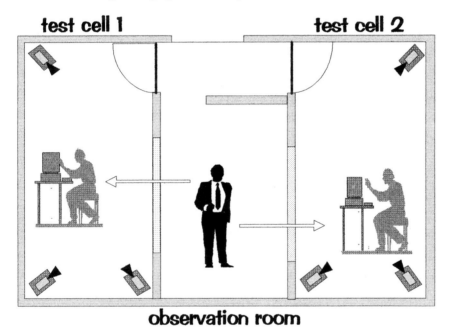

Figure 2. Layout of the Usability Laboratory

5. The Results

To date we have conducted tests on the entire range of products produced at the laboratory. These products are used for software distribution, performance monitoring, and remote computing. In addition we have also conducted tests that compare several competitors when performing equivalent tasks.

The tests have all concentrated on key tasks and scenarios, for example, installation, trouble shooting, and use of the product. These tests have confirmed the validity of placing the team in-line with the users as it increases the realism and involves the observers directly in the dynamics of the man-man interaction, because the:

- Team is "immersed" in the test
- Users are emotionally involved
- Scenarios are more realistic

We have tested the whole range of products developed at RNSL that are as follows:

- Software Distribution
- Performance Monitoring
- Remote Computing

Typically we concentrate on three key areas:

- Installation - The installation and configuration tasks are fundamental to the users perception of the product. It is vital that this task be designed minimize dissatisfaction and frustration.
- Diagnosis of software and network malfunctions - Due to the complexity and heterogeneity of networking systems problems will occur which the users must be able to solve efficiently and effectively.
- Use of the product - Depending on the type of product the actual tasks that the user expects to be able to do must be designed for ease of use and intuitiveness.

6. Products Tested

Two products that were extensively tested and designed in our laboratory were used at the Winter Olympic Games in Lillehammer 1994. These tests identified a number of key problems that would not have otherwise been highlighted.

6.1 Distributed Console Access Facility - DCAF

DCAF is used to control a network of computers remotely from a central site using various communication protocols. A typical application of this product is as a "Helpdesk" that provides support to a large group of users.

The tests we conducted identified the following problems that were resolved:

- Users need informal communication channels - The original design made no allowance for the need for users to communicate informally by chatting or exchanging information
- Installation needs to be simplified - The initial installation task did not allow for a gentle introduction to get started with the a complex system. This was solved by adding a component that helped the user set up a basic system before requiring the user to consult the user manual.

6.2 NetView Distribution Manager/2

NetView Distribution Manager/2 is used to distribute software on a network of computers connected to a central site using various communication protocols. A typical application of this product is when a new operating system needs to upgraded on the network.

The tests we conducted identified the following problems that were resolved:

- Installation process is too complex - This was simplified through the introduction of software which prompted the user for key information about the system and the introduction of a "Getting Started" manual
- Improve support for identifying network malfunctions - This was improved by providing better messages and on-line information.

7. Conclusions

The design of the laboratory with a central observation area has proved extremely successful with both test observers and users. It has permitted us to look at both sides of the coin in networking systems, namely the:

- Human-computer Interaction
- Human-Human Interaction.

This second issue is often ignored in usability testing, due to the difficulties in simulating such an environment. We believe that this approach has addressed this problem and puts us in a better position to provide complete evaluations of new networking systems. The layout of the laboratory has given very positive results both for the user and for the development process.

CUSTOMER INFORMATION SYSTEM

R. Garetti

Divisione Servizi Olivetti-Ivrea (TO), Italy

1. INTRODUCTION

We live in a super-informed world, a world in which the information givers have many different media at their disposal: the printed word and the luminous screen, for example, compete for our attention, seeming to offer more and better information.
The information consumers find themselves confused, no longer able to choose, they read more and more, watch and listen to more, but end up understanding less and becoming less discriminating. The dialogue which has traditionally developed as people draw on a source of information appears to be in decline; the consumer not only does *not* learn, but loses the aptitude to learn; the loss of a precious faculty which by right should be a fundamental part of human nature. People are becoming more and more isolated, they are under increasing pressure to achieve outstanding results more quickly than ever before, and are operating in a world in which the marketeers are constantly painting a more confident and inflexible picture.
Maybe we are failing in something. This may be the moment for us to radically change the way in which we inform, perhaps we need to rediscover more honest and more meaningful forms which are measured in terms of the help and value they give to the recipient and not in terms of their convenience to the originator and transmitter of the information.
Perhaps, for this to happen, the consumers themselves must change, they must learn to choose, to refuse and reject the information which does not help: they must **rebel**!
In considering the nature of communication today, we need to learn once again how to use symbols [1], as a means of re-establishing a dialogue between the provider and consumer of information, giving them both the chance to contribute personally.
Until now, the publisher or broadcaster has always been somehow set apart from the public. The writer or the film-maker has always been placed on a kind of intellectual pedestal.
Communication between ordinary people has always been lost, either because it is oral and never recorded or because the written note or the graffito becomes the property of the social historian or archeologist. Today however, thanks to technology, the boundaries between the "serious" and the vernacular are

becoming less well-defined. Almost anybody with something to say can become involved in the creation of a well of information.

Today Information Technology and the economic system in general are in difficulty. The world of Information Technology, after a period of great expansion based on proprietary solutions and the dominance of the products over services, pushed by the emergence of standards, is moving towards a crisis prompted by an excess of what can be offered. The economic crisis has caused a reduction in demand, further increasing the difficulties for the Information Technology sector. In order to survive, the most flexible Information Technology Enterprises are moving their core business from products to services. But these changes can become possible only if the Enterprises re-engineer their processes and empower those involved in their execution by using Information Technology tools in an effective way.

This article is about the results of our first research into CIS - an information system based on user-need and orientated around the user. To present these results in an organic fashion, we find it is necessary to first speak of information, of services, of education and training, of working methods, of the team and of learning, of rules and behaviour, of the map of roles and relationships. All are essential components and must not be undervalued if one wants to understand the evolving phenomena. We then presen the major results of our research and conclude with some suggestions on the way to procede from there.

2. GENERAL METHOD

It is necessary to follow an approach, a discipline, a methodology. It is necessary to make easy-to-use services quickly available, giving the customer immediate and concrete advantages. In a commercial context, this will generally be judged in terms of competetive advantage. In the world of services [2] the relationship between the service provider and the customer is very complex: we should not try to over-simplify it.

The provider and consumer of the service really need to understand each other and need to be able to trust each other. It is essential that the main characteristics of the service and the way in which it is to be delivered should be planned from the very start, together with the customer: it is of fundamental importance that the service provider and consumer share a common vision. One of the main characteristics of the service world is that the need for the service is normally implicit rather than explicit. All too often, the need emerges unexpectedly in a way which is difficult to forecast [3], it is expressed in most cases as an emergency, and is delivered as a *firefighting* service.

All too often, it is perceived by the customer as an added cost resulting from avoidable error, and not as an investment. By developing integrated service projects, a "Virtual" Enterprise can be implemented which allows the *"knowledge"* to accumulate in a repository, built with the co-operation of everybody and usable by everybody. The Enterprise structure comes to be regarded as highly articulated as a result of this process.

Considering the theme of *Information Systems* in more detail, it is worth remembering that they have always been with us: factories, firms and banks have always had information systems based on one instrument or another.

With the arrival of the computer, the term has taken on a technological significance which on the one hand has allowed us to rationalise its processes, and on the other has distorted its original function. Information systems are seen by some as centres of power, and by others as a sign of progress based on the influence of technology.

If we change this approach and *shift* our attention to the users we realise not only that, by definition, an information system manages information, but also that the term information can take on many different meanings.

Above all, *every user* needs a means of exchanging day-to-day information :
a mail system for notes and letters. The system must also allow *management* access to key information in a succinct format, in order for them to quickly understand what is going on, and to make sound decisions as a result of that understanding. More properly we need to talk of the Executive Information System as one of the priorities of a user-orientated information system.

Today, the information system will not necessarily cover *educational* services. However, both now and in the future education will change dramatically from what it has been (the classroom, the board, the teacher teaching and the pupils learning). Even if the information systems of the past were never considered as having an educational role, perhaps in the future they will be obliged to do so.
To be certain that any instrument is correctly used, a period, no matter how brief, must be allowed for *training*.

CIS is an instrument which has been designed to be simple to use, but *hidden* within it there are services which can be exploited to the full only after a suitable period of education and training. Education and training are both a part of the *learning process* and cannot be separated.

An Information System must obviously improve the profitability of services by making processes more fluid across the organisation, but first of all it must give greater *Customer Satisfaction.* Usually, the technological infrastructure will need to be rebuilt in order to benefit from the *convergence* of the Information Technology with the telecommunications and multimedia technologies.

3. THE METHOD OF WORK

As the individuals within the enterprise learn, so the enterprise itself becomes a more educated organism. If the individuals within the organisation are not able to learn new skills and ideas, or if they gain only a partial or unbalanced view of what is required, then a certain sort of sickness will *infect* the organisation.
The symptoms of such a sickness are various, but the most insidious of all is the lack of faith in the working group. Our ability to learn will always be affected by the time that is avaiable and the energy we have to expend during that time.

Learning requires a *continuous effort* [4] : this is generally easier at the beginning than it subsequently becomes. It starts to get really difficult when learners feel that they are expending more effort than the the knowledge they are gaining is worth. To reduce the risk of such a negative experience and to rediscover the delight of learning, we must change [5], we must face problems in a different way.

This new way of learning can be charatcterised by a few *simple rules* [6].
First of all we need to understand what it means to learn as part of a *team*, we need to learn how to create a group dialogue. This demands that we learn to suspend, for a moment, our own assumptions and become genuinely open to the thinking of others. Successful group dialogue also demands that we learn to recognise and remove behavioural traits which pose a threat to learning.

Moreover, it is fundamental that we reason in a way which is tuned to the system - *Systems Thinking*. We must endeavour to identify all relationships which exist between system components in order to help ensure that the actions needed to create new products and services are effective.

It is necessary to develop the *skills* needed as an individual to clarify and investigate the facts. We need to focus our energies and to be patient in order to look at reality objectively. It is fundamental that we discover the link between personal growth and the growth of the organisation in order to find a reciprocal sense of responsibility between the individual and the organisation.

It is also necessary to beware of deeply-rooted assumptions and generalisations of *Mental Models*. Whether consciously or subconsciously, these influence our understanding of the facts and the actions which result from that understanding. If one is not aware of these existing mental models, then attempts to enter new markets and to develop new organisational plans will fail. It is necessary to encourage an open dialogue between people who will freely express their own point of view and who are open to the influence of others. In short, we must develop the ability to create a sense of *shared vision* on which we can build.

By organising work around a shared sense of identity and purpose, people are able to learn and to achieve excellence [7] not because they are told to but because *they want* to. In practice, this means knowing how to create a vision for shared products and services which encourage *genuine* involvement rather than simply seeking consensus.

But it is not sufficient to know the rules we must learn to apply them and this happens only by *commiting ourselves* to the discipline.

As a general observation, people will stop learning when they are isolated. This isolation can occur when people feel excluded from the group, even though they may remain nominally a part of it.

In contrast to the principles of group learning, the dissemination of information via many networks which pass as information systems, *bombard* individuals with data but at the same time isolate us from our peers.

The individual today has more and more information but less and less knowledge: our individual ability to transform information into knowledge rapidly tires. *The solution* then, is to expand the knowledge of the group.

Just as the individual who works in isolation risks becoming marginalised, so the organisation which fails to make potential connections can rapidly find itself critically handicapped.

Operationally, to develop a user-orientated information system, the first thing to do is to create a team which will define a rule-based working method.
The role of the team leader or *facilitator* is to propose certain rules, which must then be accepted by all team members.

After an initial training period, the rules set the behaviour of the team. At this point, the team is ready to go into action, starting with a clean slate: they are ready to construct an activity (service) **map** (figure 1.).

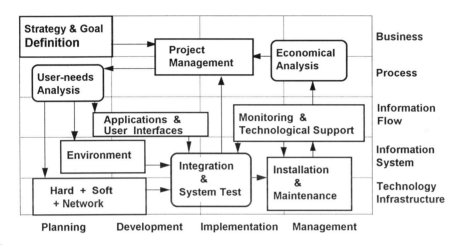

Figure 1.

The map defines the period to be dedicated to planning, development, implementation and management along the x-axis. Levels of competence are mapped along the y-axis: business, process, information flow, information system, technology infrastructure.
You place the activities on the map and plot the flows. As it represents a process, one traces the *evolutionary cycle* showing both the activity flow and the lines of reaction. After a number of meetings, the team will be able to assign individual responsibilities, plan the developments, and manage the entire process.

4. RESULTS

A team made up of people with very *different* backgrounds worked together for approximately one year. From a technological point of view, they learnt a lot from creating the first release of CIS in a relatively short time and with limited resources, but perhaps more importantly, they learnt things which would not have been possible without the team *ethic*. For example, the team learnt that with an information system based on user need, the definition of "*User-needs analysis*" on the map itself has a precise and fundamental value as the point of departure for the entire process. In addition, they learnt that if the information system needs to become the principal working instrument for an entire organisation then it must be *secure*, but security cannot be achieved simply by strengthening system test activity or by introducing higher levels of encryption: they learnt that security must be achieved at the level of system architecture and service management.

You do not achieve *ease-of-use* simply by having a clean interface and on-line support to help resolve specific problems: a real educational effort and a continuous dialogue with the users is required. It is not enough simply to use a PC regularly: it is necessary to give instruction on how best to optimise the archive structure and to collaborate in *reengineering* the work itself.

However, we feel the real problem today lies not in the technology, but in how we need to be organised in order to *use* it, *distribute* it and *keep it vital*.
Throughout the presentation, the need to find a method and then to use it in the creation of an information system was highlighted. Although all this is indispensable it is not enough. It is not enough to have the builder, it is also necessary that the *users* subsequently behave in the same way. The team is only the point of departure. The team is enabled in order to set the process in motion, and it is essential that the users themselves play a corresponding role, that they understand and participate in the invention of *a new way of using information*.
Working in this way, the end result is an information system which will genuinely serve the needs of all.
A User-Oriented Information System serves anybody who is convinced that the future will be based on the values of knowledge [8]. A User-Oriented Information System serves anybody who believes that the health of the enterprise can only be assured through the development of a workgroup culture [9].
The organisation which seeks to invest in its own culture and in the channels through which it grows is clearly one which believes in its own future.

REFERENCES

1. Douglas R. Hofstadter : GODEL, ESCHER, BACH : *an Eternal Golden Brain* (1984) Adelphi Edizioni, Milano
2. Stan Bavis & Bill Davidson : *2020 I BUSINESS DEL FUTURO* (1992) Il Sole 24 Ore Societa' Editoriale Media Economici Seme, Milano
3. Jacques Monod : *Il Caso e la Necessita'* (1970) Arnoldo Mondadori Editori, Milano
4. Francesco Novara, Mario Fulcheri : *Stress e Manager* (1992) Fondazione A. Olivetti, Ivrea
5. P. Watzlawick, J.H. Weakland, R. Fisch : *CHANGE* (1974) Casa Editrice Astrolabio - Ubaldini Editore, Roma
6. Peter M. Senge : *The FIFTH DISCIPLINE* (1990) Doubleday / Currency, New York
7. T.J. Peters, R.H. Waterman Jr. : *In Search of Excellence* (1984) Sperling & Kupfer Editori, Milano
8. Alvin Toffler : *Power Shift* (1990) Bantam Books, New York
9. Valerio Ochetto : *Adriano Olivetti* (1985) Arnoldo Mondadori Editori, Milano

WWDU '94 and impact on job content, human interaction and cooperation, work organization

F. Novara[a]

[a]Management Business School - Turin University, Turin - Italy

1. INTRODUCTION

An increasing change in the buyers of Information Technology carries out increasing problems for the functionality, usability and acceptability of the display units.
As K.D. Eason and Susan Harker[1] pointed out some years ago, "traditionally the purchasers of computer equipment were technical specialists, for example, data processing managers, who were primarily concerned with technical and economical criteria and who expected to deal with application issues themselves. As the technology has become cheaper and its potential more widely appreciated, the range of purchasers has expanded enormously. Not only do D.P. Managers buy IT products but user department managers, office managers and, in many instances, the end user him or herself".
The advanced technology proposes more and more tools with a wide range of functionality at low cost. But the pursuit of a wide functionality does not fit the needs of people who use a narrow part of it and can be mixed up.
At the same time, the opportunity of multi-user systems demand to support users who must learn to share facilities and information. J. Grudin [2], in a "Social evaluation of the user interface" proves that the failure of early multi-user system is due to the gap between designers and users. As K.D. Eason and S. Harker remark, "organisational issues play no part in the training of IT system designers and there is no explicit recognition of the need to determine organisational requirements within the design cycle". The same way, the choice of products, the systems configuration, the introduction and implementation are left to the user organisation. But, according to N. Bjorn - Andersen[3] "besides being complicated and extensive, the implementation process is also quite costly, and is increasingly getting more so .... It is going to be almost equally large as the hardware and software costs".
Conrath and Du Roure, Schmitt and Kozar, Markus proved that many systems smartly designed, perfectly programmed either turned out to be ineffective when applied or were quickly abandoned.
Hirscheeim [4] explains the 'technical bias': When new technologies are developed, their technological sophistication becomes the focal point of interest. This is partly due to enamouring effect technology has, partly to the type of person who wishes to be involved with its design ..... and partly to the reasons for considering its use (to make organisations more productive through technological means)". The same author points out the complexity of the themes: "Token social and human considerations such as user-friendly interfaces, ergonomically sound design, and the like have been thought to be sufficient considerations of the social and human realm. But are they ? ..... Simplistic considerations such as these mask the complexity of and do no justice to the reality of social organisational life".

2. BRIDGING THE GAP BETWEEN SUPPLIER AND USER

This was the topic of our contribution to the Project "Human Factors in Information Technology" of an ESPRIT Programme, and since then it has been the topic of our subsequent studies.
In summary, the results can be ordered into the following themes:
A) The definition of objectives for the introduction of information technology.
B) The involvement of management responsibility.
C) The analysis of the activities requiring automation.
D) The impact of information technology on the organisational environment and its control.
E) The definition of the product requirements.
F) The planning, the process of introduction and implementation of the information technology.
We present the outstanding data and remarks.
A) The definition of objectives for the introduction of information technology.
In general, the supplier is asked to propose the opportunities that technological advancement offers to the objectives of the user organisation (improvement of effectiveness or even generation of new objectives enabled by the technology)..
The supplier can support the user organisation in the customisation of products to his requirements (often the user lacks skill to evaluate the flexibility and adaptability of technological systems to their own aims).
The supplier is asked to avoid:
∞ pushing overselling: there are experiences with invasions of machines that subsequently hamper the acquisition of new and better adapted equipment;
∞ proposing "new for the sake of new": the buyers ask if a costly system is at risk of being declared obsolete from the same supplier after an unacceptably short time. ("if the systems are complex, the supplier should guarantee a life of at least 2-3 years for the proposed installation");
∞ the urge to replace the buyer who is not expert in choosing technological solutions: "the technological choice is a strategic choice", "to delegate this choice means putting the company in the hands of another". The user should be asked for clarification of objectives for effective introduction of the new technology.
B) The involvement of management responsibility
The directors whom we met were convinced - from the difficulty that they had experienced - that they must involve managers in the choice of automation. They recognised the need to indicate to them the opportunities offered by the technology and to involve them in the choices affecting their departments, thus encouraging them to acquire a "technological mentality" and an active participatory role in "confronting the new technology".
C) The analysis of the activities
While analysing the present is often judged a "waste of time" (why study something that is destined not to exist?), the organisations we met readjusted their present structures and functions critical to the success of technological innovation. They did not see the development of information systems as a technical process, carried out by a designer who operates in an unfamiliar world "from the outside". This approach induces the view that system design is a question of technical competence, that excludes the users from assuming any relevant responsibility in the success of the development. Markus[5] and Kumar[6] documented the failures of information systems, due to the attempts at development that conflicted with the culture and attitudes prevailing in the organisation.
The user is therefore to be involved from the first phase of analysis and rationalisation of existing procedures in order to identify what should be automated, to evaluate the costs and the benefits, and to define the specifications.
The positions of the user organisations in confronting the suppliers in this matter are di-

versified. We came across:
∞ positions of autonomy where the users perform analyses with their own analysts and then compares the offers of the various suppliers to choose which is the most appropriate;
∞ requests for technical support and provision of tools for "problem modelling" of which the supplier has experience;
∞ development in collaboration with the supplier of a new product (that can be subsequently supplied to users in similar fields).
The methods of analysis can be outlined as follows: the analysis of activity (task analysis) connects the individual tasks (methods of operating, classification of information) to the organisational interactions to which these tasks are functionally tied. The automated tasks take place within the context of a job (with various degrees of priority in each context, different timespans, continuity, modes of activation....) and the job is dependent on the requirements of the work role.
There are therefore the following points to consider:
∞ the organisational conditions: flow of information, modes of communication, forms of co-ordination and control;
∞ the users: their professional and personal characteristics, their level of experience with information technology, working interdependence and reciprocal conditioning, their inclination or resistance to the use of computer tools (due to effects on their jobs, professional outlook and status), the need for education (education to develop an "information technology mentality" in management) and for training.
The analysis can make use of objective methods (collection of data, observations, recording, in particular on critical moments or accidents) and subjective methods (interviews and analysis of their content, questionnaires, checklists, thorough investigation of human errors). These methods must allow the acquisition of knowledge of facts and results, and of their interpretation by the people who produce or make use of the results, suffer from their consequences or correct them. The issues of this knowledge can provide for the theoretical basis of experimentation on products.
D) The impacts of information technology on the organisational environment and its control.
In any organisation - more so in the complex ones - the evaluation of impacts of technological change must be considered: the impact on the organisational web (functions and their relations, forms of communication, information flow, allocation of decisions, forms of co-ordination and control, structure and content of jobs, occupational and professional level) and on the expectations of the social components (according to important factors such as professional competence, age, status).
The importance of preventing and correcting undesirable impacts was clear (for instance, passing from the standardisation of tasks to the restructuring of jobs; introducing elements of flexibility; and allowing staff rotation between peripheral and central offices).
E) Definition of product requirements
The subjects of our research agree on the critical aspects of functionally and usability of information technology tools for non-professional users: the tools often result in being difficult to be understood and used; they are provided with facilities exceeding the actual needs of use.
The increasing use of individual workstations (personal computers) poses the problem of interconnections between machines and between departments in the company.
Reported below are the requests raised by the organisations in this study, taking into account the high degree of consensus between the organisations:
∞ They ask for simpler hardware: for infrequent use, the keyboard should become as the telephone, instead of being hostile with its numerous keys, indications and contraindications.
∞ The application software is risky. There is no secure basic supplier standard: there are

reliable and non-reliable suppliers. The software is much less robust than the hardware and the users cannot afford to wait for the supplier's help. However, since they made the investment, they must collaborate.

∞ The software should be as simple and as close to natural language as possible. People are aware of the effectiveness of the information technology product, but the tools provided should be simpler and need less mental effort. The directions for use should be easy to learn and to remember. To meet with initial acceptability, the tools should not be sophisticated. They should provide hierarchical menus so that the user can get to the intended function without problems.

∞ Where the use of computer technology is continuous the user learns relatively quickly and automatically. But in offices in which use is discontinuous and in managerial work, learning is difficult and one forgets.

∞ The software applications are very diverse: standardisation is necessary but, up until recently, every supplier had his own standards. Information technology should share common features and so be easy to manage.

∞ It is expensive for the user organisations to write their own software and it prolongs the time taken to make information systems work.

∞ Where a standard methodology does not exist, it is not easy to change between programs; one should be able to integrate the products. The software should therefore be portable and integrable, since it has a great impact on the organisational structure and involves higher economic investment.

∞ There should be a standard between different classes of systems supplied by different manufacturers.

∞ Standardisation should not impose on the users a standard method of use preventing alternative modes and personal adaptation in operation and timing. It should ensure the attainment of work results for different users.

∞ Contacts with the supplier's planning and design centres proved to be very useful, and are widely encouraged for the innovation of products and systems.

Our research produced observations on managerial work coinciding with those of Mintzberg's study [7].

The successful managers do not conform to the stereotype of a mind that reflects with detachment on complex alternatives. They have an overriding preference for oral communication either on the telephone or person to person. These studies suggest the need for guidance in how to approach the study of decision- making processes - processes of problem solving in the organisation from a personal and social order perspective - and the study of their treatment and solution.

Many authors suggest that managers need more than what the traditional Management Information Systems can provide to help them to co-ordinate their activities, take on reciprocal commitments and share a visible and unambiguous behaviour.

F) The planning and the process of introduction and implementation of information technology

The organisations seen in our studies recalled their negative experiences, for example:

∞ the planning was deficient: effects of superimposition and chaos resulted:

∞ the introduction of new tools was the result of decisions from the top level that had not been adequately explained to lower level management and even less to the other employees;

∞ the need to train the older generation of employees who still have a long future working life, was undervalued or it was neglected because of cost.

These organisations confirm that two important contextual themes are relevant in the planning processes: the values concerning the aims of automation and the problems of resistance to change.

These experiences show that, in introducing new tools, it is not practical to try to predefine every element with all their interconnections in the process in detail, and to rigidly plan and implement the process in "one shot".

The discussions we had in the application environments of our study agree with the methodological guidelines of the various sociotechnical system experts who claim that, once the technical system is separated from the social system and the needs of each have been analysed, the planning proceeds by recombining the elements so that the "key variances" are fully controlled using the co-ordinating capacity of the system components.

A technique for critical specification (that is, of incomplete and non-detailed specification):

∞ defines the critical functional characteristics for the development of the system at every stage;

∞ identifies the variables that are to be included in fixed structural parameters and those that are to be excluded.

The internal variability and auto-correction mechanisms allow adaptation to environmental variability. In this way the optimal mode of autoregulation is defined.

According to this guideline, the process of implementation follows an experimental approach, that guides the evolutionary development of the system towards its final objectives. That is, the experimentation is regulated by evolutionary assumptions, that elaborate the specifications according to which the development of the system is proposed. The assumptions are verified in the auto-regulation of the system. (This constant feedback can help evolve the systems own objectives).

This methodology implies a strategy of participation (involving analysts, system managers, end-users) and of co-ordination, which assures a shared responsibility for the changes in course, exploits all experiences and makes all the human components of the process responsible.

To support this strategy, the training of staff defines:

∞ the operating skills that must be changed and relearnt

∞ the habits of interaction that must be acquired and maintained

∞ the technical and theoretical knowledge that must be acquired.

From the organisations that we interviewed, we obtained an overall agreement on the strategies for introduction and implementation of a system. They can be summarised as follows:

∞ promotion, planning and strategic control of planning by top management, with the joint responsibility of line management prepared to play an active role in the choice and introduction of information technology;

∞ integrated organisational and technical innovation: the innovation is committed to the co-operation of central skills (organisation departments, general design teams), local start-up groups, (teams for specific design), "key-men" (for passing on skills) in local offices and at key work points;

the supplier should contribute with:

∞ product customisation, suggestions for exploitation of their operational flexibility, coherent design for system integration;

∞ support during the course of implementation and evaluation of results (from which the supplier can draw conclusions on the critical factors for functionality, usability and acceptability of their own products).

3. CUSTOMER ORIENTATION

In the organisations we studied, the issues and responsibilities of information technology are managed by top Directors who have a wide perspective of their application environments: the objectives of technological change, as stated previously, have strategic relevance and the technology must be congruent with the organisational changes that the company requires.

To keep pace with the evolution of the markets and of the market sectors, suppliers are being asked to employ a multi-faceted expertise throughout the cycle extending from a realistic knowledge of the clients needs, to adequate support in the end-use of the product. They are therefore expected to develop the skills and define the responsibilities in their company activities and to integrate them after first overcoming the traditional barriers.

It was suggested that a primary objective was to acquire reliable statistical data on which to base decisions on what areas and aspects to conduct an in-depth analysis. Besides evaluating the present technological assets (the real use of the products, they weaknesses and their strengths, the possible improvements) one can realistically acquire knowledge of opportunities to define new characteristics of products. The continuous progress of technology reduces the number of problems while enriching product functionality at an acceptable price. The problem instead is definition of the actual and potential needs of the market and their sectors.

There are instances of development and design groups assigned to specific product applications, rather than to specific areas of technology. More radically, there are cases of companies that assign a line of activities to a specific segment of the market (from marketing through to after-sales service). They develop competence and competitive skills in these areas.

The ergonomics of products and the ergonomics of organisational systems ("macroergonomics") have acquired growing importance for the acceptance and success of information technology. While human factors laboratories are developed within the supplier organisations, some of the user organisations have been pushed by the suppliers to set up their own laboratories, with which the suppliers can usefully communicate and cooperate.

REFERENCES

1. Eason K.D., Harker S. - The Supplier's Role in the Design of Products for Organizations. In: The Computer Journal, Vol. 31, n. 5, 1988.
2. Grudin J. - Social Evaluation of the User Interface. In: Human-Computer Interaction, INTERACT'87. (H.J. Bullinger and B. Shackel ed.s), Elsevier North - Holland, Amsterdam, 1987.
3. Bjorg-Andersen N. - Implementation of Office Systems. In: Office Systems. (A.A. Verrijn-Stuart and R.A. Hirscheeim ed.), Elsevier North - Holland, Amsterdam, 1987.
4. Hirscheeim R.A. - Office Automation: a Social and Organizational Perspective. J. Wiley - London, 1985.
5. Markus M.L. - System in Organizations: Bugs and Features. Pitman, Boston, 1984.
6. Kumar K. - Values in Information Systems Development. Ph.D. Tesis, Waterloow University, Canada, 1984.
7. Mintzberg H. - An Emerging Strategy of Direct Research. In: Administrative Science. Quarterly, 24, n. 4, 1979.

Human information processing in man-machine interaction.

Matthias Rauterberg

Work and Organizational Psychology Unit, Swiss Federal Institute of Technology (ETH)
Nelkenstrasse 11, CH-8092 Zurich, Switzerland

Abstract
Information and information processing are one of the most important aspects of dynamic systems. The term 'information', that is used in various contexts, might better be replaced with one that incorporates novelty, activity and learning. Many important communications of learning systems are non-ergodic. The ergodicity assumption in Shannon's communication theory restricts his and all related concepts to systems that can not learn. For learning systems that interact with their environments, the more primitive concept of 'variety' will have to be used, instead of probability. Humans have a fundamental need for variety: he or she can't permanently perceive the same context, he or she can't do always the same things. The fundamental need for variety leads to a different interpretation of human behaviour that is often classified as "errors". Variety in the relationship between a learning system and his context can be expressed as incongruity. Incongruity is the difference between internal complexity of a learning system and external complexity of the context. Traditional concepts of information processing are models of homeostasis on a basic level without learning. Activity and the learning process are driving forces that cause permanently in-homeostasis in the relationship between a learning system and his context. A suitable model for information processing of learning systems must be conceptualised on a higher level: a homeostatic model of in-homeostasis. A concept to information processing is presented that derives an inverted U-shaped curve between incongruity and information. This concept leads to important design recommendations for man-machine systems.

1. INTRODUCTION

We live in a dynamic and irreversible changing world. We are information processing systems and have a huge learning potential. What happens to humans, if they have to behave in an approximately static environment? If we need growth (in a psycho-dynamic sense) and development, how long we are able to tolerate contexts that fix and constrain our activities? There is a lot empirical evidence that humans are getting bored if the context is characterized by repetitiousness, lack of novelty, and monotony (cf. [16]). Ulich [18] differentiates between boredom and monotony. Boredom emerges from the feeling of not having enough possibilities to be active. Monotony emerges from the feeling of doing always the same things. "Monotony is a consequence of standardisation of the work process" ([18], p. 8). On the other side, there is strong empirical evidence of stressed and over-loaded workers (cf. [22]).

We have to realise and to accept that humans do not stop learning after end of school. We are compelled to learn and to make experiences our whole life. Human information processing can not be independent of these life-long learning processes. In this sense, humans are open systems. In his law of requisite variety Ashby [1] pointed out, that for a given state of the environment, an open system has to be able to respond in an adaptable way, otherwise the adaptability and the ability of the system to survive is reduced. A learning system, without input or with constant input, either decays or (in the best case) remains the same. Learning and the need for variety implies, that with constant input variety the requisite variety of the system tends to decay over time. This is a strong argument against 'one best way'-solutions in work design on a structural level (cf. [18]).

We can find in the literature different interpretations of the term 'information'. Several approaches from different point of views are done to clarify 'information' (e.g., [11], [13], [17], [19]): (1) information as a message (syntax); (2) information as the meaning of a message (semantic); (3) information as the effect of a message (pragmatic); (4) information as a process; (5) information as knowledge; (6) information as an entity of the world.

Table 1
Several terms to describe the amount of information of a message before and after reception.

before reception	after reception	Author	
degree of freedom of the decision	content of the decision	HARTLEY 1928	[8]
uncertainty	certainty	SHANNON 1949	[15]
uncertainty	information	BRILLOUIN 1964	[6]
potential information	actual information	ZUCKER 1974	[23]
entropy	amount of information	TOPSØE 1974	[17]
information	exformation	NØRRETRANDERS 1991	[11]

If we try to apply information theory to human behavior, then we have to integrate activity, perception, and learning. In this proposal we are looking for an interpretation of 'information', which is compatible with concepts of activity and learning. Going this way, we hope to avoid the paradox of 'new' information. Information before and after the reception of a message is not the same! Different concepts are introduced in the literature to 'solve' this paradox (see Table 1).

The concept proposed in this paper assumes, that information processing is an interactive concept. We also try to enclose perceptual and behavioural aspects. We suppose further on, that the stimulus effects of the environment (or context) interact with the real or potential complexity of the receiver (e.g., the complexity of the mental model). The context can be the environment beyond the human skin, the neural stimuli of extremities (e.g., arm and leg movements, motor restlessness), and mental processes like 'daydreaming', etc.

In this paper we replace in a first step the term 'information' with the term 'incongruity' to incorporate novelty and other related concepts. Our second step is to define incongruity with complexity. Finally we present a suggestive relationship between incongruity and information based on behavioural activities.

2. ACTIVITY AND INCONGRUITY

Weizsäcker [21] differentiated the concept of 'information' into two dimensions: (1.) 'Singularity of the first time', and (2.) confirmation and redundancy. For both aspects we can find two different research traditions in psychology: (1) novelty and curiosity ([4], [9], [20]), and (2) dissonance theory ([7]). Both research tracks are only loose coupled till today.

Investigators of novelty assume, that living systems (like mammals, especially humans) are motivated by an information seeking behavior. In situations, which are characterized by sensory deprivation, mammals and humans are intrinsically looking for stimulation. They increase the complexity of the context or the perception of it. On the other side, mammals try to avoid situations with a high amount of stimulation, dissonance, or stress. Hunt [9] designated this amount of increased complexity as 'incongruity'. Incongruity is the difference between the complexity of the context and the complexity of the active and learning system (see Figure 1).

If the complexity of the mental model is less complex than the complexity of the context, then mammals (e.g., humans) try to optimise this positive incongruity. Seeking behavior starts, when the positive incongruity sinks below an individual threshold or changes to negative incongruity (deprivation). Behavior of avoidance can be observed, when the positive incongruity exceeds an individual threshold (dissonance, stimulation overflow). Most of daily situations can be characterized by positive incongruity.

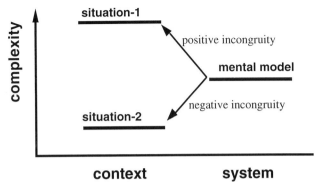

Figure 1. The difference between the complexity of the mental model and the complexity of the context is called incongruity.

The complexity of the context (e.g., the internal structure of the interactive software) can be measured (cf. [5]). The next step is to look -- from the users' point of view -- for a good measure for the complexity of the *perceived* context. This problem is difficult, because we have to differentiate between the pre-structured part of perception based on learned mental schema and the unstructured and not predictable part, which enable the human to integrate new aspects into the stored knowledge.

3. LEARNING AND ACTIVITY

Learning implies abstraction. Humans under non standardised and fixed conditions evolve during their lifetime very abstract invariants. This fact is the basis of wisdom of old humans. Actual research is done under the topic of 'meta-cognition' and 'meta-learning'. Learning as a driving force for irreversible developments is the most underestimated factor in human behaviour, especially in the work and organisational context. Bateson [3] developed a hierarchical concept of four different learning categories that reflects different levels of abstraction. The basic idea of Bateson's concept is that the variety on one level can be reduced to the invariant structure on the next higher level. This invariant structure forms the next higher, more abstract level of the memory.

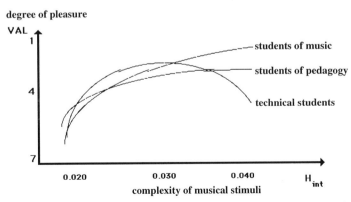

Figure 2. The inverted U-shaped function between 'informativeness' (degree of pleasure) and complexity of stimuli (H_{int}) (reproduced from [12]).

Learning is a permanent process that changes our long-term knowledge base in an irreversible way (the schemata, see Figure 3). Learning increases the complexity of the mental model [14]. The structure of our long-term memory changes to more complexity and higher abstraction. This dependency was empirical investigated by Raab and Ebner [12]. Raab and Ebner presented musical stimuli of different complexity to three groups of different experience with music: (1) technical students with low experience, (2) students of pedagogy with medium experience, and (3) students of music with large experience. Raab and Ebner got two important results: (1.) The 'informativeness' of the stimuli (degree of pleasure) has an inverted U-shaped function in relation to the complexity of the stimuli, and (2.) the optimum of this curve depends on the amount of experience (i.e. the complexity of the mental model; see Figure 2). Boreham (1993, personal communication) described the different reactions of nurses and high qualified physicians in a monitoring task during anaesthetisation. Humans with lower cognitive complexity (e.g., nurses) are more able to be satisfied informational in a context with constant variety than humans with higher cognitive complexity (e.g., physicians). The optimal incongruity level depends on the complexity of the cognitive structure.

If the complexity of the context is fixed then -- caused by learning -- the positive incongruity must decrease (see Figure 1). If the positive incongruity remains under an individual threshold then learning systems try (a) to increase the contextual complexity through activities, (b) to reduce their learning rate, or (c) to increase their perception of the contextual complexity (i.e., going into details, fantasy, hallucination, day dreaming, etc.). Neisser [10] was one of the first researcher, who tried to integrate learning, perception, and activity (see Figure 3). He emphasised that human experience depends on the stored mental schema, which guide exploring behavior and the perception of external context. This is an irreversible process. One consequence is, that the contextual complexity must increase appropriately to fit the human needs for variety and incongruity, resp.

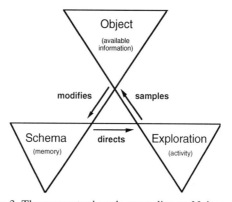

Figure 3. The perceptual cycle according to Neisser [10].

We are able to measure the complexity of human behavior (e.g., exploration activities; see [14]). The next step is to look for a good measure for the complexity of the perceived context. This problem is difficult, because we have to differentiate between the pre-structured part of perception based on learned mental schema (available information, [10]) and the unstructured and not predictable part, which enable the human to integrate new aspects into the stored knowledge (potential available information, [10]).

4. ACTIVITY AND INFORMATION

A context with sensory deprivation has not enough positive incongruity or even negative incongruity. On one side, a human will leave a context with very low incongruity (to little difference to context complexity), and on the other side with very high incongruity (to much context complexity; see Figure 4). In between we have the range of positive emotions with behavior, which increase novelty on one side, and on the other side that increase confirmation and redundancy, or reduce dissonance, resp.

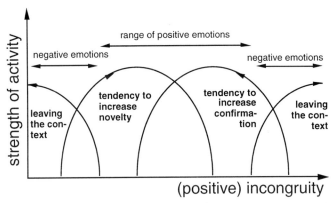

Figure 4. The coherence between positive incongruity, emotions and observable behavior.

Overall we assume a reverse U-shaped function as the summarised coherence between incongruity and information (see Figure 5). If a human has to behave for a while in a total fixed and stabile context and he has a normal learning rate, then he must start to increase the incongruity. This can be done on two different ways: (1) increasing the complexity of the context or the perception of it, and/or (2) reducing the complexity of the mental model. Way (2) implies the possibility of "forgetting", the decrease of the learning rate or the manipulation of the perception mechanisms (suppression).

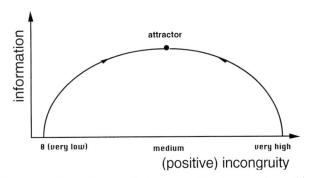

Figure 5. The summarised coherence between positive incongruity and information.

Different authors describe very clearly the problems arising when an operator has to take over a complex process during a monitoring task (the vigilance problem). To take-over process control is especially problematic when the system runs into an unknown state. Training in a simulator is one possible consequence, better is permanent on-line control in the real process. High skilled operators tend to lose the potential to be aware of the whole process. They need a special qualification to get open minded. In inescapable situations with information under-load we can interpret human failures as a subconscious strategy to increase external complexity.

5. CONSEQUENCES FOR THE DESIGN OF MAN-MACHINE SYSTEMS

Bainbridge [2] describes very clearly the problems arising when an operator has to take over a complex process during a monitoring task (the vigilance problem). To take-over process control is especially problematic when the system runs into an unknown state. Training in a simulator is one possible consequence, better is permanent on-line control in the real process. High skilled operators tend to lose the potential to be aware of the whole process. They need a special qualification to get open minded. If incongruity is too low, then humans try to increase the contextual complexity. This perspective allows us to have an alternative interpretation of human 'failures' in inescapable situations with information under-load (e.g., process monitoring in a steady-state). To increase the signal rate of the machine system artificially is not an appropriate design strategy for man-machine systems [2]. Job rotation and job enrichment can help to reduce information under-load, but not for along time. Depending on the learning rate of the worker, we have to be aware of the monotony problematic. The best solution is to involve the worker in the task solving process, especially when the task is a 'complete task'. Operators should have on-line control over the real process [2]. To satisfy the human need for variety (and optimal information) the work system must be flexible and individualisable. Of course, this demand leads to difficulties in complex system design. But, neglecting this demand we run directly into most of the ironies described by Bainbridge [2].

6. REFERENCES

[1] Ashby, R.W. (1958): Requisite variety and its implications for the control of complex systems. Cybernetica, 1(2), p. 83-99.
[2] Bainbridge, L. (1982): Ironies of Automation; in: G. Johannsen & J.E. Rijnsdorp (eds.): Analysis, Design, and Evaluation of Man-Machine Systems. (International Federation of Automation Control, p. 151-157), Düsseldorf: VDI/VDE-Gesellschaft Mess- und Regelungstechnik.
[3] Bateson, G. (1972) Steps to an Ecology of Mind. Chandler Publ.
[4] Berlyne, D.E. (1960) Conflict, arousal, and curiosity. McGraw Hill.
[5] Bennett, C. (1990) How to define complexity in physics, and why? in: W. Zurek (ed.): Complexity, Entropy, and the Physics of Information. (pp. 137-148), Addison-Wesley.
[6] Brillouin, L. (1964) Scientific Uncertainty and Information. Academic Press.
[7] Festinger, L.A. (1957) A theory of cognitive dissonance. Stanford University Press.
[8] Hartley, R.V.L. (1928) Transmission of information. Bell System Technical Journal, 7(3), p.535-563.
[9] Hunt, J.M.V. (1963) Motivation inherent in information processing and action. in: O.J. Harvey (ed.): Motivation and Social Interaction: Cognitive Determinants. Roland.
[10] Neisser, U. (1976) Cognition and Reality. Freeman.
[11] Nørretranders, T. (1991) Mærk verden. Gyldendal.
[12] Raab, E. & Ebner, H. (1982) Rhythmus und musikalisches Erleben: der affektive Eindruck einstimmiger rhythmischer Strukturen von variierender Komplexität. Zeitschrift für experimentelle und angewandte Psychologie, 29(2), 315-342.
[13] Rauterberg, M. (1989) Über das Phänomen "Information". In: B. Becker (Hrsg.) Zur Terminologie in der Kognitionsforschung. (Arbeitspapiere der GMD Nr. 385, pp. 219-241), Gesellschaft für Mathematik und Datenverarbeitung.
[14] Rauterberg, M. (1993) AMME: an automatic mental model evaluation to analyze user behaviour traced in a finite, discrete state space. Ergonomics, 36(11): 1369-1380.
[15] Shannon, C. (1962) The mathematical theory of communication. Urbana.
[16] Smith, R.P. (1981) Boredom: A Review. Human Factors, 23(3), pp. 329-340.
[17] Topsøe, F. (1974) Informationstheorie. Teubner.
[18] Ulich, E. (1987) Umgang mit Monotonie und Komplexität. Technische Rundschau, 5, pp. 8-13.
[19] Völz, H. (1991) Grundlagen der Information. Akademie.
[20] Voss, H.-G. & Keller, H. (Hrsg.) (1981) Neugierforschung: Grundlagen, Theorien, Anwendungen. Beltz.
[21] Weizsäcker von, E. (1974) Erstmaligkeit und Bestätigung als Komponenten der pragmatischen Information. in: E. von Weizsäcker (Hrsg.): Offene Systeme, Band I. Beiträge zur Zeitstruktur von Information, Entropie und Evolution. Klett.
[22] Wickens, C. (1992, 2nd edition) Engineering Psychology and Human Performance. HarperCollins.
[23] Zucker, F. (1974) Information, Entropie, Komplementarität und Zeit. in: Weizsäcker von, E. (Hrsg.): Offene Systeme, Band I. Beiträge zur Zeitstruktur von Information, Entropie und Evolution. Klett.

A study on VDT work and psycho-physiological load

Takao Ohkubo[a] and Keun Sang Park[b]

[a]College of Industrial Technology, NIHON University,
1-2-1, Izumi-cho, Narashino-shi, Chiba, 275 JAPAN

[b]Graduate School of Industrial Technology, NIHON University,
1-2-1, Izumi-cho, Narashino-shi, Chiba, 275 JAPAN

abstract

A series of experiments was carried out while using totally six female subjects in order to evaluate their psycho-physiological variations during their work with VDT both subjectively and objectively compared to those of ordinary office type work and speech communication type work. The results led by the experiment were as follows; the effects with data input work on the subjects from the view point of psychological load was larger than those with the ordinary office work. Oral communication between subjects gave the positive effects upon each subjects to reduce their psychological and mental burden.

Key word : VDT work, Female worker, Accommodation time, Heart rate, CFF

1. INTRODUCTION

The application of VDT systems into work places in various kinds of industries has rapidly been spreading in the past few years in proportion to the evolution of micro-electronics [1]. But, on the other hand various fatigue or health problems for VDT workers to be solved have also become serious [2]. Japan industrial Safety Health Association has announced and published and encouraged to adopt the guidelines of occupational Health in VDT operation since 1985 that covers working environment, work practice, Maintenance of VDT equipment and furniture and control of the working environment [3].Various kinds of improvement for activities VDT work environment have been carrying out among big industries since then. Namely, they are buying new chairs for VDT work, or new VDT-related products with lower noise level and smaller sized, or tables, or glare prevention screen on CRT, preparing wider working area or improving visual environment including increase in illumination level, education of VDT workers in terms of health care and health care system of mental disorders or eye related.

For these reasons, work load on workers caused by the VDT works is changeable depending on the content of tasks they must do. We, therefore, should take those factors into consideration when we plan to build up the optimum working environment for VDT workers. The main purpose of this study is to to compare and evaluate psycho-physiological load of VDT workers who are engaged in two different types of work such as data input and information guidance with that of ordinal clerical works.

2. METHODS

All subjects for the experiments consisted of healthy women whose visual sufficient skills in all works used for the series of experiments. The average age of the in totality 6 middle-aged women was 34.8 years. 3 of them used spectacles for myopia. As for the contents of the work for the experiments, the following three different kinds of tasks were given to the subjects. (1) Clerical work in which the subject must post the information for the experimental use directly to a ledger. (2) Data input work in which the subject must put the inquiry information into the computer with using keyboard and write the answer displayed on the CRT screen to a ledger. (3) Information offering work in which the subject must receive an experimental inquiry via receiver from a customer, input it into computer to get it's correct answer for the customer, that is obtainable from the CRT screen, and respond to the customer. Work intensities between the three experimental conditions were programmed to be equal. The total amount of work and errors were checked by the words written on the ledger and was recorded automatically in the computer memories.

One continuous work time setting up were two hours and an hour. Each subject was requested to perform one work period of two hours work with 105 minutes as lunch rest in the morning and two work periods of one hour work with 75 minutes as rest interval in the afternoon, so that the total CRT display work time per a day was 240 minutes for both experiments with 80 minutes rest.14 inches conversational mode CRT display with Chinese characters input was used in this study. The luminance of character was 135 cd/m2 and of background was approximately 35 cd/m2. The contrast between character and back ground was 3.8:1. The display polarity was classified into the following groups, namely, green letters on dark background and orange letters on dark background for negative picture,and black letters on light background for positive picture. The illuminance on the CRT display was 200 lx and that on the key board was 550 lx.

As to the environmental condition in the laboratory, indirect diffused light by rubber was adopted, thus preventing direct entrance of the light from the light source into the eyes of the subjects. In order to avoid the influence of direct sun light, all the windows of the laboratory were completely covered by thick curtains to block the sun light. The mean temperature and humidities in the laboratory were almost consistent throughout the experiments and 26.3° C, 46.4% at the point of subjects' shoulder, 25.5° C,48.0% for their knee point respectively. The mean noise levels during their work were 43.4 phone for the clerical work and 45.3 phone for the other two VDT works.

The measurements of visual functions and fatigue of subjects were carried out before the experiment and between the continuous work. They were work intensity, visual acuity, near point and accommodation time (contraction and relaxation time), CFF towards white, red blue color, eye movements, heart rate and motion and time analysis including subsidiary behaviors.

3. RESULT AND DISCUSSION

In visual tasks such as VDT or clerical work , the maintenance of visual control functions for the accurate recognition of information is important. The

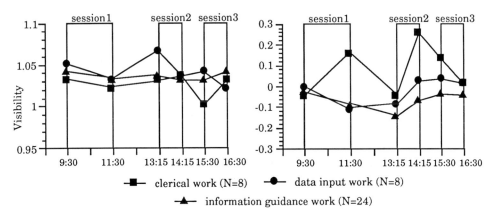

Fig.1 Variations of the near point distance for the three different works.

Fig.2 Variations of accommodation time (CT) for the three different works.

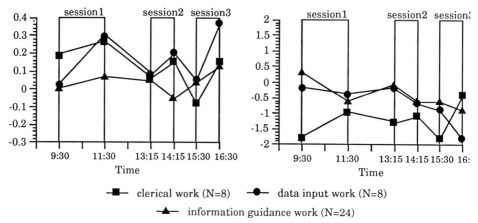

Fig.3 Variations of accommodation time(RT) for the three different works.

Fig.4 Variations of CFF value for the three different works.

control function of the near point was measured before and after three different kinds of tasks. Although there appeared only small difference between each tasks, a fall and the variation of control function of the near point were the greatest for the data input work, followed by the clerical work and then information offering work. The result of the comparison of three different polarities in terms of he different colors such as the green, orange and the black showed the orange as the least deterioration of visual function (Fig.1). Fig.2 and Fig.3 show the change rate of eye accommodation time (Fig.2 for the contraction time and Fig.3 for the relaxation time) of each type of works. The contraction time and its variation are the biggest in case of clerical work whereas the other two remaining fairly stable through the working times. The relaxation time for the different three conditions shows mostly increase after the working session and decrease after the rest hour.

When the variations of CFF values according to the difference of the work were determined, a maximum fall of 2.1% was obtained for the data input work after the first working period that remains almost within the optimum range.

Especially, after the noon recess the maximum rate of increase reached nearly 2.0% indicating a clear resting effect. CFF value for the other two types of work showed gradual deterioration as the work hours proceeding but less values compared to the data input work (Fig.4).

Heart rate measurement is thought to be one of the effective ways of evaluating or working the variation of the psycho-physiological function of

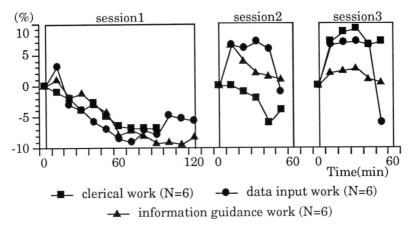

Fig.5 Variations of Heart rate for the three different works.

workers relating to the autonomic nervous systems. But, on the other hand it varies depending on many factors such as the individuals differences, working hour or time, working postures, body movements and etc.. Despite that, the pattern of heart rate variations for the three different works all showed gradual decrease during the first work, period in morning, then increase at the second and the third work period in the afternoon (Fig.5).

As for the subsidiary body movements for workers who are engaged in three different types of work, the results are as follows; Information guidance work shows the least occurrence with less of upper limb movements compared to the other two works. Data input work shows no subsidiary behaviors except for upper and lower limbs for the first 20 minutes after starting the work. No head movement can be seen in this type of work. Workers who are engaged in the information guidance work show rather frequent occurrence of subsidiary behaviors of all parts of the body from the beginning of the work. In spite that a slight increase of movements can be seen until the end of work they show not much difference between the first and the last period.

Relating to the subjective assessments of fatigue for the workers during their working hours, the results show that the rank orders among three groups of subjective feelings are group 1 as the biggest, group 2 as the second and group 3 as the least in case of clerical work. Due to our experiences, this type can typically be observed among workers who are engaged in neuro-sensory work night work.

Data input work shows the most frequent occurrence of group 1 symptoms, and the same occurrence rate for group 2 and group 3 symptoms. This type is typically seen among the workers who are engaged in muscular and neuro-sensory work. Information guidance work shows the most frequent occurrence of group 1, then group 3 and finally group 2. This type can be observed among workers who are engaged in either psychological or muscular work. The contents of fatigue feelings observed in the experiments among all works are "Feel heavy in the head", "Become rigid or clumsy in motion", "Get tired in the whole body", and "Give a yawn". "Feel strained in the eyes" is observed particularly in clerical work and data input work when work is finished. "Unable to straighten up in the posture" is the least among information guidance workers whereas the most for clerical workers. "Feel brain hot or muddled" and "Feel thirstily" are frequently observed for data input workers and information guidance work.

5. CONCLUSIONS

In conclusion, (1) work load for data input workers is the highest among the 3 different work, (2) clear rest effect as well as last input can not be observe in case of data input work, (3) clear deterioration for various functions in particularly seen in the end of data input work.

Reasons of various VDT work related disorders are not simple at all but are very complexes. Although recommendations are set and proposed, improvements of VDT work environment have not so advanced.

REFERENCES

1. Cakir A., Hart D.J. and Stewart T.F.M., Visual Display Terminals, Jhon Wiley and Sons Ltd. 1980.
2. Laubil T., Hunting W. and Grangjean E., Visual impairments related to environment in VDT operators, Ergonomic aspects of VDTs, ed. Grandjean E and Vigliani E., 85-94, Taylor and Francis, London, 1980.
3. Japan Industrial Safety and Health Association, Guidelines to Occupational Health in VDT Operations, 1985.
4. Okubo T. et al., A study of diurnal variations in fatigue of shift -workers, Proc. of the 4th ICPR, 1977.
5. Okubo,T. et al., Some fundamental problems of applications of industrial robots introduction line, Human-computer Interaction, ed. Salvendy G., Elsevier Science Publishers, Amsterdam, 1984.

Psychophysiological Investigation of System Response Times and of Different Break Schedules in Highly Demanding Work With Display Units

W. Boucsein and M. Thum

Physiological Psychology, University of Wuppertal, 42119 Wuppertal, Germany

Abstract

The psychophysiological approach which combines physiological, subjective, and performance recordings can be used to quantitatively investigate stress-strain processes in both, laboratory and field settings. A series of studies on system response times and different break schedules have consistently differentiated between two types of strain. Mental strain resulting from work density and from task difficulty has its main impact on the cardiovascular system, while emotional strain resulting from time pressure together with inadequate temporal structures in human computer interaction mainly increases spontaneous electrodermal activity. Psychophysiological recordings can be used to objectively quantify early indications of such stress-strain processes, in order to make predictions of their long term consequences for the development of psychosomatic disorders that could be related to work with display units.

1. INTRODUCTION

Formerly, strain experienced in workplaces was primarily due to physical reasons. More recently, with the introduction of computers nearly everywhere, stress-strain processes turned out to have a significant mental component, and it is this *mental strain* or workload that has been the focus of contemporary research. Furthermore, psychological or social factors can result in excess mental workload generating a further effect that one might think of as *emotional strain*. This is because people, unlike computers, can get upset when they are faced with excessive mental work. Moreover, there are features of work like increased task complexity, which may result in merely mental strain, whereas a feature like the imposition of deadlines, i.e., time pressure, may result not only in mental but also emotional strain.

However, although it may seem plausible enough to distinguish conceptually between merely mental and additional emotional strain, the distinction itself is difficult to make in empirical terms. The questions for the psychophysiologist who wishes to contribute to the problem really resolves itself to that of whether there are *psychophysiological markers* for those different kinds of strain? Our working hypothesis, based on an examination of the literature, is that *cardiovascular* activity varies most significantly with mental strain, while *electrodermal* activity (EDA) is most closely related to emotional strain (Boucsein, 1993).

Using this working hypothesis, several laboratory studies and one field study on work with display units have been performed by our group. As a general result, our work indicates that psychophysiological methods can provide information that both complements, and is different from, information provided by performance and questionnaire-based methods. Our work generally focusses on inadequate temporal structures during human computer interaction. This context has proved to be a reliable source of both kinds of strain, mental and emotional. Inadequate temporal structures may result from *involuntary breaks* of unpredictable length caused by system response times, or from unfavorable *break schedules* due to organizational procedures.

2. LABORATORY STUDIES

We started our laboratory studies in 1982, focussing on *system response times* (SRTs) caused by hardware and software features of the computer system. The interest of ergonomists was considerable, because it was apparent that SRTs are not only a source of added costs, but also of considerable strain. However, we found that negative consequences for performance, subjective well being, and autonomic functioning resulted not only from *too-long* but also *too-short* SRTs. This complex outcome serves to remind us that the general recommendation "the faster the better" does not seem to be appropriate for human computer interaction.

In most of our studies, we used an easy to learn detection task. In a row of random letters and spaces presented in the center of a visual display, a space surrounded by identical letters had to be targeted. SRTs were varied systematically between 1.5 and 8 sec. Additional *time pressure* was induced by using incentives for working as fast and as correctly as possible. Keystroke numbers and errors were taken as performance measures. The frequency of non-specific electrodermal responses (NS.EDR freq.), systolic blood pressure (SBP), and heart rate (HR) were used as physiological recordings. Ratings of mood and physical symptoms served as subjective measures. Table 1 gives a brief summary of the results from eight studies with more than 400 subjects (Ss).

The clear negative effects of *too-short* SRTs were confirmed in several studies. Since our Ss were not experienced computer users, they may have been rushed by the tasks being presented in a too fast a sequence. If *time pressure* was present, they developed considerable strain, being mainly reflected by an increase of their cardiovascular activity (HR and SBP). Their error rate also increased markedly, and more subjective complaints of the sort made in computerized workplaces were reported. When *no time pressure* was imposed, no specific physiological and subjective strain emerged with short SRTs. However, the Ss spontaneously increased their working speed, showed a tendency to higher error rates, and reported more subjective arousal as well as physical symptoms in general.

A different picture emerged when SRTs were *too long*. At first glance, it may seem that over-long SRTs simply resulted in Ss rationally adopting a more relaxed and careful work style when under *time pressure*. So the Ss made less errors, presumably because error correction was much more time consuming. However, any increased relaxation was more apparent than real, because Ss experienced their working situation as being more uncomfortable, and their increasing NS.EDR freq. suggested an augmentation of emotional strain.

Table 1.
Psychophysiological strain resulting from SRTs and time pressure

System response time	Parameter category	Incentive (time pressure, bonus)	
		present	absent
too short	physiological	SBP ↑, HR ↑ (arousal) (mental strain)	no marked changes
	performance	errors ↑ while maintaining speed (unprecise workstyle)	speed ↑, errors (↑) ("harassed" workstyle)
	subjective	neck-, head-, and eye pain ↑ (task specific strain)	arousal ↑, report of symptoms ↑ (general complaints)
too long	physiological	NS. EDR frequency ↑ (emotional strain)	development of EDA ↑ during SRT (increasing emotional strain)
	performance	errors ↓ (precise workstyle)	errors ↓ (precise workstyle)
	subjective	general well being ↓ (uncomfortable work situation)	general well being ↑ (only at the beginning)

Results *without time pressure* were pretty much the same with respect to performance. At the beginning, subjective well being was present, but during the course of work emotional tension seemed to develop, as suggested by an increasing amount of EDA.

Our recommendation was to determine *optimal* SRTs for the task in question. The criterion for optimal that we used was the following combination: Best performance, no marked increases of cardiovascular activity, low NS.EDR freq., and the lowest reports of pain symptoms. With our particular task and sorts of Ss, this optimal SRT turned out to be around 5 sec. That optimum would probably be shorter with Ss who are trained and who are familiar with the task, as well as being shorter with other kinds of tasks. The main point, of course, is not what the optimum is, but that what is optimal be determined by using dependent variables that are additional to performance criteria, and a realization that considers both, the nature of the Ss and of the task.

3. FIELD INVESTIGATION

The psychophysiological approach used in our laboratory has been recently applied to a field study performed by the second author. The purpose was to investigate the *optimal break schedule* for a complex and highly demanding computer task. Based on previous research on less complex, short cyclic mental tasks such as data typing, 10 min of break after each hour of work were introduced for most German computer work places. However, work with display units has become a lot more complex now, and it is not clear that this sort of break schedule remains appropriate for what is now a more complex task.

One reason for a possible inappropriateness may be that the process of thinking is interrupted (e. g., being forced to have a 10 min break at the end of every hour while writing a paper). Another reason could be that adequate *recovery* of stress related physiological changes during complex work with display units may require more than a short break. Therefore, we decided to perform a field study to directly compare *short* and *long break* conditions with respect to recovery from mental and emotional strain by means of a psychophysiological approach.

The study was conducted at the European Patent Office in The Hague, The Netherlands. Our Ss were 11 *patent examiners* who were members of a prototyping group using a computer workplace with two display units (12 and 24 inch). Instead of working with paper documents, these examiners have access to patents on a laser disk which can be displayed on a 24 inch computer screen. On the basis of a search through granted patents, the examiners have to write a report about the novelty of the current application. Each of the examiners performed his/her work under two different break schedules on different days, the order of which was balanced: a long break schedule with 15 min break after 100 min of work and a short break schedule with 7.5 min break after 50 min of work. The total break time on each day was 82.5 min, including a lunch break.

Physiological recordings of HR, EDA, electromyogram (EMG; neck lead), respiration, pulse wave transit time, and gross body movements were taken continuously using an *ambulatory monitoring* device (VITAPORT). The Ss indicated the beginning and the end of each break with a marker. They were instructed to sit relaxed in their chair during the first 2 min of each break and during the first 2 min after each break, in order to obtain artifact-free physiological recordings of the recovery during the break. The three points of time selected for the present evaluation were 11 am, 3 pm, and 5 pm. Subjective variables were acquired 8 times each day by an adjective checklist and ratings of physical symptoms.

No *performance* variables had been acquired because the keyboard action did not correlate with either task difficulty or performance quality. The only indicator of performance quality is the final report about the patent application. The quality of this report could not be measured objectively during our study, because objections against the report can be filed even years after the report was written. So, from a simplistic point of view, our study may have contained no informative dependent variable. However, as can be inferred from our results, psychophysiological recordings may well fill in that gap.

For the *physiological* variables, three *change scores*, calculated as "relaxation period after the break minus relaxation period at the beginning of the break" were calculated. The amount of total break time under both conditions was exactly the same at all three points of evaluation. The amount of body movements was very low (avg .003 g per 2 min) and did not differ significantly between the different break schedules and the points of measurement.

Figure 1 shows the results for heart rate variability (HRV). Although failing to reach significance, there was a trend for HRV to decrease during the working time. A significant main effect of the factor "Break Duration" indicated an increased variability under short-breaks condition. Moreover, HRV became increasingly more reduced during the long break in the late afternoon. We interpret this as *increased mental effort* while struggling against fatigue (cf., Boucsein, 1993, Tab. 1). In the morning, there was an increase of HRV during short breaks, pointing to a more effective reduction of mental strain compared to the long break schedule.

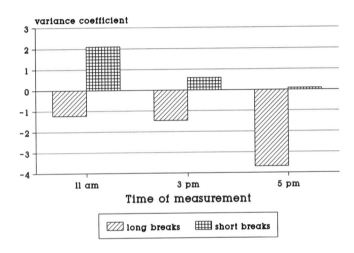

Figure 1. Heart rate variability under the different break schedules.

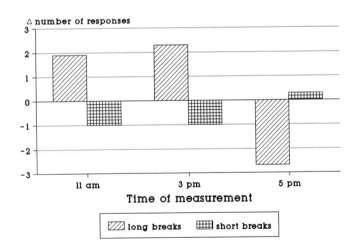

Figure 2. Electrodermal activity under the different break schedules.

The analysis of the NS.EDR freq. resulted in a significant interaction "Break Duration by Time of Measurement". While an increase of the NS.EDR freq. during the 11 am and 3 pm breaks and a decrease during the 5 pm break could be observed under the long break schedule, the reverse pattern was found under the short break schedule, namely a decrease in the morning and an increase in the late afternoon (see Fig. 2). The electrodermal pattern of results suggests that the long break schedule actually increases *emotional strain* during the 11 am and 3 pm break. This is analogous to the laboratory experiments presented in Table 1, where we found detrimental effects of too-long SRTs. In contrast, the longer break schedule during the 5 pm break was associated with a reduction of emotional strain. This could be due to the fact that the 5 pm break was very close to the regular end of the working day at 5:30 pm so that an interruption of thinking processes was less likely, because the Ss knew that they would leave the workplace a few minutes after the end of this break. A comparison of the differential HRV and NS.EDR freq. results (see Figs. 1 & 2) strongly supports our working hypothesis that these parameters reflect *different aspects* of *strain* during work with display units that may be labeled as mental and emotional strain (Boucsein, 1993).

With respect to the factor "Break Duration" in connection with this particular real-life task that involves complex mental work, our preliminary *recommendations* are as follows. In order to minimize loss of efficiency during the course of a workday, a *prolongation* of the *break* time in the *late afternoon* may be of great benefit. Since a 50 minutes work/ 7.5 minutes break schedule was associated with less mental strain, as indicated by an increased HRV, and also associated with less emotional strain during the 11 am and 3 pm reading, as indicated by the NS.EDR freq., such a short break schedule should be applied until the late afternoon.

However, the more effective reduction of fatigue and stress symptoms under the long break schedule during the last point of measurement, as indicated by the decrease of the NS.EDR freq., gives evidence that *fewer* but *longer breaks* should be taken in the *late afternoon* to counteract the loss of resources. Our results show that break schedules have a considerable impact on the resources of the individual during complex work with display units. Even though we could not measure performance, we could make recommendations based on our psychophysiological approach. Since performance quality is dependent on the resources of the individual, the use of an appropriate break schedule apparently contributes to the maintenance of high performance quality. Our next step will be to extend this approach to find out about appropriate break schedules during overtime work, which is very common in highly skilled workers with display units.

Another aim of our field study was to compare psychophysiological changes during *system breakdowns* with those during *regular breaks* and *consultations* by other examiners, either by phone call or in person. A total of 12 system breakdowns happened, all except one before noon, three under the short-break schedule and 9 under the long-break schedule. Since no significant differences between those particular short and long breaks were found, the system breakdowns were compared with the nearest regular break and the nearest consultation. Physiological variables before, during, and after the interruptions were compared for the three types of interruptions.

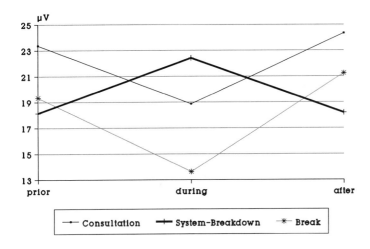

Figure 3. Neck-EMG during the different types of interruptions.

Figure 3 shows the EMG results. Neck muscular tension was lowest during regular breaks. Consultations yielded the same course, though emerging higher muscular tension in general, while neck EMG was considerably increased during system breakdowns.

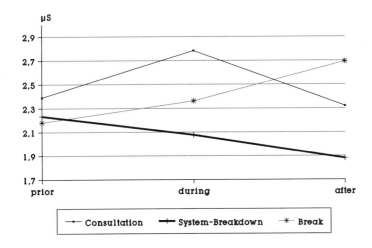

Figure 4. Electrodermal activity during the different types of interruption.

Interestingly, EDA showed a steady decay after system breakdowns but a steady increase during the regular breaks. HR decreased, indicating a decrease of mental strain that persists after the break. The increase of EDA during consultations may be a speech artifact (see Fig. 4). However, the steady increase in EDA during the regular breaks points to the possibility of increasing *emotional* load, as opposed to a decrease in *physical* and *mental load*. This could be an effect of interrupting the complex reasoning task the examiners might have been in the midst of. Maybe a *rigid break schedule*, independent of short or long breaks being applied, is *not adequate* for highly complex work with display units at all.

In summary, physiological recordings within a psychophysiological approach appear to be useful tools for investigating stress-strain processes that may result from inadequate temporal structures in human computer interaction, in both laboratory and field settings. This has been shown for both, relatively short intervals such as SRTs, and for long intervals as the duration of breaks during a whole working day performing complex computer tasks.

REFERENCE

Boucsein, W. (1993). Psychophysiology in the computer workplace - goals and methods. In H. Luczak, A. Çakir, & G. Çakir (Eds.), Work With Display Units 92 (pp. 135-139). Amsterdam: North-Holland.

The effect of anticipatory mismatch in work flow on task performance and event related brain potentials

F. Schaefer [a] and O. Kohlisch [b]

[a] Physiological Psychology, University of Wuppertal, 42119 Wuppertal, Germany

[b] Institute of Occupational Physiology at the University of Dortmund, Ardeystrasse 67, 44139 Dortmund, Germany

1. INTRODUCTION

The introduction of the interactive human-computer dialogue in the workplace has caused important changes of temporal work flow. The worksteps done by the computer system are not perceivable for the user and thus are not experienced as an integrated part of the work process. Thus, these system response times (SRTs) play an important role in software ergonomics.

In general, SRTs are regarded as causing a reduction of work efficiency by slowing down the human-computer system. It could be shown in several experiments using subjective and physiological measures that long SRTs additionally decreased the users' work satisfaction and increased their emotional strain [1]. Consequently, a widely accepted recommendation is to make SRTs as short as possible.

However, some studies have shown that working under very short SRTs can decrease performance accuracy [1, 2]. This supports the assumption that an optimal SRT may exist for every task depending on its demands [3]. Duration and variability of SRTs determine the users' temporal anticipation of the work flow. Without accurate anticipation of the work steps the subject will not be able to prepare for action in an optimal way. It could be shown by psychophysical studies that the end of long SRTs is difficult to anticipate, thus preventing the development of correct expectations about the work flow. On the other hand, the user is able to establish distinct temporal expectations if a certain SRT duration is not exceeded [4]. There is evidence that SRTs cannot be simply regarded as breaks for the user but are filled with task relevant mental processes between the actions.

Psychophysiological indicators for the mental processes can be derived from EEG recordings. Event related potentials recorded at a certain scalp area are regarded to be a manifestation of neuronal stimulus processing in the cortex below. Because the event related potentials are superimposed by spontaneous potentials, the recordings of several stimulus repetitions must be averaged to obtain the event related typical pattern of positive and negative deflections. The negative peak with a latency of 120-180 ms (N1) and the positive peak after 280-450 ms (P3) have proved as reliable indicators over different conditions being sensitive to variations of complex mental demands as the evaluation of abstract material in memory [7]. These potentials can be used as indicators for the analysis of mental processing stages in the sense of a "mental chronometry" [6]. While the N1 wave was found to indicate the detection of the relevant stimulus features, the P3 latency varied with the recognizability of a target [8] and is regarded as indicator of a "post decision closure" [9]. A high P3 amplitude was typically observed when an event failed to match expectation [7].

The present study was based on the assumption that SRTs are used for mental preparation for the subsequent work step. If a SRT is shorter than expected, the user's preparedness has not reached its maximum. Thus, it is hypothesized that N1 and P3 latency on presentation of the subsequent task is increased. Additionally, task completion time should be prolonged. On the other hand, if SRTs exceed the expected duration, additional effort will be required from the user keeping preparedness at the maximum level [5]. Since this demands additional neural activity, P3 amplitudes should be increased and performance should be deteriorated for the subsequent worksteps.

2. METHOD

In the present study fifty-four subjects performed a series of 396 target recognition tasks each. The tasks were considered to be a model of the evaluation of abstract material in memory as it occurs at the computer workplace, i. e., during database retrieval. As illustrated in figure 1, each task started with the presentation of a target word in a small fixation window centered at the computer screen. All words consisted of random sequences of six alternate vowels and consonants making them pronounceable. Target presentation was terminated by the subject pressing the space bar with the index finger of the left hand. Before the display of the recognition list, a SRT of a fixed standard duration occurred, during which a moving bar was displayed in the fixation window to support the subject's temporal anticipation. Then the recognition list was shown in the same fixation window. It consisted of three words including the target, preceded by the numbers 1 to 3. The subject had to detect the target and to mark it by pressing an appropriate key using one finger of the right hand. The chosen item was marked by a dark background bar for 500 ms. Afterwards a blank screen was displayed for 1s until the beginning of the next trial.

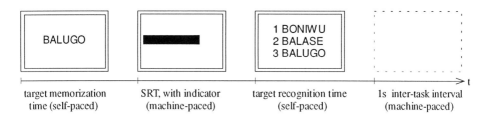

Figure 1. Screen display during the four steps of one task.

The match of SRT with the subject's expectation was varied as one experimental factor: In 60 cases the standard SRT was either diminished or enlarged by 25% causing a discrepancy between the moving bar indication and the occurrence of the recognition list. The deviant SRTs were completely balanced across the whole sequence of items, but their occurrence was unpredictable. Standard SRT duration was either 1, 2, or 4 s, and was varied between the subjects as a second experimental factor.

The duration of memorization and the response time for recognition were recorded, and event related brain potentials were sampled above the frontal and parietal association areas of the cortex at Fz and Pz with ear lobes as reference, according to the international 10-20 system. Additionally, vertical EOG was taken from the right eye for artifact control.

All variables were averaged separately for the experimental conditions. The tasks preceding those with a deviant SRT were used as the "SRT as expected" control for statistical analyses. To detect possible after-effects of deviant SRTs, the subsequent tasks were also analyzed. Latencies and amplitudes of N1 and P3 were taken from individual EEG averages as parameters for statistical analysis. Effects were tested by analyses of variance with match of expectation as repeated measures and duration of standard SRT as between-subjects factor (SPSS/PC+ module MANOVA, using Greenhouse-Geisser correction for DF).

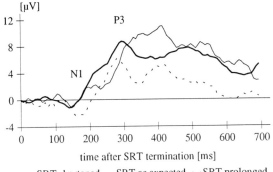

Figure 2. Averaged event related potentials for the different "matches of expectation" for one subject.

3. RESULTS

Figure 2 shows the event related potentials of a typical subject averaged separately for SRTs with a standard duration of 1s, SRTs diminished to 0.75s, and SRTs prolonged to 1.25s.

Standard SRT duration as well as deviant SRTs yielded significant main effects on task performance and event related potentials. Both effects appeared to be statistically independent, since no interactions could be observed.

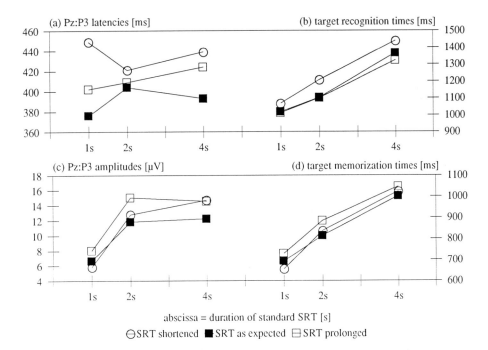

Figure 3. P3 amplitudes and latencies, target recognition times and target memorization times of the subsequent task.

As shown in the upper part of figure 3, central as well as behavioral responses were delayed after unexpectedly short SRTs: Compared with normal SRTs, P3 latency was enlarged 20-75 ms for Pz ($F(2,71)=5.84$, $p<.005$), and target recognition time was increased about 75 ms ($F(2,93)=26.77$, $p<.001$). Additionally, N1 latency showed a mean delay of 15 ms at Fz ($F(2,47)=3.52$, $p<.05$). Performance of the subsequent task was not affected by unexpectedly diminished SRTs.

As shown in the lower part of figure 3, an increase in P3 amplitude at Pz ($F(2,77)=4.20$, $p<.025$) reflected the anticipatory mismatch caused by unexpectedly prolonged SRTs. While performance of the actual task remained unaffected, work speed was reduced for both steps of the subsequent task (memorization: 50 ms, $F(2,79)=7.33$, $p<.005$, recognition: 30 ms, $F(2,99)=4.72$, $p<.05$).

Additionally, there was a tendency for increased P3 amplitudes for Fz ($F(2,60)=2.41$, $p<.10$), and the P3 latencies during the subsequent tasks were significantly delayed for 30-50 ms, if the SRTs did not match the expected duration.

As can be inferred from figure 3b and 3d, performance speed decreased linearly with increasing standard SRT duration (memorization: $F(2,50)=5.03$, $p<.01$, recognition: ($F(2,50)=8.88$, $p<.001$). In contrast, the relation between P3 amplitude at Pz and standard SRT duration showed a marked difference between the 1s and 2s conditions (fig. 3c): compared with the shortest SRTs, P3 amplitudes were highly increased under the longer SRTs ($F(2,43)=6.63$, $p<.005$).

4. CONCLUSION

In the present study different effects due to the direction of the mismatch could be distinguished. Unexpectedly diminished SRTs caused a retardation of central information processing and motor response. Apparently the preparatory processes were still in progress when the next task step was presented on the screen. This was indicated by the observed prolongation of N1 and P3 latencies as well as by delayed target recognition times.

The mismatch caused by unexpectedly prolonged SRTs was indicated by an increased P3 amplitude, but performance was not affected directly. However, performance speed was slowed down during the execution of the subsequent task. Similar changes in performance speed and P3 amplitude could be observed as a main effect of standard SRT length. Since the end of long SRTs is difficult to anticipate [4], mental preparation of the users has to provide for a security interval in order to be prepared in time. Consequently, from the user's point of view there is no difference between generally long SRTs and unexpectedly prolonged SRTs: In both cases preparation has to be completed before the end of SRT. The observed decrease of performance speed for the subsequent tasks leads to the conclusion that mismatches caused by SRT prolongation are consciously perceived causing an interference with task execution. For diminished SRTs on the other hand, this could not be found. This could be an explanation for the generally decreased work satisfaction under long SRTs reported in the literature [2, 3].

The results indicate that SRTs should not be regarded as wasted time that can be reduced as much as technically possible, but their duration has to be considered under ergonomic aspects. Apparently, the user generates expectations about temporal work flow and adapts his mental processes using SRTs for preparatory processes. Thus, task performance is negatively affected by any anticipatory mismatch.

Thus, software engineering should not result in diminishing SRTs as far as technically possible at any price, but in optimizing their distribution in a way that work flow is predictable for the user. Short predictable SRTs can be used for task relevant mental processes improving work efficiency. Thus, before making efforts for a further reduction of mean SRT, it should be considered if predictability is possibly affected by an increase of SRT variability, since even short SRTs deteriorate work if they occur unexpectedly.

REFERENCES

1. Kuhmann, W., Boucsein, W., Schaefer, F., & Alexander, J. (1987). Experimental investigation of psychophysiological stress-reactions induced by different system response times in human-computer interaction. Ergonomics, 30, 933-943.
2. Barber, R.E., & Lucas, H.C. (1983). System response time, operator productivity, and job satisfaction. Communications of the ACM, 26, 972-986.
3. Kohlisch, O., Kuhmann, W., & Boucsein, W. (1991). Auswirkungen systembedingter Arbeitsunterbrechungen bei computerunterstützter Textverarbeitung. Zeitschrift für experimentelle und angewandte Psychologie, 38, 585-604.
4. Schaefer, F. (1990). The effect of system response times in temporal predictability of work-flow in human-computer interaction. Human Performance, 3, 176-183.
5. Bertelson, P. (1967). The time course of preparation. Quarterly Journal of Experimental Psychology, 19, 272-279.
6. Kutas, M., McCarthy, G., & Donchin, E. (1977). Augmenting mental chronometry: The P300 as a measure of stimulus evaluation time. Science, 197, 792-795.
7. Donchin, E. (1981). Surprise!...Surprise? Psychophysiology, 18, 493-513.
8. Parasuraman, R., & Beatty, J. (1980). Brain events underlying detection and recognition of weak sensory signals. Science, 210, 80-83.
9. Desmedt, J.E. (1980). P300 in serial tasks: An essential post-decision closure mechanism. In H.H. Kornhuber & L. Deecke (eds.), Motivation, motor and sensory processes of the brain (pp. 682-686). Amsterdam: Elsevier.

DESIGN AID TOOLS FOR USER INTERFACE DESIGN

Harald Reiterer[a+b] and Stefan Schäfer[a]

[a] German National Research Centre for Computer Science (GMD), PO. Box 1316, D-53731 St. Augustin, Germany

[b] University of Vienna, Institute for Applied Computer Science and Information Systems, Liebiggasse 4/3-4, A-1010 Vienna, Austria

1. INTRODUCTION

To reach high ergonomic quality Graphical User Interfaces (GUIs), human factors knowledge has been developed and expressed as guidelines (for example [Mayhew,1992]), style guides (for example [IBM,1992]), and standards (for example [ISO,1994], [EN,1993]). The volume of these available sources is huge. Simultaneously, GUI designers need today more and more competence, knowledge, and experience to handle this great amount of information. This means for most of them that executing their jobs requires taking into account far more information than they can possible keep in mind or they can possibly apply.

Empirical results have shown that most of the software designers have no or only very limited knowledge about human factors [Molich and Nielsen,1990]. Therefore most of them were not able to apply human factors knowledge in the design process, even though they have information or get information about their existence. In this study, designers were asked what kind of support they prefer to overcome their lack of human factors expert knowledge. A great amount of them replied that they would prefer computer based design aids integrated in their development tools. However, the problem is how to capture and encode human factors knowledge relevant to designers' tasks and how to present it to them in formats that support their mode of work. This results into a need for GUI development tools with domain competence based on human factors knowledge that may be encountered, learned, practised, and extended during ongoing use - in other words, tools in which users *learn and use on demand*. An important research goal in GUI development tools is therefore to discover helpful, unobtrusive, structured, and organised ways to integrate the use of this human factors knowledge into the tools without stifling creativity [Hartson and Boehm-Davis,1993]. These research issues should include methods and tools for providing the designer assistance in understanding, searching, and applying this knowledge. This leads to following questions: what is the best presentation format for communicating human factors knowledge and how could we ensure that it will be observed?

2. DESIGN AID TOOLS FOR COMMUNICATING HUMAN FACTORS KNOWLEDGE

This last thought was the starting point for the GMD project IDA (User **I**nterface **D**esign **A**ssistant) [Reiterer 1994]. The primary goal of this project is to explicitly incorporate domain competence in user interface development tools to empower GUI designers. This means those development tools and designers are bringing complementary strengths and weaknesses to the job. Rather than communicating with tools, designers should perceive the use of the development tools as communication with an application domain [Fischer and Lemke,1988]. To shape the tools into a truly usable and useful medium, the tools should let the designers work directly on their problems and their tasks.

2.1 Basic design issues for design aid tools

To develop design aid tools, several issues have to be resolved. Lemke [Lemke,1989] defined basic design issues, which should be taken into account during the development of design environments. This section discusses these basic design issues for the area of user interface design.

- The *design domain*: The design domain GUI design is a sub domain of the whole software development process. As a field, GUI design includes GUI hardware and software, user and system modelling, cognitive and behavioural science, human factors, empirical studies, methodology, techniques, and tools. This is a wide area of knowledge and typical GUI designers do not necessarily have competence in all these areas. Design aid tools are a good chance to give them support required for their task, designing usable interfaces.
- The *elementary building blocks*: They are a collection of interaction objects like controls or widgets that are available for creating GUIs. The elementary building blocks for the design can either be taken directly from what is available in the tool (e.g. generic interaction objects of the UIMS) or a special higher-level building block can be created that is closer to the problem domain of the design environment (e.g. application domain specific interaction objects as templates).
- The *designers and their domain model*: It is important to identify the designers using the design environment. Knowing the types of designers will have important consequences for how the design environment will be shaped, the level of functionality provided, and how that functionality will be delivered to the designers. Typical properties of the GUI designers that should be considered are: known GUI programming languages, experience with previous GUI development tools, available learning time, etc.
- *Cognitive processes* in the use of design environments: Using a design environment remains a complex cognitive activity. This problem solving activity requires special needs for a design environment. It must support the designer's attention, comprehension and search activities. Attention is specially important if designers are unaware of some of the design issues. They do not search for something they are not aware. Therefore, the design environment must bring all important issues to the designer's attention. Comprehension means, that all information presented to the designer will be interpreted and integrated into his conceptual model of the domain.
- Supporting the *whole design process*: The design phases of problem structuring, solution generation, and solution evaluation should be supported by the design environment. The support of the whole GUI design process is a necessary precondition, but today seldom found in available development tools.

The consideration of all these basic design issues led to a multifaceted architecture for design aid tools assisting the GUI designers during the design, implementation, and evaluation process. They following have been developed in the IDA project and have been connected with a UIMS:

- An adviser (*Advice Giving Tool*) that supports design and implementation activities presenting human fac¬tor's knowledge for GUIs.

- A library of reusable ergonomic GUI software (*Construction Tool*) that supports implementation activities considering human factors.
- An evaluation tool (*Quality Assurance Tool*) evaluating the ergonomic quality of GUIs based on human factors knowledge.

2.2 Typical use of the design environment

The following design scenario gives an impression of the use of the IDA design aid tools. A designer is implementing a GUI for a specific application domain. The transient control panel, called IDA-Toolbar, enables the designer to launch design aid tools represented as icons in the toolbar, and is placed over the UIMS (Figure 1).

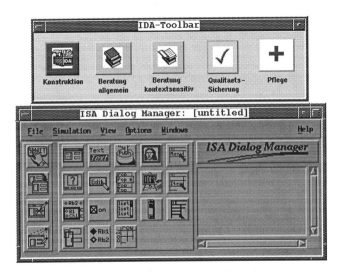

Figure 1. Presentation of the IDA design aid tools.

To reduce the implementation work load, the designer can use predefined ergonomic GUI templates. For this purpose, the *Construction Tool* is launched by clicking on the icon in the IDA-Toolbar. The construction tool then offers domain-oriented templates, contained in an object-oriented library, from which the designer specialises a required instance. This instance will be further integrated in the interface under design. Therefore the designer constructs the GUI by extracting predefined templates from the library and placing them into the working area of the UIMS. Now the designer can modify the instance of the template, based on specific application requirements. This allows a "design by modification" approach. If the designer needs advise the *Advice-giving Tool* is launched by clicking on the context-sensitive advice icon or the global advice icon in the IDA-Toolbar. This on-line advice giving system presents GUI design and human factors knowledge with the help of multimedia documents. The aim of the advice giving system is to determine a pattern matching between the examples of the adviser and the current task of the designer. The designer is aided in building an analogy by assuming that the presented example or information is relevant to his current task. If the designer now wants to evaluate the ergonomic quality of the GUI under design, the *Quality Assurance Tool* is launched by clicking on the icon in the IDA-Toolbar (see section 3). The quality assurance tool analysis the conformance of the GUI with the human factor's knowledge included in a knowledge base.

3. Quality Control of the User Interface Design Results

Several research projects in the domain of knowledge-based support for user interface designers have been carried out in the last years. Most of them tried to design the user interface automatically with the help of a rulebase in which styleguide rules were included. One result of these projects was the experience that this approach has its limits caused by the immense part of semantic knowledge used during the design process. Considering this experience we tried to find another way to support the designer during the design of a user interface. The main idea behind the *Quality Assurance Tool*, called QUID is to support the designer with a knowledge based system that could be putted into the statement "critiquing instead of solving". Therefore the main aim of the system QUID is to check a design for styleguide conformance and whether the main ergonomic ideas where taken into account during the design process.

QUID is an object-oriented knowledge-based system and was implemented with the help of the expert system-shell Kappa© (from Intellicorp). As input, the system takes the Dialogue Definition Language (DDL)-file of the UIMS, in our case ISA Dialog Manager©. The DDL-file contains all information about the "look" and "feel" of the GUI. Because the "feel" includes a great part of semantic information, the check made by QUID concerns only the "look". Using a c-interface, QUID asks for each object in the design and gets all information that is needed to check the ergonomic quality of an interface. All interface objects coming out of the c-interface are represented internally in QUID and the rules are chained over them. The results of QUID are shown in a window, that contains all information needed to understand the ergonomic deficiencies detected by QUID. Figure 2 shows an example window.

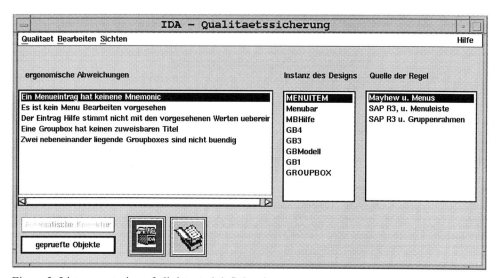

Figure 2. List presentation of all detected deficiencies.

In addition to this result presentation a second possibility was developed, presenting the results after every detection of an ergonomic deficit in the design. This presentation form is based on the common spell-checker metaphor. Figure 3 shows an example window, which will be presented directly after the detection of each deficit.

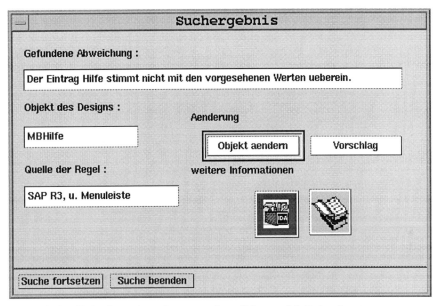

Figure 3. Spell checker oriented presentation of detected deficiencies.

The detected ergonomic deficits are documented with different information in both cases (Figure 2 and Figure 3). First of all there is a short comment given to the user, describing the kind of deficit that has been detected (labelled "ergonomische Abweichungen", "Gefundene Abweichung"). The second information identifies the faulty object, giving out the name of the object created by the designer (labelled "Objekt /Instanz des Designs"). Using this information, the designer can easily understand the output of QUID and can identify the problem and the object that has to be changed. The last information shown in the output-window concerns the source of the rule. Considering the output of QUID, the designer has several possibilities to continue his work:
1. If further explanation of the short comments are needed, the advice-giving tool can be activated (clicking on the icon , see Figure 2).
2. If a specific template is available, the construction tool can be activated (clicking on the icon , see Figure 2).
3. If the designer selects the identifier of an object, the object editor of the UIMS will be activated by double-clicking on the identifier or by pushing the push button labelled "Objekt aendern". Now the interaction object containing identified ergonomic deficiencies can be improved.
4. In some cases, detected deficiencies can be changed automatically. In this case the designer can activate a separate dialogue box (by pushing the push button labelled "Automatische Aenderungen" or "Vorschlag") which gives him the opportunity to correct the deficiency.

The benefit for the designer is that he has not to branch into the object editor of the UIMS.
Putting it all together, the idea of QUID is a promising approach to provide knowledge-based support for a user-interface-designer. The combination of taking into account the limits of knowledge-based systems and maximising the abilities in analysing only the output of the UIMS and taking only those rules that concern the "look" of an interface, enables the system to give the optimal support that can be given by a knowledge-based system.

3. CONCLUSION

Based on co-operations with scientific (Fachhochschule Darmstadt; University of Bonn) and industrial partners (Software AG, Darmstadt; SAP AG, Walldorf; Hoechst AG, Frankfurt) prototypes of all design aid tools have been developed and connected with a commercial UIMS (ISA-Dialog Manager from ISA GmbH, Stuttgart). The usefulness and usability of these prototypes have been evaluated from GUI designers in the realistic context of their application domains. The following benefits for the designer using design aid tools could be shown:

- Designers will be able to learn human factors knowledge during their daily work using their development tool ("learning and use on demand").
- Designers will be enabled to apply ergonomic style guides and guidelines ("usability").
- Designers will be able to use predefined ergonomic interaction objects ("reusability").
- Designers will be able to evaluate the ergonomic quality of their design during the design process ("quality assurance").

REFERENCES

[EN,1993] EN 29241. Ergonomische Anforderungen für Bürotätigkeiten mit Bildschrimgeräten, 1993.

[Fischer and Lemke,1988] G. Fischer and A. Lemke. Construction Kits and Design Environments: Steps Toward Human Problem-Domain Communication, Human-Computer Interaction, Vol. 3, 1988, pp. 179-222.

[Fischer et al.,1991] G. Fischer, A. Lemke, T. Mastaglio and A. Morch. The role of critiquing in cooperative problem solving, ACM Transactions on Information Systems, Vol. 9, No. 3, 1991, pp. 123-151.

[Hartson and Boehm-Davis,1993] H. Hartson and D. Boehm-Davis. User interface development processes and methodologies, Behaviour & Information Technology, Vol. 12, No. 2, 1993, pp. 98-114.

[IBM,1992] IBM. Object-Oriented Interface Design, IBM Common User Access Guidelines. Que Corporation, Carmel, 1992.

[ISO,1994] ISO 9241. Ergonomic Requirements for Office Work with Visual Display Terminals, ISO, 1994.

[Lemke, 1989] C. Lemke. Design Environments for High-Functionality Computer Systems, Doctor Thesis, University of Colorado, 1989.

[Löwgren and Nordquist,1992] J. Löwgren and T. Nordquist. Knowledge-Based Evaluation as Design Support for Graphical User Interfaces, in Proc. of CHI'92, Addison-Wesley, Reading, 1992, pp. 181-188.

[Mayhew,1992] D. Mayhew. Principles and Guidelines in Software User Interface Design, Prentice Hall, Englewood Cliffs, 1992.

[Molich and Nielsen,1990] R. Molich and J. Nielsen. Improving a human-computer dialogue. Communications of the ACM, Vol. 33, No. 3, 1990, pp. 338-348.

[Reiterer, 1994] H. Reiterer. User Interface Evaluation and Design, Research Results of the Projects Evaluation of Dialogue Systems (EVADIS) and User Interface Design Assistance (IDA), GMD-Berichte Nr. 237, Oldenbourg, München, 1994

Problem solving strategies in shop-floor control systems

G. Zülch[a] und K. Grießer[a]

[a] ifab - Institute of Human and Industrial Engineering, University of Karlsruhe (TH), Kaiserstr. 12, D-76128 Karlsruhe, Germany

Abstract

Two series of experiments were carried out to get more information about different problem solving strategies in the field of shop-floor control systems. Depending on the complexity of the task and on personal preferences, the subjects chose either a structured way of solving the problem or chose a „trial and error"-strategy. In general, the subjects who chose a structured way of solving the problem gained better results, but nevertheless both strategies should be supported by the system. For solving rather simple and rather complex tasks most subjects chose a „trial and error"-strategy. Tasks of intermediate complexity were mostly solved in a structured way. Display colours had no influence on the efficiency of the problem solving process.

1. INTRODUCTION

Due to the increasing use of data processing in the field of production, user-friendly software-design is becoming more and more important. In the last years a lot of tasks were moved from other departments to the shop floor hence employees are confronted with new software-products to support tasks like order control, quality control or maintenance. In future all these computer-supported tasks will probably be integrated into work places for high skilled workers. One big problem is, that in future these programs will be used by people who are no experts in this field. Especially the differences in education, knowledge, experience etc. of people using the same software-products were the motivation to make investigations on the design of user-friendly interfaces in the field of production.

The experiments were carried out on several typical tasks in the field of production planning and control systems, especially the short-term planning of shop orders. These problems are characterised by several jobs having to be processed on several machines. Each job consisted of a sequence of operations which had to be done on different machines. The scheduling problem was to find a feasible machine loading. The subjects of the experiments had to optimise the mean flow time and had to react on special events like urgent orders or engine troubles. The scheduling problems varied due to different types of information representation (coloured versus monochrome display) and due to the complexity of the presented problem.

The aim of the experiments was to find out if there is a relationship between the complexity of a task, different kinds of information representation, personal preferences and the choice of a special problem solving strategy. Figure 1 shows an interface which was used in this study. The example shows the Gantt-chart of orders with their lead times.

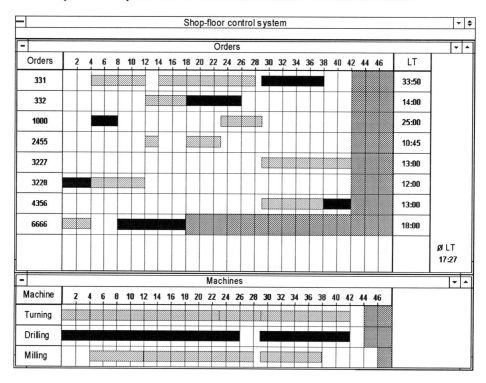

Figure 1: Interface of a shop-floor control system

2. METHODS

To obtain information about the behaviour of the subjects during the problem-solving-process the eye mark registration method, video-recording, key-stroke-recording and structured interviews were used (Figure 2).

2.1. Eye mark registration method

In order to achieve the desired results, the eye mark registration method with the NAC Eye Mark Recorder Model V (NAC 1986) was very important. Eye mark registration serves as a method to find out where the subject is looking at and which type of information representation he prefers. The freedom of head movement is not restricted during the experiments. Both the visual field and the fixation points (produced by near-infrared LEDs) of each eye can be overlayed (NAC-camera-controller). The video signal can be observed on

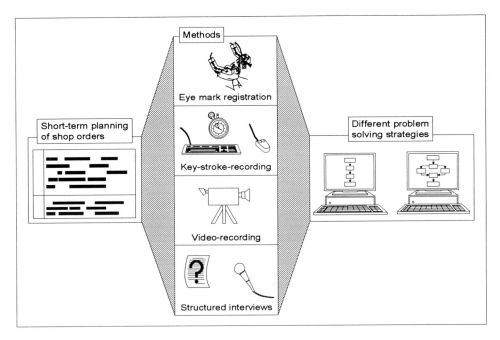

Figure 2: Methods of the investigation

a control-monitor, to be analysed by the image-analysing system S.A.M. (ENDERLE, KORN, TROPF 1982) later on and recorded on-line on a video recorder. Though the freedom of head movement of the subject was not restricted during the experiments, the head movement has to be eliminated by on-line calculation in order to achieve the objects of fixation. The experiments were controlled and statistically analysed by a personal computer. With the computer-based equipment it is possible to analyse for instance the duration of fixations and sequences of gazes.

Figure 3 shows the equipment of the "Laboratory for Human-Machine-Interaction" at the Institute of Human and Industrial Engineering (ifab) at the University of Karlsruhe.

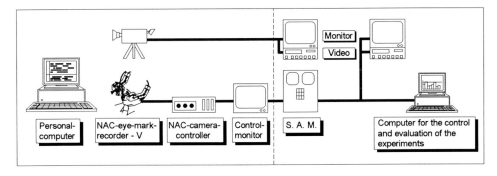

Figure 3: Laboratory for Human-Machine-Interaction

2.2. Key-Stroke-Recording

The method of key-stroke-recording was used to store the interactions of the subjects. Based on this data the behaviour and the strategies of the subjects can be analysed. With this method it is possible to record for instance the time the subject needs to solve a problem, the key-strokes, the mouse movements or the interaction-rate (keystrokes per time) etc.

3. RESULTS

Two series of experiments were conducted in order to achieve the results. Fifteen subjects ranging in age from 23 to 35 years (mean = 27,6 years) took part in the first series of experiments. They were all familiar with a personal computer and had a wide cross-section of experience with scheduling problems. They all had to solve five scheduling problems differing in their complexity. In the second series of experiments ten subjects took part. Each one had to solve five tasks differing in complexity of the task and representation of information.

The plan of variables comprised independent variables like the colour representation, the number of orders or the occurance of special events like rush orders or machine break downs. Furthermore, the dependent variables like the operation time, the amount of interactions, the work speed etc. were fixed in the plan of variables.

In general the results confirmed earlier experiments that there are two main strategies to solve the given kind of problems (ZÜLCH, GRIEßER, REUß 1992; ZÜLCH, GRIEßER 1991). There are subjects who tend to play („trial and error"-strategy) and others who chose a structured way of solving a problem (e.g. by mental calculation). As there are different problem solving strategies, all of them should be allowed or even be supported by the software product.

Variables	Initial trend for increasing task complexity	Trend due to further increase in task complexity
Operation time	↘	↗
Amount of interactions	↘	↗
Distance of eye movements	↘	↗
Strategy: trial and error	↘	↗
Strategy: mental calculation	↗	↘

Figure 4: Trends of different variables

Figure 4 shows the trends of different variables and problem solving strategies. In the first column the initial trend for an increasing complexity of the tasks can be seen. The operation time the people needed was decreasing even though the complexity of the tasks was increasing. The amount of interactions and the distance of eye movements was going down, too. The explanation of this phenomenon is the change of strategy the subjects used to solve the problems. In solving tasks of higher complexity, the subjects used more and more the strategy of mental calculation. When the task seemed to be too complex to solve it by a strategy of mental calculation the subjects switched over again to the „trial and error"-strategy. The operation time was now increasing as well as the amount of interactions and the distance of eye movements. Especially the complexity of the task was the deciding factor for the choice of the strategy.

For solving rather simple tasks and rather complex tasks most subjects chose a „trial and error"-strategy. The intermediate tasks were mostly solved in a structured way.

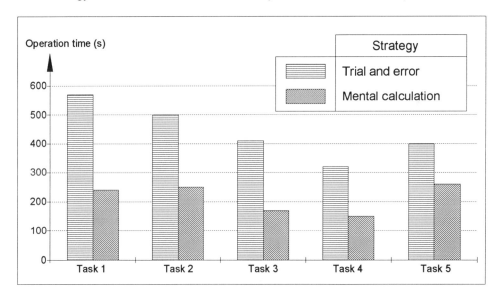

Figure 5: Operation time

Some dependent variables gave hints about the problem solving strategy which was used. A longer time from the start of the experiment till the first interaction was an indicator for a structured way of solving the problem ($r_s=.93$; $p<.01$). Furthermore the experiments showed a significant correlation between a low interaction rate and a structured way of solving the problem ($r_s=.81$; $p<.01$).

The analysis of the strategies indicated that those subjects who chose a structured way of solving the problem gained better results ($r_s=.91$; $p<.01$). In comparison with those who chose a „trial and error"-strategy they needed in general approximately half of the time to solve the problem (Figure 5).

Another interesting result was that colours had no influence on the efficiency of the problem solving process, even though all subjects preferred a coloured display in the structured interviews after the experiments.

REFERENCES

1. E. Enderle; A. Korn; H. Tropf, Echtzeit-Registrierung von Blickbewegungen bei frei beweglichem Kopf, FhG-Berichte, München, (1982)3, S. 12 - 15.
2. NAC Inc., Operation Manual - Eye Mark Recorder Model V - Tokyo, 1986.
3. G. Zülch; K. Grießer, Untersuchungen zur Informationsdarstellung bei komplexen Planungsaufgaben mit Hilfe der Blickregistrierung, Jahresdokumentation 1991 der Gesellschaft für Arbeitswissenschaft, Gesellschaft für Arbeitswissenschaft (Eds.), Schmidt, Köln, 1991, S. 15.
4. G. Zülch; K. Grießer; S. Reuß, Informationsdarstellung bei rechnerunterstützten Planungssystemen, Zeitschrift für Arbeitswissenschaft, Köln (18NF)(1992)3, S. 150 - 154.

Additional sound feedback in man-computer interaction: two empirical investigations.

M. Rauterberg, E. Styger, A. Baumgartner, A. Jenny, and M. de Lange

Work and Organizational Psychology Unit, Swiss Federal Institute of Technology (ETH)
Nelkenstrasse 11, CH-8092 Zurich, Switzerland

Abstract
Two experiments were carried out to estimate the effect of sound feedback: (1) operating an assembly line simulator (Experiment-A with sound feedback of hidden events), and (2) queries in database search (Experiment-B with sound feedback of the search result quality). Experiment-A: Relevant information of hidden events (e.g., disturbances and machine break downs) was given only in a visual, and in visual and audible form. The results indicate, that additional sound feedback improves significantly the user performance and increases positively some mood aspects. Experiment-B: Individualised sound patterns (music, speech, noise) inform the user about the amount of correspondence between the requested data and the actual output on the screen (result feedback). The results of this empirical investigation indicate, that additional sound feedback does not improve the user performance, overall. But, if we differentiate between users, who prefer sound, and those, who do not, we can find significant improvements. We can conclude that sound feedback is necessary, but must be eligible.

1. INTRODUCTION

Sound feedback can be utilised to improve the user's understanding of visual predecessors or can stand alone as independent sources of information. (E.g., sound as action feedback [2]; sounds as diagnostic support applied with the direction of a process simulation [3].) The following examples help to illustrate the important kinds if information that sound can communicate [5]: (1) Information about *physical events* – We can hear whether a dropped glass has bounced or shattered. (2) Information about *invisible structures* – Tapping on a wall is useful in finding where to hang a heavy picture. (3) Information about *dynamic change* – As we fill a glass we can hear when the liquid has reached the top. (4) Information about *abnormal structures* – A malfunctioning engine sounds different from a healthy one. (5) Information about *events in space* – Footsteps warn us of the approach of another person.

The parallel use of different media and the resulting parallel distribution of information, for example by simultaneously showing a predecessor through a concrete representation and its explanation through audio distribution, leads to a denser sharing of information. In this case, the user can dedicate his attention solely to the visual information, that has parallel audio support. This reduces the need to change the textual or other visual delivery and prevents the overflow of visual information. By comparing audio signal patterns with visual signal patterns Gaver [3] could not show the different advantages of each. He describes only some global impressions of different user reactions to sound feedback in a collaborative environment.

Our main interest was to test the hypothesis that people in the real world monitor multiple background activities simultaneously through sound. So, in the first experiment we use auditory cues to help users to monitor the status of ongoing processes. Diagnosing and treating problems with a simulated plant were aided by alert sounds (see also [3]). In difference to [3] we used individual sessions, and not a collaborative environment. We carried out the experiment-A (feedback of hidden events), that allows us to test our hypothesis with the methodology of applied statistics (cf. [6]). As stated in [8] dialog systems should offer the user alternative procedures for accomplishing his or her goals (flexibility) and allow the user to tailor the system according to his or her needs. These criteria take into account both inter-individual and intra-individual differences of the users. So, in the second experiment we tested the hypothesis that customisation of sound feedback supports the usage of interactive software.

2. EXPERIMENT-A: FEEDBACK OF HIDDEN EVENTS

2.1 Method

Subjects: Eight male students of computer science at the ETH (mean age 24 ± 1 years) were instructed to operate an assembly line simulator.

Material: This simulator was implemented with a direct-manipulative interface under Windows on an IBM compatible PC. The audible feedback was continuos sound, that was similar to the special events (normal operating sound, stopping of coolant, no coolant, pneumatic tear off, etc.). The simulation is based on a flexible manufacturing system in Switzerland [4], that produces cases made of aluminium (see 'work pieces' on assembly line in Figure 1). The whole system consists of eight computer-numeric-controlled (CNC) manufacturing centres and eight loading robots for these centres. In the input directing station all work pieces are automatically directed on the assembly line. The assembly line transports each work piece through different stations to the CNC manufacturing centres and back to the output directing station. The whole plant was deliberately designed to be too large to fit on the computer screen, so users could only see about half the CNC machines at any time (see Figure 1 as an 'actual screen clipping' of the whole plant with scroll bar on the right side).

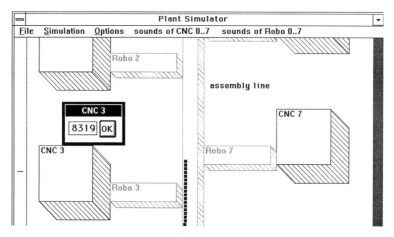

Figure 1. Example of screen clipping with the repair dialog box of CNC-3 (cf. [4]).

We designed our simulator so that each of the machines made sounds to indicate its status over time. Each sound was designed to reflect the semantic of the actual event. For instance, a splashing sound indicated that cooling liquid was being spilled. Because of the complexity of our system, as many as 38 sounds made be placed at once. We attempted to design the sounds so that none would be masked (rendered inaudible) by other sounds. There are two strategies to be useful in avoiding masking. First, sounds were spread fairly evenly in frequency, so that some were high-pitched and others lower. Second, we avoided playing sounds continuously and instead played repetitive streams of sounds, thus maximising the chance for other sounds to be heard in the gaps between repetitions. CNC 0 and CNC 4 are characterised by a high-pitched sound. CNC 3 and CNC 7 are low-pitched.

Tasks: Normal running of a machine was coupled with a characteristic sound pattern. Each machine breakdown generated instead of the normal sound a specific alert sound. If a robot or a CNC centre breaks down, then this centre can not process the pallet of four work pieces further on. The first consequence of a breakdown is a jam on the assembly line. The second consequence is the productivity of the plant decrease.

Subjects were instructed to operate a plant simulator and to take care for a high productivity rate. The task was to trouble-shoot the whole manufacturing system. First, each subject had to detect that a breakdown happened. Then he has to find the interrupted machine (robot or CNC machine). The actual breakdown event shows the operator how to repair the machine. The operator can get this information visually in a modal dialogue box with the status report at the control station or in an auditory form through sound feedback.

Each interrupted machine could be repaired by entering an appropriate repair code (a four-digit number, e.g. '8319', see Figure 1) in a repair dialogue box at the machine. The operator sees only a part of the whole plant (see 'actual screen clipping' in Figure 1). He moves the actual screen up and down by clicking with the mouse in the scrollbar area to 'go to' the interrupted machine. A mouse click on the machine symbol pops up the repair dialogue box. Entering the correct repair code transfers the interrupted machine in the normal state. If an incorrect repair code is entered, then no internal state change happens and the user could hear only a short beep.

Procedure: Test condition-1 was only visual feedback at the operator control panel. Test condition-2 was visual and audible feedback. We used a follow up test design (Latin square). Both task trials lasted exactly 20 minutes each. Before and after each task trial the user has to answer a mood questionnaire (eight scales with overall 36 items as monopolar rating scales). After each task trial we measured the subjective satisfaction with a semantic differential (11 bipolar items). Each individual session took about 90 minutes.

Measures: A work piece could have one of the following status: (1) loading on the assembly line at the input directing station, (2) transportation on the assembly line, (3) fixation on the carrier at the reset station, (4) final fixation and twist on the carrier, (5) fixation on a pallet with three other work pieces at the robot, (6) processing one of two sides in the CNC station, (7) change from one side to the other at the reset station, (8) to be provided with a serial number at the labelling station, (9) loading off the assembly line at the output directing station. Steps (3) to (7) are carried out twice, once for each side of the work piece.

Our *first dependent variable* is a point scale that measures the productivity of the plant. Each work piece, that entered the assembly line at the input direction station, counts one point. One point is counted additionally for each side, that was processed at a CNC machine. Each work piece, that left the assembly line at the output direction station, counts an extra point. Each work piece on the assembly line counts one to four points. The productivity score after 20 minute's simulation time is the sum over all work pieces that entered the assembly line (productivity score). The *second dependent variable* is the number of requested status reports at the control station (# of status reports). The *third and fourth dependent variables* are number of correct and number of incorrect repairs (# of correct repairs, and # of incorrect repairs). The eight scales of the mood questionnaire and the 11 items of the semantic differential are control variables to measure users' satisfaction.

2.2 Results

The results of this experiment showed, that the performance of operating an assembly line simulator could be significantly improved, when feedback of machine break downs and other disturbances was continuously given in an audible form, too (see Table 1).

We can also observe a significant increase of two different aspects of the user's mood. Users felt significantly more self-assure and more social accepted after working with sound feedback than without sound (see Table 2). Their readiness for endeavour, restfulness, and mood increased in the test-condition with sound. On one side, we can observe a significant improvement of performance through sound feedback, on the other side we can find, that users perceive the simulation with sound more in-transparent and feel more or less confused than without sound (see Table 3).

Table 1.
Results of the four dependent variables that measure users' trouble-shooting activities.

Variable (0)	(77)	With sound	Without sound	P sign.
productivity score		70 ± 5.6	65 ± 5.3	.052
# of status reports		17 ± 5.8	23 ± 4.0	.032
# of correct repairs		36 ± 2.5	36 ± 2.3	.999
# of incorrect repairs		16 ± 11.0	9 ± 7.1	.184

Table 2.
Results of the differences (after score – before score) of two of eight scales of a mood questionnaire (monopolar rating scale [1 ... 6]) that show significant differences.

Variable (-5)	(+5)	With sound	Without sound	P sign.
self assurance		+1.8 ± 2.0	-0.6 ± 1.7	.022
social acceptance		+0.1 ± 1.0	-1.1 ± 1.0	.031

Table 3.
Results of two of eleven items of a semantic differential (bipolar rating scale: -2, -1, 0, +1, +2).

Variable (-2)	(+2)	With sound	Without sound	P sign.
intransparent - transparent		+0.4 ± 1.1	+1.4 ± 0.6	.064
confuse - unequivocal		+0.1 ± 2.7	+1.1 ± 1.0	.179

3. EXPERIMENT-B: CUSTOMISED RESULT FEEDBACK

We carried out a second experiment to test the hypothesis that sound feedback is particularly helpful, if the user can choose his or her individually preferred sound pattern.

3.1 Method

Subjects: Twelve subjects (4 female, 8 male; mean age 22 ± 2 years) were instructed to define queries on a database.

Material: The database has a direct manipulative interface and contains 350 different cocktail prescriptions. The database was implemented under HyperCard on an Apple Macintosh IIfx. The user could choose his or her preferred sound feedback with the customisation interface (see Figure 2). Each discrete result feedback was one of 49 different sound pattern for the following six output conditions: 'fit exactly', 'fit except one part', 'fit except 2 parts', 'fit except 3 parts', 'fit except more than 3 parts', 'does not fit'.

Tasks: The task was to search an appropriate cocktail, when the components are given (e.g., type of liquor, type of juice, etc.). Each user had to search four different prescriptions.

Procedure: The users chose individually the most convenient sound for each output condition from one of the three sound classes (result of this personal selection: speech in 42%, music in 25%, and noise in 33%). Factor-A was 'feedback' ('with sound' versus 'without sound' condition). We used a follow up test design (Latin square). Both task-solving trials lasted maximally 15 minutes each. Each individual session took about 60 minutes.

Measures: The *first dependent variable* is the total search time (in seconds). The *second dependent variable* is the search time per prescription (in seconds). The *third dependent variable* is the number of dialog operators ('# of dialog operators'; e.g., mouse clicks). Before and after each task trial the user has to answer a mood questionnaire (eight scales with overall 36 items as monopolar rating scales as control variables). After the task trial with sound feedback we measured each personal opinion (subjective 'sound preference' questionnaire with five monopolar rating scales).

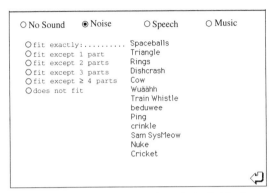

Figure 2. The customisation interface to select the individual sound feedback.

3.2 Results

The results of Experiment-B showed, that the performance of direct manipulative database queries could not be significantly improved, when feedback was given in an audible form (see Table 4). This result can be explained by the uncontrolled factor 'individualisation'. Most of the users' sound selections did not reflect the ordinal structure of the result feedback (7 sound selections without ordinal structure, 4 sound selections with ordinal structure).

Table 4.
Results of the three dependent variables that measure users' performance of database queries for both test-conditions 'with sound feedback' and 'without sound feedback'.

Variable	With sound	Without sound	P sign.
search time total	685 ± 193	649 * 288	.709
search time per prescr.	201 ± 99	182 ± 113	.627
# of dialog operators	98 ± 38	112 ± 60	.577

In the analysis of subjective sound preferences we distinguished between those users that prefer sound (N=5) and those users that do not prefer sound (N=7). For a post-hoc analysis we constructed the Factor 'preference' with two levels: 'sound preferred' versus 'sound refused'. Overall both test-conditions, when sound was preferred, the mean search time is 633 ± 248 sec; mean search time, when sound was not preferred (refused, resp), is 692 ± 241 seconds. This difference is not significant (F(1,10) = 0.28, p ≤ .609).

Table 5.
Results of the three dependent variables that measure users' performance of database queries only for the test-condition 'with sound feedback' and both users' groups.

Variable	Sound preferred	Sound refused	P sign.
search time total	544 ± 215	786 * 95	.023
search time per prescr.	136 ± 54	246 ± 99	.046
# of dialog operators	71 ± 26	117 ± 32	.029

But, if we analyse only the test-condition 'with sound feedback' then we get the following result for the variable 'search time total' between the two groups 'preferred' versus 'refused': mean search time for 'sound preferred' is 544 ± 215; mean search time for 'sound refused' is 786 ± 95. This difference is significant (F(1,10) = 7.18, p ≤ .023). Similar results are found for the two other dependent variables, too (see Table 5).

The significant difference of the variable 'total search time' can be explained by the significant interaction term between the Factor 'test-condition' and the Factor 'preference' (mean search time for 'with sound' and 'sound prefered' is 544 ± 215 mean search time for 'without sound' and 'sound prefered' is 721 ± 270; mean search time for 'with sound' and 'sound refused' is 786 ± 95; mean search time for 'without sound' and 'sound refused' is 570 ± 310; F (1,10) = 5.04, p ≤ .049).

4. DISCUSSION AND CONCLUSION

The results of Experiment-A showed, that the performance of operating a plant simulator could be significantly improved, when feedback of machine break downs and other disturbances was continuously given in an auditory form, too. We can also observe a significant increase of different aspects of users' mood. We found that sound feedback was effective in the following way. Sound feedback helped users keep track of the ongoing processes. Sounds allowed users to track the activity, rate, and functioning of normally running machines. Without sound feedback, users overlooked machines that were broken down. With sound feedback these problems were indicated either by the machine's sound ceasing or by the various alert sounds. Continuos sound feedback allowed users to hear the plant as an integrated complex process. Integrating the results of Experiment-B, we can conclude that sound feedback is necessary, but must be eligible.

Most of all user interfaces stresses the visual perception. Sound feedback can probably help to reduce eye strain. New possibility for the interactive representation of complex sound generating events and processes are possible, especially in multimedia interfaces [7]. Simulations with the utilisation of audio data will in future also have their application in the training of people with impaired senses, in particular of people with damaged vision.

5. REFERENCES

[1] Cohen, J. (1993) "Kirk Here:" Using Genre Sounds To Monitor Background Activity. in S. Ashlund, K. Mullet, A. Henderson, E. Hollnagel and T. White (eds.) Interchi'93 Adjunct Proceedings. (pp. 63-64), ACM.
[2] Gaver, W. (1989) The Sonic Finder: an interface that uses auditory icons. Human Computer Interaction 4:67-94.
[3] Gaver, W., Smith, R. & O'Shea, T. (1991) Effective sounds in complex systems: the ARKola simulation. in S. Robertson, G. Olson & J. Olson (eds.), Reaching through technology CHI'91. (pp. 85-90), Addison-Wesley.
[4] Kuark, J. (1988) Der Informationsaustausch zwischen Operateuren und einer Fertigungsanlage. Nachdiplomarbeit in Mechatronik. Eidgenössische Technische Hochschule, Zürich.
[5] Mountford, S. & Gaver, W. (1990) Talking and Listening to Computers. in B. Laurel and S. Mountford (eds.) The Art of Human-Computer Interface Design. (pp. 319-334), Addison-Wesley.
[6] Rauterberg, M. & Styger, E. (1994) Positive effects of sound feedback during the operation of a plant simulator. In: B. Blumenthal, J. Gornostaev & C. Unger (Eds.) Human Computer Interaction. (Lecture Notes in Computer Science, Vol. 876, pp. 35-44), Berlin: Springer.
[7] Rauterberg, M., Motavalli, M., Darvishi, A. & Schauer, H. (1994) Automatic sound generation for spherical objects hitting straight beams based on physical models. In: T. Ottmann & I. Tomek (Eds.) Eductional Multimedia and Hypermedia. (Proceedings ED-MEDIA'94, pp. 468-473), Charlottesville: Association for the Advancement of Computing in Education.
[8] Ulich, E., Rauterberg, M., Moll, T., Greutmann, T. & Strohm, O. (1991) Task Orientation and User-Oriented Dialog Design. International Journal of Human-Computer Interaction 3(2):117-144.

Designing multi media user interfaces with eye recording data.

M. Rauterberg, P. Berny, G. Lordong, A. Schmid, M. Zemp & T. Zürcher

Work and Organizational Psychology Unit, Swiss Federal Institute of Technology (ETH)
Nelkenstrasse 11, CH-8092 Zurich, Switzerland

Abstract
An eye movement recording experiment has been carried out to test the hypothesis that fixation patterns contain design relevant information. Eight users solved ten tasks with a multi media information system. During this task solving process all eye movements were continually recorded. The following aspects should be considered to come up with design relevant knowledge: (1) pictorial versus textual objects, (2) explicit versus implicit design, (3) task relevant information, and (4) the object area size. We present and discuss empirically proved approaches to solve several design problems for multi media information systems.

1. INTRODUCTION

One important problem in interface design of multi media interfaces is making appropriate design decisions regarding the positioning of visual feedback on the screen (e.g., messages, animation windows, icons, etc.). While highlighting techniques can aid the user in locating important messages, it is not always possible to predict what may be important to the user at a given time. The traditional solution is a mask layout that allows the user to easily find any of the information on it by adopting a consistent format for all masks of a character user interface (CUI, cf. [3]). In the context of the design of graphic user interfaces (GUIs) important messages are often placed in the centre of the screen (cf. [10]). This solution is based on the strategy of minimising the distance between the unknown locus of the *primary attention focus* (PAF) of the user and the locus of the message on the screen. Some open questions are: What is an *optimal* screen layout (e.g., 'picture' versus 'text')? Where is the *best* place to put visual feedback on the screen? A 'hotspot' is a mouse- or touch-sensitive area on the screen. How can a user discriminate among 'explicit' and 'implicit' hotspots?

Table 1.
Survey of variables that control dynamic visual attention (from [4] and [5]).

1.)	The rate at which the display varies: the greater the bandwidth is, the more frequently is the display sampled.
2.)	The value of the information: the more the information is worth, the more frequently is the display sampled.
3.)	The cost of observation: the more costly an observation is, the less frequently is the display sampled.
4.)	Forgetting: as the time since the last observation elapses, the user becomes less certain of the value of the last observed information even if it varies only slightly or not at all.
5.)	The coupling between displays can control the dynamic of visual attention.

One major determinant is *attention* both of the context and quality of perception [7]. It is known that at least the five variables in Table 1 play a role in controlling dynamic visual attention. To investigate the causes of visual attention control in man computer interaction we have to measure eye movements in the context of different conditions. Yarbus [15] convincingly demonstrated how a person's intention affects the way he or she looks at a picture. The intentions or strategies governing fixation patterns are under the voluntary control of subjects. One strategy choice available to subjects when they have limited time to look at a picture is wether to make many brief eye fixations, or fewer but longer-duration eye fixations. Graf et al [6] could show the interdependencies between training, fixation-time, and task complexity.

To determine the point of visual attention, several studies measured eye movements. There are much unsolved problems to correlate eye movements with higher psychological processes. But, 'eyes as output' are one of the best empirical sources. Kahneman [8] distinguishes three types of eye movements that correlate with mental processes: (1) Spontaneous looking, (2) task-relevant looking, and (3) looking is a function of the changing orientation of thought. Thus, the location where a person is looking provides a ready prima facie index of what they are interested in, where they are going visually to gain needed or wanted information, and their overall cognitive set.

We try to test the hypothesis that fixation patterns give us design relevant information. To do this we carried out an eye movement recording experiment. One plausible assumption is that the visual focus measured with eye movement recording can be controlled by popping up windows and boxes at several positions on a screen. Another plausible assumption is that all fixations are concentrated on average at specific areas of the screen. To investigate the orienting process on the change of the fixation patterns we analyse the eye fixation pattern in two different situations: (a) place of first fixation on a screen, and (b) place of second and third fixation on a screen.

2. EMPIRICAL VALIDATION
2.1 Method

Subjects: A total of 8 subjects participated. Group A consists of 4 men with the average age 25.0 ± 1.1 years. Group B consists of 4 men with the average age 26.8 ± 3.1 years. All subjects were students working as a probationer at the German enterprise DORNIER Inc.

Experimental setting: We used the eye tracking system (ETS, accuracy $\leq 1°$) of DORNIER Inc. The subject sat in a normal distance (30"-50") in front of a computer screen (17") without any contact to the eye recording measurement unit (pupil/corneal reflection method based on infrared illuminated eye images).

Material: The experiment was run on a PC (Olivetti M386) with colour screen (VGA, 17"). The standard Windows 3.0 environment with a multi media information system of a German bank association was used. The original version was developed by the German multi media software house ADI Inc. in Karlsruhe. This version consists of 62 different screens (masks) with on average 11.6 ± 5.1 objects per screen (number of all objects is 721). The second version of this multi media system was redesigned and programmed at our usability laboratory. This version consists of 51 different screens (masks) with on average 13.2 ± 4.9 objects per screen (number of all objects is 672). Due to the fact that the original interface version and the adopted version differ in the dialog structure and not primarily in the screen layout, we will present results only of four screens of the original version (see Figure 1, 2, 3, and 4).

Tasks: Subjects were instructed to solve 10 tasks: (1) Search a house for a price of 450,000.– DM. (2) Who is responsibly for the sales talk about an estate? (3) Where is the office of this person located in the building? (4) To buy the house you need a mortgage. Where can you get this? (5) Where can you get information about buying and selling of securities? (6) The bank offers different events of entertainment. You have a free day (April, 7th, 1993). Which events are offered? (7) You have not enough cash and you are nearby the main station. Where is the next cash service? ('Hbf.' is an abbreviation of the German word 'Hauptbahnhof' -- 'main station' in English; c.f. Figure 4) (8) Where is the cash counter located in the building? (9) Which spectrum of services are available at the cash service desk? (10) Look for the next estate, which you can find?

Procedure: Factor A is the 'object type' ('picture' versus 'text'; all objects with more than two ASCII symbols are 'text objects', except the picture with title of screen 3; see Figure 1, 2, 3, and 4). Factor B is the 'design type' of each object ('explicit' versus 'implicit' design; e.g. hot spots like buttons have explicit design, all other hotspots (e.g., logo, picture, signs) have an implicit design; see [12]). Factor C is the 'task relevant information' of each object ('relevant' versus 'not relevant'; only the following objects have task relevant information: the big arrow in the lower right corner of screen-2; the big 'EC-symbol' nearby the symbol 'Hbf' and the 'Hbf'-symbol itself in screen-4; all text with 'Info-Center' and the 'red point' nearby 'Foyer' in screen-3). We used a 'Latin-square' test design.

Measures: The visual fixation point is given by the ETS as a crossing point of two white lines on the video and as absolute values (x-, y- co-ordinate) in a log file. The frequencies of eye positions were counted with time increments of 20 ms. We defined visual areas as representations of objects (e.g., button, logo, picture, etc.). Each object is characterized by its position and its screen space or area size. We present in this paper the analysis of the first three fixations of all eight users looking on one of four different screens each time, when they came to one of these screens during their task solving process. We differentiate the variable 'number of first fixations' ('# of first fixations') from the variable 'number of total fixations' per object (cf. Figure 1, 2, 3, and 4). The variable 'number of rest fixations' is defined as '# of total fixations' minus '# of first fixations'. The variable '# of relative first fixations' is the ratio of '# of first fixations' divided by 'object area' (measured in dots^2). This was done to eliminate the influence of the object area size on number of fixations.

2.2 Results

We analysed all presented data in Figure 1, 2, 3, and 4 with analysis of variances and correlation analysis. The screen-1 in Figure 1 is characterized by 12 different objects, 30 first fixations (top number at the right side of each object), and 186 total fixations (bottom number at the right side of each object). The screen-2 in Figure 2 is characterized by 9 different objects, 30 first fixations, and 249 total fixations. The screen-3 in Figure 3 is characterized by 15 different objects, 21 first fixations, and 252 total fixations. The screen-4 in Figure 4 is characterized by 19 different objects, 16 first fixations, and 104 total fixations.

Table 4.
Results of three analyses of variances for the six dependent variables.

dependent variable	Factor A 'Object'			Factor B 'Design'			Factor C 'Task'		
	df	F-Value	P-Value	df	F-Value	P-Value	df	F-Value	P-Value
# of first fixations	1, 53	5.075	.028	1, 53	0.558	.458	1, 53	0.169	.683
# of rest fixations	1, 53	10.186	.002	1, 53	4.518	.038	1, 53	4.557	.037
# of total fixations	1, 53	10.832	.002	1, 53	4.071	.049	1, 53	3.813	.056
# of relative first fix.	1, 53	1.664	.203	1, 53	1.386	.244	1, 53	20.644	.0001
# of relative rest fix.	1, 53	0.784	.380	1, 53	0.242	.625	1, 53	71.512	.0001
# of relative total fix.	1, 53	0.985	.325	1, 53	0.414	.523	1, 53	61.669	.0001

Factor-A 'object type' -- picture versus text: We find a significant difference for the benefit of objects with a textual content (mean of 'first fixations' 2.5 ± 2.5) compared to objects with a pictorial content (mean of 'first fixations' 1.1 ± 2.2; $P \leq .028$, see Table 4). There are also significant effects for the variable 'number of rest fixations' (17.1 ± 9.2 for 'text' versus 8.3 ± 11.2 for 'pictures'; $P \leq .002$) and for the variable 'number of total fixations' (19.6 ± 10.4 for 'text' versus 9.4 ± 12.6 for 'pictures'; $P \leq .002$). These advantages of textual objects disappear completely if we take the influence of the area size of the objects into consideration (variables 'number of relative ... fixations').

Factor-B 'design type' -- explicit versus implicit: We find a significant difference for the benefit of objects with an explicit design (mean of 'rest fixations' 18.2 ± 10.1) compared to objects with an implicit design (mean of 'rest fixations' 10.9 ± 10.9; $P \leq .038$, see Table 4). A similar effect can be shown for the variable 'number of total fixations' (20.4 ± 10.2 for 'explicit design' versus 12.5 ± 12.8 for 'implicit design'; $P \leq .049$). These advantages of explicitly designed objects disappear completely if we take the influence of the area size of the objects into consideration (variables 'number of relative ... fixations', see Table 4).

Factor-C 'task relevant information': If we compare the mean fixation rate of objects with task relevant information with objects without task relevance then we can find significant differences for the variable 'number of rest fixations' (20.7 ± 8.3 fixations for 'relevant' objects versus 11.4 ± 11.0 fixations for 'not-relevant' objects; $P \leq .037$) and 'number of total fixations' (22.8 ± 7.7 fixations for 'relevant' objects versus 13.2 ± 12.7 fixations for 'not-relevant' objects; $P \leq .056$). If we take the influence of the area size of the objects into consideration then we find highly significant differences for the benefit of objects with task relevant information's ('number of relative first fixations': 0.27 ± 0.37 for 'relevant infos' versus 0.03 ± 0.05 for 'not-relevant infos', $P \leq .0001$; 'number of relative rest fixations': 1.63 ± 1.08 for 'relevant infos' versus 0.20 ± 0.22 for 'not-relevant infos', $P \leq .0001$; 'number of relative total fixations': 1.90 ± 1.40 for 'relevant infos' versus 0.23 ± 0.25 for 'not-relevant infos', $P \leq .0001$).

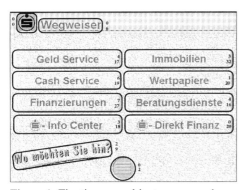

Figure 1. Fixations per object on screen 1.

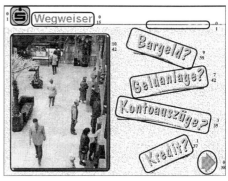

Figure 2. Fixations per object on screen 2.

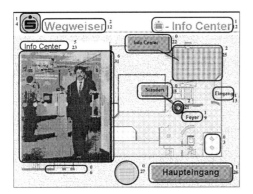

Figure 3. Fixations per object on screen 3.

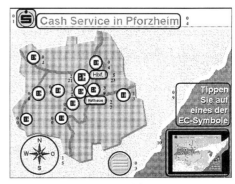

Figure 4. Fixations per object on screen 4.

Orienting phase: We find two significant product moment correlations (R): one between 'number of first fixations' and 'number of rest fixations, $R_1 = .53$ ($P \leq .0001$, N = 55), and the other between 'number of relative first fixations' and 'number of relative rest fixations, $R_2 = .83$ ($P \leq .0001$, N = 55). If we exclude all data points with 'task relevant information', then both correlations change ($R_1 = .62$, $P \leq .0001$, N = 48; $R_2 = .45$, $P \leq .001$, N = 48). Objects that have a high attractiveness for the first time tend to keep their attraction over time.

Power of the center: If we count the number of all fixations in the center of different screens (e.g., see Figure 1, 2, 3, and 4), then we have an empirical indicator of the attractiveness of this central region. We defined an area of 200 dots by 200 dots (13%) of total screen space (640 dots by 480 dots) in the middle of each screen. We counted 56,350 fixations (26%) in this area of all 217,920 measuring points. This analysis was done with all data points of 62 screens of the original version and of all 51 screens of the adopted version.

3. DISCUSSION AND CONCLUSION

It is worth bearing in mind that no-one knows how perception – with its complexity – really functions. Anyone who works with design uses his powers of perception and possibly also refers to the perceptions of other people. Patterns of seeing are extremely tenacious (and vitally necessary) and extend far beyond the area of design. One methodological approach – to overcome these obstacles' – is eye movement recording during real task solving processes. Results of our eye recording experiment can be used to optimise the strategy to control and to influence the user's primary attention focus (PAF). First, we have to analyse the fixations as one parameter of attention.

Picture versus text: Pictorial objects (e.g. icons) are better than textual objects if the user has to solve a search task on a static screen (c.f. [2] [8] [14]). The generalisation of these empirical findings to our design problem is questionable (c.f. [13]): (1) In our case the user does not know what he or she is really looking for (semantically uncertainty), (2) the user has to solve a task in a more complex sense (search time is a minor part of the whole task solving time), and (3) the user deals with different and changing screens (orientation and navigation uncertainty). Due to these three conditions we have to interpret our results. The high attractiveness of textual objects -- measured with number of fixations -- can be possibly explained by their strong impact on the reduction of semantically uncertainty. Otherwise, if we control the influence of the object size, then we can not find anymore a difference between pictorial and textual objects.

Explicit versus implicit design: One important advantage of multi media screen design is the unconstrained design space: every type of textual or pictorial structure can be used. The designer is not fixed to use only rectangular windows or buttons, etc. as in the context of Ms Windows, SAA/CUA, OSF/Motif, etc. We call the design of a hotspot, that looks like a traditional button, the 'explicit' design, because the user has explicitly information about the hotspot. On the other side, if we relate hotspots with different shapes to any area on the screen, then we call this approach the 'implicit design' (see [12]). Most of all multi media information systems have a mixed design. In these cases the user has to find out, where the hotspots are on the screen, especially the implicit ones. Our results support an explicit design strategy.

Task relevant information: For the design process it would be very helpful, if the designer would know all task relevant information, so that he or she can design appropriate objects on the screen. This can be done with a task analysis during the design phase. On the other side, the results of our variables 'number of relative ... fixations' lead us to the interpretation that these variables are very sensitive measures of objects with task relevant information. All objects with a value above 1.0 [$100*fixations/dots^2$] are candidates to have a look on.

Power of the center: Arnheim [1] could show the influence of the whole picture composition on the process of interpretation. One important aspect is the design of the center. The center has a high attraction on the visual attention process. Our results are totally congruent with Arnheim's analysis and composition strategy.

Left above placement: Graf [5] found out that the upper part of the screen is an appropriate feedback area. In an additional investigation we could show [11], that the best result for feedback location can be obtained in left above area of the PAF. This feedback placement strategy depends on the actual place of the PAF.

Location of the PAF: One of our design goals is the control of the user's PAF. What we need, is a good indicator, that can be used by the interactive program, to determine where the PAF is actually on the screen. We found the actual position of the mouse cursor as such an indicator [11]. We are now able to present the actual information, feedback, etc. nearby the actual focus on the screen (left above placement). This solution is not possible, if we have a touch screen. For this case we have to steer the attention flow of the user. This steering can be done by popping up information, one after the other (or other dynamic factors: video clips, etc.).

Orienting and dynamic aspects: Analysing the recorded videos we have to differentiate two situations: (1) the user comes to an unknown screen, (2) the user looks on a known screen. In case (1) a user tries to orient himself. After this orientation phase he is looking for the task related or other interesting information. A new element, that appears dynamically on the screen, interrupts the users' search behavior. If the new information is not task related, then the user is disturbed. In case (2) he has a strong expectation about the dynamics on the screen. If a user expects a specific information appearing on a certain place, then his eyes jump several times to the place, where the information should appear on the screen. In these cases a reduction of time to pop up information could be helpful. Analysing the videos we can observe the strong influence of dynamic screen processes on eye movements. To solve the instructed tasks, most of the users are looking around on the screen to find the right information or a hotspot (mouse sensitive area). If something appears on the screen during this search process, then the normal reaction is to look on this new element. One important condition is the size of appearing elements. If the size is too small, then most of the users have no chance to react on this signal (cf. [11]).

4. ACKNOWLEDGEMENTS

We have to thank the following persons for their generous support: Dr. Karl Schlagenhauf (ADI Software Inc., Karlsruhe, D) and Dr. Scherbarth (Dornier Inc., Friedrichshafen, D).

5. REFERENCES

[1] Arnheim, R. The Power of the Center. Regents of the University of California, 1982.

[2] Arend, U., Muthig, K.-P. & Wandmacher, J. Evidence for global feature superiority in menu selection by icons. *Behaviour and Information Technology,* 6(4), (1987) 411-426.

[3] Burroughs Corporation. InterPro (TM) user interface standards, Version E (March 20, 1986).

[4] Foley, P. & Moray, N. Sensation, perception, and systems design. In: G. Salvendy (ed.), Handbook of Human Factors. (pp. 45-71), John Wiley, 1987.

[5] Graf, W. Ergonomische Beurteilung der Mensch-Computer-Interaktion anhand von Blickbewegungen. Dissertation ETH Nr. 8707, Eidgenoessische Technische Hochschule, 1988.

[6] Graf, W., Sigl, F., van der Heiden, G. & Krueger, H. The applicability of eye movement analysis in the ergonomic evaluation of human-computer interaction. In: B. Knave and P.-G. Widebäck (Eds.) Work With Display Units 86. (pp. 803-808), Elsevier, 1987.

[7] Groner, R., d'Ydewalle, G. & Parham, R. (Eds.) From Eye to Mind: Information Acquisition in Perception, Search, and Reading. North-Holland, 1990.

[8] Kahneman, D. Attention and Effort. Prentice-Hall, 1973.

[9] Larkin, J. & Simon, H. Why a diagram is (sometimes) worth ten thousand words. *Cognitive Science,* 11, (1987) 65-99.

[10] OSF/Motif Style Guide. Open Software Foundation. Prentice Hall, Revision 1.1 (1991), p. 4/44.

[11] Rauterberg, M. & Cachin, C. Locating the primary attention focus of the user. In: T. Grechenig & M. Tscheligi (Eds.) Human Computer Interaction. (*Lecture Notes in Computer Science,* 733, pp. 129-140), Springer, 1993.

[12] Rauterberg, M. Explizites und implizites Design multimedialer Informationssysteme. *multiMEDIA,* 8, (1993) 11-14.

[13] Scott, D. Visual search in modern human-computer interfaces. *Behaviour and Information Technology,* 12(3), (1993) 174-189.

[14] Scott,D. & Findlay, J. Future attractions: a visual search study of computer icons and words. In: E. Lovesey (Ed.) Contemporary Ergonomics 1990. (pp. 246-251), Francis & Taylor, 1991.

[15] Yarbus, A. Eye movements and vision. Plenum Press, 1967.

Ergonomic aspects in designing automotive displays with route guidance information

R. den Buurman,

Faculty of Industrial Design Engineering, Delft University of Technology,
Jaffalaan 9, 2628 BX Delft, The Netherlands

1. INTRODUCTION

Substantial extra car driving occurs because of inefficiency in trip planning and route following. In-vehicle computer systems can guide the driver by audible and visible instructions to a preset destination. The visual instructions can be displayed on a screen on the dashboard, or in a head-up display (HUD). Basically a HUD consists of a small cathode ray tube or other type of electronic display, a collimating lens and a transparent mirror, the combiner. In cars, the combiner is usually integrated into the windscreen. The collimated screen image from the combiner provides a virtual image superimposed on the outside road scene in front of the driver (Figure 1). To see the virtual image, the driver's eyes have to remain within the exit pupil of the optical system.

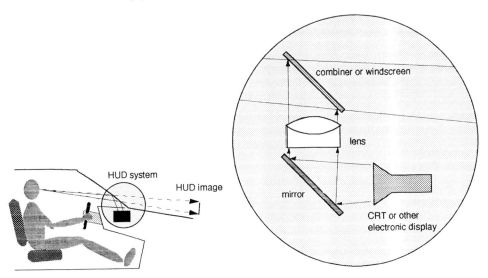

Figure 1. Basic arrangement of an automotive HUD (1)

This is a limited 3-D area, determined by the size of the collimating lens and the combiner. With a head-up display, the driver can see the information without the need to look down at the dashboard, and without having to adapt visual accommodation substantially.

Less visual distraction from the road scene increases safety, particularly for older drivers where eye fixations are slower and the speed and range of accommodation is smaller.

However, there are a number of factors in producing a well designed head-up display. One problem is that the driver will completely lose the displayed information with too far a change of head position. Another problem is how to prevent the displayed information from being confused with elements in the outside world. There are also ergonomic questions, such as luminance and contrast, and their control by day and night. In addition the optimum viewing distance of the displayed information must be determined and it's position in the driver's field of view. What is the best form of presentation so that the driver can match the information with features in the outside world? And there is also the question of acceptance of such display systems by their intended users.

2. DISCUSSION OF LITERATURE

The driver population differs greatly in height. To bring the driver's eyes into the "eye box" as required for seeing the display, an adjustable driver seat could be used or an adjustable HUD or both. Preference should be given to easily adjustable seats as they ensure that all drivers, big or small, get about the same eye reference point and consequently the same good view of the road outside. At the same time all drivers will have the HUD image identically positioned in their field of view. To allow for head movements and for changes in sitting posture, the "eye box" of the HUD should be as large as possible. There is some agreement in the literature that its dimensions should not be less than 10 x 10 x 10 centimeters (2,3,4).

For the displayed information a field of view of 5° vertically and 10° horizontally is more than adequate, normally a field of 1.5° vertically and 3.0° horizontally will suffice (5,6,7). According to Goesch (6) the image should be located at minimum height above the bonnet line, right in front of the driver. With an optical distance of about 2 meters from the windscreen such a HUD image would not cause accommodation problems even for older drivers (8). And it would not disturb the driver's view on the road and his control as, in normal driving situations, this near region does not contain relevant traffic cues (9). In addition such a HUD image, standing stable against a quickly changing background, integrates with the car and not with the world outside. Thus good discriminability can easily be obtained. From Labiale (7) it is clear that, although visual information can be scanned very rapidly by the driver, and relevant information picked out, too complex a display may distract the driver's attention, as may irrelevant use of too many colours (10). So simple information should be presented. Alternatively, the driver's attention may be attracted to a critical display by a short auditory signal or speech message. The message should disappear as soon as the system can be sure that the vehicle has passed the intersection, otherwise the driver could get confused (1).

Quick responding automatic luminance control is necessary to prevent the driver from being blinded and the displayed information from becoming invisible with changing outside circumstances. A contrast ratio of 1.20, meaning an intrinsic display luminance of 0.20 of that of the outside world, is generally considered to be acceptable for HUDs in daylight circumstances (2,3,6). This means HUD luminances controllable up to 4000 cd/m^2 in daylight circumstances. At night or at entering a dark tunnel the HUD luminance must be under 300 cd/m^2. In addition the driver should be able to switch off the system during the journey, or to position it in a "no display" state.

3. USER TRIALS AND DESIGN

User trials were done using a car simulator with a video projector showing the "outside world". The HUD was provided by a VGA colour monitor with a horizontal screen. It was mounted just in front of the car below the height of the bonnet and not visible to the driver. Images were viewed through a slightly reflecting, transparent perspex plate, acting as the combiner and placed over the monitor at an angle of 45 degrees (Figure 2).

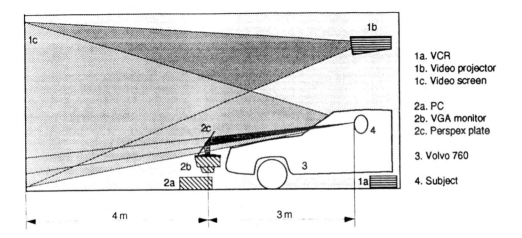

Figure 2. The car simulator (1)

Six subjects took part in the experiments which consisted of six session for each subject with six different design concepts, presented in a balanced order. The route guidance information was presented either on a flat panel display (FPD) mounted on the dashboard or on the HUD as described. The subjects "drove" through a video projection of an urban scene. They were required to control the steering wheel, accelerator, brakes and indicators, although there was no interaction between the driver and the video projection.

The time was recorded between the appearance of a new route guidance message and the reaction of the driver pushing a button. Furthermore subjects were asked to "think aloud" about the six route guidance concepts presented to them. They were asked to comment on what it meant and what they liked and disliked about it. A questionnaire was also completed after every session, which covered colours, form of direction indication, highlighted roads versus highlighted side roads, perspective in the graphics and 2-D versus 3-D indications. Every experiment (six sessions) ended with a final interview. The study did not look at luminance and contrast, or optimal optical distance and location of the HUD image, as these had been satisfactorily established previously from the literature.

The results of the study revealed good acceptance of the HUD and a strong preference for it over the FPD. Reaction times on HUD messages were shorter and some FPD messages were even missed by the subjects. A thing that didn't happen with HUD messages.

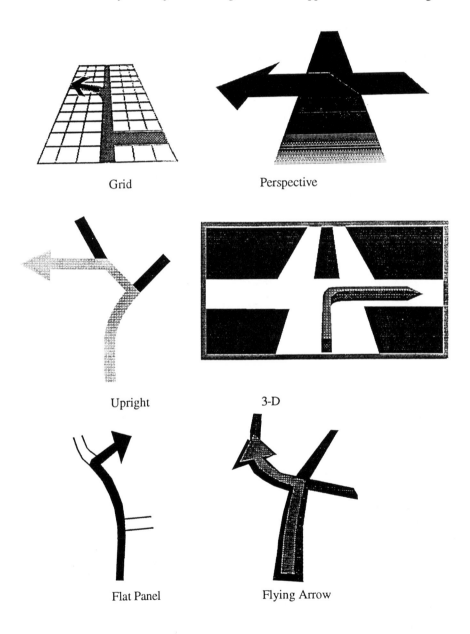

Figure 3. Black and white examples of the tested design concepts (1)

Subjects preferred the design concept "Grid" to the other ones, with the concept "Upright" second best. Figure 3 shows black and white examples of all tested concepts.
The relative comprehensibility of the concepts was assessed by studying the questionnaires and the subjects verbal reactions during the trials. "Upright" scored best with "Grid" and "Flying Arrow" sharing a close second place.

As subjects came with some interesting suggestions for improving the "Grid" concept and such recommendations were not made for "Upright", "Grid" was chosen as the basis for the final design.

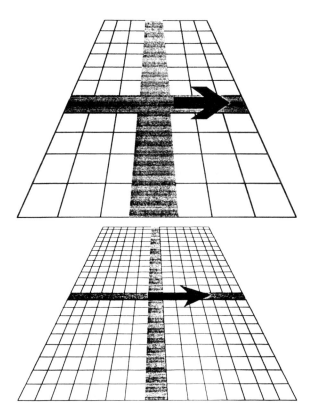

Figure 4. "Grid" concept (top) versus final design (Weishut 1991)

The fineness of the grid, the perspective, and the form and starting point of the arrow were adapted. Figure 4 shows the "Grid" concept versus the final design.
The final design was worked out in three luminance levels of green, a colour for which the human eye is very sensitive in day-light conditions. In the experiments multi-coloured designs were found more distracting than monochrome ones. It also became clear that, in order not to confuse the driver, the displayed road image at the bottom of the grid should always coincide with the actual heading of the car and start in the middle of the grid.

4. CONCLUDING REMARKS

From the literature review, and the results of the study, there are some general features for HUD which should be incorporated for ergonomically well designed displays.
- The projected image of the HUD should be located just above the bonnet line right in front of the driver
- The images should be stable, without vibrations, and covering a field of view of at least 1.5° vertically and 3.0° horizontally
- The images should be projected at a perceived distance of about 2 meters in front of the windscreen
- The "eye box" of the HUD should measure at least 10 x 10 x 10 centimeters
- Easily adjustable seats should enable the drivers to bring their eyes within the "eye box"
- The contrast ratio of HUD versus road scene should be at least 1.2 in day-light conditions; the luminance of the HUD should not exceed 300 cd/m^2 at night
- The HUD should be equipped with a, quick responding, automatic luminance control
- Use of different colours for the HUD should be minimised; there is preference for the use of colours with wavelengths near the day-light sensitivity peak of the human eye (green and yellow).

Acknowledgement

The author is very much indebted to G.M.R. Weishut M.Sc. in Industrial Design Engineering for his major contribution to this project during his work at Philips Systems Project Centre, Eindhoven, in the framework of his study.

REFERENCES

1. G.M.R. Weishut, Automotive Head-Up Displays, M.Sc.Thesis, Faculty of Industrial Design Engineering, Delft University of Technology, The Netherlands, 1991.
2. S. Patterson, e.a., Automotive Head-Up display. In Jin Chang, B. and T.M. Lemons (eds.) *Automotive Display and Illumination,* SPIE, Vol.958, Washington, 1988.
3. R.B. Wood and M.E. Thomas, Head-Up display for Automotive Applications, In Jin Chang, B. and T.M. Lemons (eds.) *Automotive Display and Illumination*, SPIE, Vol.958 Washington, 1988.
4. R.W. Evans e.a., Head-up displays in motor cars, *2nd Int. Conf.on Holographic Systems, Components & Applications,* Bath, 11-13 Sept. IEEE, London, 1989.
5. D.W. Swift and M.H. Freeman, The Application of Head-Up Displays to Cars, in A.G. Gale e.a. (eds.) *Vision in Vehicles*, Elsevier, Amsterdam, 1986.
6. T.C. Goesch, HUD hit the road, *Information Display,* 6, (1990)7.
7. G. Labiale, *Visual Displays*, Yard Consulting Engineers Ltd., Glasgow, 1990.
8. A. Çakir e.a., *Head-up display Terminals,* Wiley & Sons, New York, 1989.
9. J. Norman and S. Ehrlich, Visual Accommodation and Virtual Image Displays: Target Detection and Recognition. *Human Factors,* 28, (1986)2.
10. R. den Buurman, The Role of Colour in Designing Computer Displays, in Quéinnec, Y. and F. Daniellou (eds.), *Designing for Everyone, Proc. of the 11th Congr. of the Int. Ergonomics Soc.*, Taylor & Francis, London, 1991.

"ALTERNATIVE KEYBOARDS" and "ALTERNATIVES to KEYBOARDS"

Karl H. E. Kroemer, Dr. Ing.
Professor and Director, Industrial Ergonomics Laboratory
Industrial and Systems Engineering Department, Virginia Tech
Blacksburg, Virginia 24061-0118, USA

1. DESIGN ASPECTS

Since a commercially viable typewriter was developed by Sholes and Glidden in 1868, there have been innumerable proposals to reduce operator effort and to improve typing performance by changing the keyboard layout (Kroemer, 1994). Figure 1 illustrates major design features.

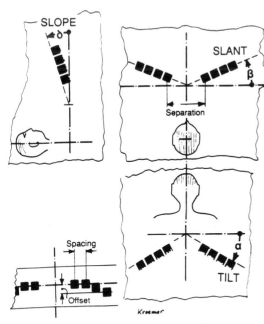

Figure 1. Terminology to describe major design features of keyboards

Originally, the keys were arranged alphabetically in two straight rows. Keys for letters that frequently follow each other were spaced apart, probably to avoid type bars getting entangled if struck in rapid sequence. The columns of keys run diagonally across the keyboard because of the mechanics of the type bars on early typewriters. The QWERTY layout, patented in 1878, was adopted as international standard (after many modifications) in 1966 and is still used, even with computers.

With today's technology there are many different ways to place keys relative to each other. Keys may show rather different features, not only in size and appearance, but also in displacement (travel) and the energy (force) needed to activate them. Yet even today, measurements of key activation travel and force are done statically, although the force-displacement characteristics of keys during their dynamic use are important for the operator.

There have been many suggestions for redesigning the QWERTY keyboard, by various criteria and for various purposes. Physiological/biomechanical reasoning led to the proposal of separating the keyboard into left and right halves and of declining them sideways. This "split and tilted" keyboard was first proposed by Klockenberg in 1926, further researched by Kroemer in the 1960s and patented (German Patent 1,255,177) in 1968. After the patent expired, various takeoffs have come on the market. Re-arrangement of the keys on the keyboard has been proposed often, prominently by Dvorak in the 1940s, to avoid supposed overloading of the left hand, of certain digits of the hand, and to avert excessive finger and hand motions.

Another set of proposals relies on the idea that keying should not be carried out by separate pressing of one key for each letter, but by simultaneously operating two or more keys to generate a character. This is called chording. Chord keyboards have been developed for sorting mail or for speed typing, such as in recording verbal discussions, or for general use (Kroemer, 1993).

Currently, nearly all keys used on keyboards are tapped down and then released. Each key is binary because it has two state conditions: OFF when not activated, ON when tapped down. A different design is the ternary chord keyboard "TCK" (U.S. Patent 4 775, 255, of 1988) where each key has three states: pushing it forward or pulling it back from the intermediate OFF position generates two separate ON conditions. Each character is generated by a "chord," that is by activating two or more keys simultaneously. This results in a keyboard with only eight keys.

Other concepts dispose of the traditional key altogether. For example, the "data hand" has wells (holes) into which the tips of the fingers are inserted. Switches respond to down, fore/aft, and right/left motions to activate characters. Even more radical is the "data glove" which is equipped with sensors for spatial displacement of each digit.

2. BIOMECHANICS OF THE HAND

Design and operation of keys and keyboards should take the biomechanics (mobility, strength, posture) of the upper extremity, especially of the hand and its digits, into account. Unfortunately, even a general discussion of hand biomechanics using the traditional anatomical/medical terminology is rather cumbersome. To specify positions, motions, and strengths in three dimensions, a coordinate system is necessary and a precise terminology is desirable to verbally describe conditions. Such a taxonomy is now available (Kroemer, Marras, McGlothlin, McIntyre, and Nordin, 1990). Consistent with engineering and physics terms, it has a Cartesian reference, with three planes at right angles to each other. For the whole body, the system origin is usually located at the lumbosacral junction of the spine or at the center of mass, but it can be moved to any location, such as to the wrist or to a joint in the hand.

Keyboarding requires specific motoric activities and their complex neural control, a classic domain of information processing and motor-skill research. Although the anatomical and biological properties of the hand are well known, the biomechanical modeling of the functioning of the hand is still incomplete. Layout and structure of the bony skeleton are mechanically complicated and its control and use in movements are very complex. Muscles may originate in the forearm or within the hand, and they attach to various sections of the hand and the digits via tendons which may be guided in sheaths, and lubricated by synovial fluid. There is great variability in the location and strength of these motion elements. Their biomechanical strains due to activities, such as keyboarding, are only qualitatively known. The control of digit actions by the nervous system is not well understood and far from being successfully modeled.

3. MOBILITY

It is commonly assumed that mobility (also called flexibility) of the hand and its digits is related to complex performance capabilities. Anthropometrically, mobility is assessed in terms of angular displacement, measured as flexing/extending and as pivoting the digits laterally (Kroemer, 1993).

We measured the "radial and ulnar pivoting" capabilities of digits 2, 3, 4, and 5 in their knuckle joints of ten subjects participating in TCK experiments. They spread each finger left and right by voluntary internal muscle effort, without help from the experimenter or pushing the fingers against a support; care was taken to keep other fingers out of the way. As expected, the digits showed various mobility capabilities: the index and the little finger pivoted laterally nearly twice as much as the middle and ring fingers. Pivoting capabilities were affected by the posture of the digit: mobility decreased as the PIP joint angle increased. No difference was found between the mobilities of the index finger of the preferred hand and the index finger of the other hand.

Keying performance in the TCK experiments for each individual was ranked, as was each person's average straight-digit mobility. The Spearman rank-order correlation coefficient between keying performance and lateral digit mobility was calculated to be 0.1. Thus, measured mobility was not related to performance on the TCK.

4. DIGIT FORCE CAPABILITIES

The relationship between digit strength and force required for key displacement is also commonly assumed important for keying performance, with stronger digits believed to be better performers, or at least less strained by the keying activity.

A specific instrument, technique, and procedure to reliably measure isometric strength capabilities of the digits was developed. On the same ten subjects, the forces exerted with the fingertip in the down direction, as in tapping a QWERTY key, at several finger flexion angles, were measured as well as the forces in fore (horizontal push) and back (horizontal pull) directions, such as in rocking a TCK key (Kroemer, 1993).

For each subject, the strength data were ranked and the Spearman rank-order correlation coefficient between strength and keying performance data computed: it was -0.2. This indicates that digit strength, measured in down, fore, and aft directions, was not of value for predicting performance on the TCK.

5. DIGIT "REACTION" TIME OR "TAPPING" SPEED

Digit keying performance is commonly believed to be associated with the so-called reaction time following an external stimulus, often a light or sound. Another often used measure is tapping speed, the number of repeated digit movements performed in a unit of time. Results of previous experiments are listed in Table 1, abstracted from Kroemer (1993). The table indicates a great variety of findings and surprising inconsistency in the conclusions about performance capabilities of the individual digits.

Table 1.
Overview of the Rankings of Finger Performance (1 Best) by Several Authors

AUTHOR	LEFT HAND					RIGHT HAND					FASTER HAND
	L5	L4	L3	L2	L1	R1	R2	R3	R4	R5	
KIESOW (1920)	2	9	6	10	5	4	7	1	3	8	DOMINANT
*GATEWOOD (1920)	10	7	9	6	8	1	3	5	4	2	RIGHT
JACKSON	NOT USED					4	2	1	3	5	N/A
HAYES & HALPIN (1978)	8	7	6	5	NOT USED		4	3	2	1	RIGHT
**LACHNIT & PIEPER (1990)	NOT USED					1	2	2	2	1	NA

*Perceived difficulty (no speed data collected).   **Dominant hand used.

Given the inconclusiveness of the findings gleaned from the literature, we decided to measure finger performance consistently. For this, we placed a standard key (Honeywell Hall Effect, SE Series) below the fingertip to measure performance in the down direction (as in tapping a traditional binary key); we placed it in front and behind the fingertip to assess performance both in the fore and aft directions (as in rocking a TCK key); and we placed it left and right of the fingertip to assess pivoting performance to either side. The wrist was fixed, as was the PIP joint. The frequency of key operations was measured over a period of 10 seconds each, on the same 10 subjects who had completed the TCK experiments and the mobility and strength measurements described earlier (Kroemer, 1993).

The findings indicated that the traditional down tapping performance was similar to either the fore or aft rocking operation, which was significantly faster than pivoting a finger to the left or right. For each of the 10 subjects, the finger movement performances in the various directions were ranked and correlated with the ranked performance on the TCK. The results were as follows: For down tapping frequency and TCK operation, the coefficient of correlation was 0.4; in back and fore rocking, the correlation was 0.1; in left and right pivoting, 0.2; the differences among the correlations were not significant.

These experiments on digit mobility, strength, and movement speeds, in relation to performance on a modern (TCK) keyboard, indicate that possibly many traditional ideas about correlations between digit biomechanics and performance on a keyboard may not apply to modern input devices. What may have been true for the 19th century QWERTY keyboard is not necessarily true for modern input devices.

6. OVERUSE DISORDERS

Since the 1920s, physical disorders of typists have been reported, often related to tendons and tendon sheaths (tendonitis or tenosynovitis). Repetitive trauma were also associated with muscles, and with the carpal tunnel syndrome. This was well documented in the 1950s and 60s.

The "force-displacement" characteristics of keys have changed significantly: today's keys require less displacement, and less energy. This development has gone hand-in-hand, however, with more key strokes executed per day, and with more people "keyboarding" than were typing decades ago. Waves of overuse disorders have swept through populations of operators, with the "RSI epidemic" in Australia in the early 1980s best known; a surge of cumulative trauma disorders (CTDs) runs currently in the USA. While the biomechanical origins of the disorders are obvious (energy and force; posture and movements; repetitiveness and duration), their exact contributions to specific ailments need further research. While displeasurable psychosocial circumstances may aggravate the situation, it is the physical activity that strains the biomechanical properties of the key operator's hand/wrist/arm/shoulder.

7. ERGONOMIC CONCLUSIONS

Apparently, the QWERTY keyboard, developed more than a century ago, has reached its limits of usability. There are many reasons for this condition, among them:
- The "one key/one character" design principle has resulted in too many keys, distributed over too large an area.
- The many keys on large keyboards overly stress biomechanical and physiological digit-hand-wrist-arm capabilities of the keyboarder.
- The arrangement of the keys, and their operating requirements, are not well matched with motion and posture capabilities of digits, hand, wrist, and arm.
- The force/displacement characteristics of keys generate use habits that are harmful to some keyboarders.
- The spatial arrangement of the keyboards generates wrist/arm/shoulder/ neck/trunk postures unsuitable for many users.

Thus, it is time to re-think a number of issues. One is the question of whether we need as much information transferred via keyboards as we practice now. A second question is whether that transfer must indeed be done with digits of the hand touching and moving input switches. A third question concerns whether or not better software might facilitate the information transfer. Finally, one wonders whether our ideas about the length of the working day, the distribution of the working hours during the day, and the locating the operator within a office (or other workplace) are still appropriate, or whether these customs are outdated.

For many keyboard operators it is neither desirable nor biomechanically suitable to perform tens of thousands of key strokes per day, occasionally even per hour. One direct way of improving that situation is by ergonomic re-design of input devices. This concerns the choice of binary or multiple-state keys, their operational characteristics, their arrangements on keyboards, and their spatial arrangement with respect to the body. Re-designing the hardware should be accompanied by "smart" software that is able, for example, to complete words or sentences or to generate tables and graphs, according to pre-programmed or adaptive (learning) programs. Furthermore, improvement could be achieved by reducing the amount of information that is transferred via keys by using instead more "mouth-to-ear" and of "mouth-to-eye" communications.

A promising approach is to rely less on physical activities of the digits of the hand to transfer information via some sort of key switch; a variety of other input devices can be used, such as mouse, trackball, light pen, graphic tablet, and touch screen. Yet, these devices are limited in their applicability, and may cause their own overuse disorders, such as musculoskeletal complaints related to mouse use, called "mousitis".

Instead of mechanical interaction between the operator's hand and equipment, other means are available to generate inputs to a computer. Voice recognition is obviously a suitable method, but others can be employed that utilize, for example:
- hands and fingers for pointing, gestures, sign language, etc.;
- arms for gestures, making signs, moving or pressing devices;
- feet for motions and gestures, for moving and pressing devices;
- the legs for gestures, moving and pressing devices;
- the torso, including the shoulders, for positioning, moving, and pressing ;
- the whole body for positioning, moving, pointing;
- the head, for positioning, moving, turning and pointing;
- the mouth for lip movements, use of the tongue, or breathing;
- the face for making expressions;
- the eyes for tracking.

Combinations and interactions of these different input methods are feasible, many of which we use unconsciously in our everyday communications (Kroemer, Kroemer, and Kroemer-Elbert, 1994; Chapters 8 and 11).

REFERENCES

Due to space limitations, only four references are listed which, however, contain listings of the related literature.

1. K. H. E. Kroemer (1993) Ternary Chorded Keys and Keyboard. *International Journal of Human-Computer Interaction*, Vol. 5 267-288.
2. K. H. E. Kroemer (1994) "Alternative Keyboards" and "Alternatives to Keyboards", *Proceedings of the 4th WWDU*, Vol. 3 C1-C7.
3. K. H. E. Kroemer, H. B. Kroemer, and K. E. Kroemer-Elbert (1994) *Ergonomics: Designing for Ease and Efficiency* Englewood Cliffs, NJ: Prentice Hall.
4. K. H. E. Kroemer, W. S. Marras, J. D. McGlothlin, D. R. McIntyre, and M. Nordin (1990) On the Measurement of Human Strength. *International Journal of Industrial Ergonomics,* Vol. 6 , 199-210.

Do Split Keyboards Help to Reduce Strain?

A.E. Çakir

ERGONOMIC Institut für Arbeits- und Sozialforschung, Forschungsgesellschaft mbH
Soldauer Platz 3, D - 14055 Berlin

1. INTRODUCTION

The keyboard, currently the primary input device for most computers, did not substantially change its principal layout for more than one century. Once designed to achieve optimum operation under the restrictions imposed by the design legacy of the mechanical typewriter with type bars, the keyboard layout of Sholes from the year 1873 survived most of its critics. Historically, the attempts to change its linear arrangement of the keys like that of Klockenberg (1926) failed due to conservative attitude of the users as it was the case with the proposal of Dvorak to simplify it.

The major shortcomings of the standard keyboard are well-documented in literature; e.g., the linear layout that forces the user to hold both hands pronated and deviated, or the key allocation that yields unequal loads for the hands and also a higher load on the little fingers compared with the other fingers. In spite of the fact that these shortcomings are claimed to be responsible for fatigue and even for injury („RSI") the new International Standards for keyboards (ISO 9995, ISO 9241-4) are still based on the linear layout. However, alternative layouts are acceptable if the keyboard conforms with the goals of the standards (user performance and comfort). This paper describes the results of a comparative study which was designed to compare an adjustable split keyboard (Apple Adjustable Keyboard, „AAK") with a standard keyboard with regard to user comfort and acceptance. The performance (throughput and errors) was also evaluated since a keyboard is unlikely to be accepted by users if they fail to achieve their normal speed and accuracy.

2. DESCRIPTION OF THE TEST OBJECT AND DESIGN OF THE STUDY

2.1 Relevant features of the Apple Adjustable Keyboard

The AAK resembles a computer keyboard with QWERTY-layout with two detachable palm rests. The only but significant difference is the adjustability of the alphanumeric part of the keyboard that is split into two halves. The angle between them is user adjustable between 0° and 30°. This unique feature helps the user to reduce the lateral deviation of the hands, but it does not influence the pronation of the hands.

The numeric pad of the keyboard including its palm rest is separated from the main part and connected to it with a flexible cable. This feature enables the user to place the numeric pad widely independent from the alphanumeric keyboard. The effects of this feature were not tested since they may be highly task dependent.

2.2 Standard keyboard for comparative testing

The responses of the test panel can only be evaluated in comparison with a standard keyboard. The standard keyboard selected for this study fulfilled all requirements of the standards of Germany and ISO/DIS 9241 part 4. In addition, the technical characteristics of the key switches that may influence user comfort and/or performance were selected to be nearly the same as those of the test object.

2.3 General design of the study

The general design of the study as a one-day comparative test was determined by the manufacturer. According to ISO/DIS 9241-4, it is permitted to give the subjects a prolonged period of training if the design of the test object is new. The rationale behind this is to give new keyboard designs a fair chance since negative transfer effects from prior use of standard keyboards may last days or even weeks. However, the market and the users have always been reluctant to give a fair chance to new keyboards if their benefits are not perceptible within a short time period. With sufficient training, a new design may pass the test but fail in practice.

The test design corresponds to the test procedure as recommended in ISO/DIS 9241-4. According to this design, the test objects - the Apple Adjustable Keyboard and a standard PC-keyboard - were used in consecutive typing periods at the end of which the subjects were questioned.

In contrast to ISO/DIS 9241-4, the task consisted of text input only, since the main benefit of a split keyboard is seen in this type of task. (*Note: The design of the Adjustable Keyboard with a separate numeric pad also offers substantial benefits for numeric data entry tasks.*)

For the study, 26 skilled typists with an experience between 2 and 30 years and good visual ability were selected for participation in the test. The composition of the test panel corresponds to that of German typists with regard to sex, age, typing performance etc. All subjects had experience with typing texts on computers and typewriters.

To avoid an influence of prior experience with the software, the subjects were asked not to correct any detected errors. The entire task was organized so that all required actions could be performed without any knowledge of the respective software (Word for Macintosh and WinWord).

The subjects were given no special training on the Adjustable Keyboard although the unfamiliarity of the subjects with this new design may affect both comfort and performance in a negative way. Thus, the findings of this study are "***conservative***", meaning that any shortcoming of the test is disadvantageous for the test object.

2.4 Test procedure

Each subject was given sufficient test material for twelve consecutive typing sessions of 20 minutes (six typing sessions on each keyboard). The order of presentation was balanced. As required in ISO/DIS 9241-4, each keyboard was used in six consecutive 20-minute sessions with a five minute break after each session. The subjects were given a period of 30 minutes in the test environment for familiarization with the test equipment. The workstations were adjusted during this period to achieve maximum comfort for each subject.

In the first session after familiarisation with both keyboards, the Adjustable Keyboard was used with an angle of 0° in order to test the overall performance of the subject (throughput and error rates) in comparison with the performance on the standard keyboard. In session 2, the subjects were asked to adjust the keyboard according to their individual preference. Most subjects claimed, however, the best setting would be that with straight rows of keys (opening angle of 0°).

For this reason, the test object was adjusted by the test staff, the subjects were forced to use the test object with half of the maximum angle - or 15° - in session 3 and 5, and with maximum angle in session 4. This session corresponds to a hypothetical session with a split keyboard whose angle cannot be adjusted. In the last typing session, the subjects were asked to adjust the keyboard according to their preferences again.

At the end of the last typing session, the subjects were asked to set the Adjustable Keyboard to their preferred angle which was then measured.

2.5 Questionnaires

Following questionnaires and tests were used in this study:
- **Personal data**
- **General comfort**: Questionnaire with 24 items, part of a standard questionnaire used in various studies to evaluate work with computers in general. This part consists of statements related to general fatigue, postural discomfort, somatic symptoms and visual workload.
- **Stress/Strain**: Scale on personal assessment of general strain. This scale, called the "Bartenwerfer-Test" has been used to assess the strain caused by work in general.
- **Postural comfort**: Assessment of postural comfort (or discomfort), i.e. strain in different parts of the human body (wrists, forearm, upper arms, shoulders, back, neck) that may be affected by the use of a keyboard.
- **Design**: Questionnaire for the assessment of the keyboard. This questionnaire was developed to test different products, including keyboards, computers, other office equipment, etc. (Çakir and Çakir, 1983). The questionnaire contains 22 bipolar scales for the following "semantic dimensions" or factors: *"Functionality of Design"*, *"Complexity of Appearance"*, *"Aesthetics"* and *"Potency"*. These factors have been derived from numerous product tests and help to make an assessment of the product on "Look and Feel".

3. ON PRIOR WORK WITH A FIXED ANGLE SPLIT KEYBOARD

Since the results of an earlier study (unpublished) are of interest for the work reported here, a brief description is inserted.

The test object was a split keyboard which was ergonomically optimized after extensive testing in laboratory (Grandjean et al., 1981). The most important features were *"low forearm-hand position, a hand-conformal key arrangement, a 25° angle between the two half-keyboards, and a lateral tilt of 10° to the half-keyboards"*. The final test was carried out with 20 typists. The authors have reported that skilled typists preferred the keyboard after only 45 minutes of typing test.

The study was undertaken to prove the claim that the optimized keyboard, though not in conformance with existing standards in some respect, improves postural comfort. In case of a positive proof, the keyboard would be treated like a standard keyboard from legal point of view.

The study was carried out at three locations with 30 subjects who worked with a VDT. About half of the test panel consisted of typists, the other half were clerical workers. The questionnaires used were the same as described above. The main difference was the test design. The subjects were asked to use the keyboard for an unlimited time period. They were questioned on the beginning of the first day, after two days, two weeks, six weeks and (partly) after six months.

For the first two days, the subjects and their employers were asked to accept a possibly reduced performance. However, the performance of the subjects was not recorded.

The results of this study were only partly encouraging for the designers of new keyboards. Postural comfort was improved significantly. Moreover, not only typists experienced the benefits of the ergonomic design but also clerical workers. However, the training period was extremely long compared with the time span of 45 minutes that was reported to be sufficient for skilled users to accept the keyboard. Most users needed up to two weeks to feel more comfortable while keying. Some users did not feel as proficient as on a conventional keyboard even after some months of use.

4. ASSESSMENT OF USER COMFORT

4.1 Assessment of postural comfort

The assessment of postural comfort (or discomfort) can help predict possible long term effects of using the test object since this study is a one-day experiment. Additional information from earlier studies in which long term effects have been studied is needed to evaluate the results.

Using a keyboard can influence the wrists, forearms, neck, shoulders and back directly, whereas other parts of the body may be influenced indirectly, e.g. by forcing a person to sit in an awkward position. For this reason, the overall postural comfort was assessed with another questionnaire (questionnaire "General comfort").

Since a keyboard represents an object that is manipulated under steady visual control, changing the layout of a given keyboard may also influence visual load. A keyboard designed to minimize the ulnar deviation and pronation may yield a comfortable arm and hand position, however, the visual control of keying can be substantially impaired. For this reason, testing a new design must include the assessment of visual comfort.

4.2 Postural discomfort in back

Backache can result from prolonged sitting or keying, thus, after the keying sessions the reported backache was expected to increase. This was the case both with the Apple Adjustable Keyboard and standard keyboard, however, for users of the Apple Adjustable Keyboard the progress was much slower.

For the standard keyboard, backache on the left side of the body was rated equivalent to backache on the right side. There was no significant difference to the rating for the Apple Adjustable Keyboard on the left side of the body. Postural discomfort on the right side of the body increased slightly when the subjects used the Apple Adjustable Keyboard while it was rated significantly higher after the first and second half of the test for the standard keyboard.

4.3 Postural discomfort in wrist

The subjects reported only a slow increase of discomfort in the wrist of the right and left hands. While the reported discomfort did not significantly change during the sessions with the Apple Adjustable Keyboard, the increase in wrist pain reported by the users of the standard keyboard was significantly higher.

4.4 Postural discomfort in other parts of the body

Reported pain in neck and shoulders, forearms and upper arms increased during the typing sessions, however, there were no significant differences between the two objects.

Also the assessment of visual load showed no differences. This may be due to the fact that the test room and test equipment was better equipped than the usual work environment of the subjects.

4.5 Somatic symptoms

Somatic symptoms, e.g. backaches, neckaches, reported at the beginning of the test and after using each keyboard were differently rated. The result of this part of the study must be interpreted with some caution, since the subjects were asked to assess how the somatic symptoms would be if they used the specific keyboard for their entire work. While they should be able to judge whether using a keyboard would cause backaches, it is questionable whether the assessment of headaches is of the same quality.

After using the Adjustable Keyboard, the subjects reported to experience less headaches than at the beginning of the test. In contrast to this, backaches in the lower and upper back show the expected progress towards worsening. On three of four scales, the Adjustable Keyboard was judged significantly better.

4.6 Assessment of fatigue

The assessment of fatigue, measured on seven scales, was also in favour of the Adjustable Keyboard: The subjects rated the work with the standard keyboard more fatiguing, and their desire for rest or sleep after work showed a bigger increase after using this object.

5. PERFORMANCE (THROUGHPUT AND ERRORS)

5.1 Throughput

The throughput with the Adjustable Keyboard, adjusted to personal preference at the beginning of the test, was slightly smaller than the throughput with the conventional keyboard. Although the difference was not statistically significant. When the angle between two parts of the keyboard was opened to 50% of the maximum angle (session 3), the throughput slumped to 95% of the initial value. In session 4, when the subjects were forced to work with maximum angle the throughput was less than 80%.

While the subjects did not detect the somewhat reduced performance at the beginning of the test - they even claimed to be able to type faster -, the reduced performance in session 4 was obvious. In the final session the subjects achieved 95% of the throughput they had in the first session. This means, that the test duration was not long enough to cause positive training effects with regard to throughput. However, according to the performance test as described in ISO/DIS 9241-4, the Apple Adjustable Keyboard would pass the performance test without an additional training since the observed difference of about 5% is not significant. (*Note: Statistically significant by means of the test described in ISO 9241-4 is a difference of about 15%*).

Since no typist in real working life would accept her or his performance reduced by about 20% by any type of equipment, they are not likely to start working with the Apple Adjustable Keyboard at the maximum angle. This means, that the difficulties split keyboards with fixed angle have experienced in practice will remain. This also means, that the design decision for a user adjustable angle has much better prospects of being successful than previous alternative keyboard designs.

5.2 Error rates

The recorded six types of errors occurred with different intensity, with „omissions and random errors" being the most important. The order of presentation was very important: The groups which typed on the Apple Adjustable Keyboard in the afternoon produced more errors than the groups which started the test with the Apple Adjustable Keyboard in the morning.

Forcing the users to work with full opening angle of the Adjustable Keyboard increased all six types of errors. Using the Adjustable Keyboard with a moderate angle slightly reduced the throughput and increased the errors by a small margin. Forcing the (untrained) users to use it at maximum angle led to a substantial slump in performance with the throughput reduced more than

20% and the errors almost tripled. The overall effect was somewhat worse since some subjects had much more difficulties especially in the afternoon; their performance was reduced to about 60%, while others made much more errors.

6. CONCLUSIONS

The results of this study confirm the assumption that new adjustable keyboard design may improve postural comfort and reduce fatigue. However, the familiarisation with a new design may last longer than most users could accept. Thus, former split keyboards have not been accepted in practice. In contrast to this behaviour, the Apple Adjustable Keyboard was immediately accepted by the test panel; and the main obstacle for broad acceptance, increased error rates caused by the "unfamiliar" keyboard design, could be taken by the adjustability that is one of the main features of the test object. This feature is in agreement with the conclusion of the study conducted by Hertting-Thomasius et al.: *"The most important result of the study is, that it is difficult for skilled typists to change keyboards, because they have to learn new motoric patterns. The authors see this as the most important hindrance for the introduction of ergonomically designed keyboards. ... Therefore, ergonomically designed keyboards should not only comprise anthropometric aspects but also to take into account their users' habits. They have to be adaptable so as to allow a continuous and slow change for skilled persons."*

To our surprise, the assumed benefits of a split keyboard were experienced by the subjects within a short test period. In our former studies, the users needed between two weeks and three months to profit from the ergonomic features of split keyboards; and during the first or second day of use they had even experienced a higher postural discomfort in the shoulder and neck region. This was caused by abducted upper arms since raised arms increase the muscular strain on the neck and shoulder muscles (cf. Ericson and Fernström, 1992). The absence of such negative effects and the positive overall acceptance of the Adjustable Keyboard in a short-term test can be interpreted as an indication for good prospects. The limited approach of the Apple Adjustable Keyboard may limit the potential benefits users could have compared with radical design changes. However, the discouraging experience of almost a century of attempts to improve the keyboard gives us the lesson that in this respect less is more.

REFERENCES

Çakir, A. E.; Çakir, G.: Comparative study on visual display terminals. ERGONOMIC, Berlin, 1983

Ericson, M. O.; Fernström, E.: Upper arm elevation during office work. In: Luczak and Çakir: Work With Display Units '92, Technical University of Berlin, Berlin, FRG, 1992

Grandjean, E.; Nakaseko, W.; Hünting, W.; Läubli, Th.: Ergonomische Untersuchungen zur Entwicklung einer neuen Tastatur für Büromaschinen. Zeitschrift für Arbeitswissenschaft, 35, 4, 1981, 221-226

Hertting-Thomasius, R.; Steidel, F.; Prokop, M.; Lettow, H.: On the introduction of ergonomically designed keyboards. In: Luczak and Çakir: Work With Display Units '92, Technical University of Berlin, Berlin, FRG, 1992

ISO/DIS 9241-4: Ergonomic requirements for office work with visual display terminals. Keyboard requirements. To be published

Klockenberg, E. A.: Rationalisierung der Schreibmaschine und ihrer Bedienung. Bücher der industriellen Psychotechnik, Vol. 2, Berlin, J. Springer, 1926

Evaluation of seated posture in VDT works

Hiroyuki Miyamoto[a], Chyi-Shiun Wu[b] and Kageyu Noro[b]

[a]Department of Computer Science, Chiba Institute of Technology,
2-17-1, Tsudanuma, Narashino 275, Japan

[b]School of Human Sciences, Waseda University,
2-579-15, Mikajima, Tokorozawa 359, Japan

In the modern offices, people pass more and more time in seated position to work with display units. A lot of research has been performed concerning chairs and seated posture, but most of them have been directed at the shape of the seat and the back rest. The pelvis provides a great deal of influence over variations in seated posture. There are few studies on how the pelvic motion in seated posture develops along with time. The purpose of the present study is to clarify the relationship between the chair and seated posture from the view point of pelvic and thorax movements during seated posture.

1. METHOD

A torque balance inclinometer was used as a sensor for the temporal variation of the pelvic and thorax angles[1]. This sensor can measure continuously the angle of pelvic inclination with a precision of 0.5 degrees over a range of ±40 degrees. The sensors are attached onto the ilium and the thorax of the subject with polyurethane spacers and belts. Also to help analyse the data obtained during subject motion, a video camera was set up and audio recorded with a microphone as shown in Figure 1.

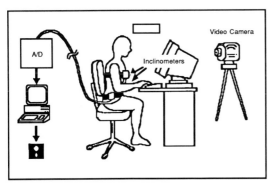

Figure 1. Experiment system

2. EXPERIMENTS AND RESULTS

Two kinds of experiments were conducted to investigate differences in micro movements of the body, pelvis and thorax, which are difficult to measure by other methods.

2.2 Experiment 1

This experiment is to clarify how pelvic motion is influenced by the choice of chair. A subject was seated in either an OA work chair or a wooden classroom chair the seat height of which are the same. The subject was indicated to do a typewriting exercise on the VDT, which simulates a typical CRT-based VDT work. Eight subjects repeated one-hour exercise for three times with a 1-hour of intermission between two exercises by changing chairs in one of the patterns shown in Figure 2.

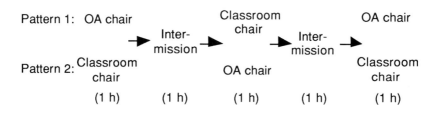

Figure 2. Experiment patterns

Figure 3 shows experimental results. While seated in the classroom chair, the pelvis moved more frequently: it inclined backward every 2 to 5 minutes with a step of 2 or 3 degrees after 30 minutes of work. This backward inclination was compensated by a larger forward step to return to the initial angle of pelvic inclination. As shown in Figure 4, the pelvis moves forward gradually after 30 minutes of work. This causes a backward rotation of pelvis to avoid muscular fatigue at lumber. This tendency was not observed with the OA chair. It was thus found that the VDT work results were better in the OA chair and that the pelvic angle very rarely went in backward so that the pelvis was well supported. It is considered that the frequent pelvic movement is due to the fatigue.

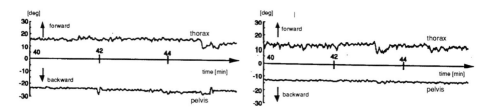

Figure 3. Inclination of thorax and pelvis in classroom chair (left), and OA chair (right) during VDT works: after 40 min

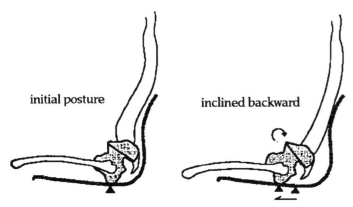

Figure 4. Inclination of pelvis: along with the time, pelvis moves forward gradually and inclines backward.

2.2 Experiments

This experiment is to investigate how the seated posture is influenced by work detail. Also with the subject sitting only in the OA chair, the influence of the work details was compared for VDT work and general work. Sitting in the OA chair used in experiment 1, five subjects were indicated to do two kinds of tasks: one was the same typewriting exercise as that used in experiment 1, the other was a typical spreadsheet calculation using a calculator and a pencil, which simulates a conventional desk work. In this experiment, the seat height, keyboard and VDT support heights were accommodated according to the anthropometric data of each subject. Figure 5 illustrates experimental results.

It was clear that the posture had a greater tendency to be fixed during VDT work, while the thorax and pelvis moved frequently during the conventional desk work. This results suggests that VDT work lacking micro movements forces users to remain in a constrained posture, and is easy to bring muscular fatigue.

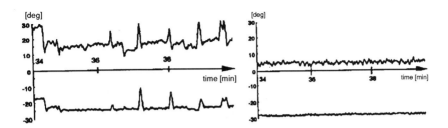

Figure 5. Inclination of thorax and pelvis during conventional desk work (left), and VDT work (right): after 34 min

3. DISCUSSION

Small movements were observed during the above experiments: the movements observed with the wooden classroom chair (Experiment 1) were due to muscular fatigue, and this kind of movements is not desirable. There were, however, much less frequent movements during VDT work in the OA chair (Experiment 2). In this case, micro movements were not allowed because hands and arms of the subject were fixed to keyboard, and eyes to VDT. It is desirable to be free from constraint posture during VDT work in order to avoid muscle fatigue.

4. CONCLUSION

We have measured the temporal variation of pelvic and thorax angles by using inclinometers, and evaluated them in function of seat parameters and work details. Although the variations are little in amplitude, they reflect some characteristics of seated posture and comfort. There are more variations in angle while seated in a classroom chair due to its discomfort. VDT users tend to remain in a certain constraint posture because of seat-keyboard relation and the VDT work environment. More frequent micro movements are observed during conventional desk work. VDT users lack micro movements in order to be free from back pain. VDT work is easy to bring muscular fatigue. It is thus advisable to use an ergonomic chair and take a short pause every 45 to 60 minutes.

REFERENCE

1. C.S. Wu, H. Miyamoto and K. Noro, Micro movements in seated working, Japanese J. of Ergonomics, 5(1994)375-321.

Seated work posture: A comparative study of two chair types*

M. Graf and H. Krueger

Institute for Hygiene and Work Physiology; Swiss Federal Institute of Technology, Clausiusstrasse 25, 8092 Zurich, Switzerland

> This investigation was undertaken to test the effects of a seatbase profile in which only the front section was sloped downwards (forward sloping) leaving the main supporting surface, i.e., the portion underneath the ischial tuberosities, parallel or backward sloping. The profile was mounted onto a chair with a synchronised backrest/seatbase mechanism. The effects of the profile on postural behaviour and comfort were measured and compared to a traditionally moulded profile. The study took place at a real VDU workplace and postural behaviour was monitored over a prolonged period. Postural behaviour differences between the two profiles were mostly insignificant. A tendency was found that the test profile initially increased the frequency of kyphotic postures but these reduced again after one month. It also tended to produce a more even distribution of upper body positions (forward/middle/backward). All but one of the subjects preferred the test profile.

1. INTRODUCTION

Over the last decade the advantages and disadvantages of forward sloping chairs have been tested and debated at length. It has been claimed that these chairs increase the angle between the thigh and the torso compared to traditional chairs (1). When the thigh-torso angle is opened over 90° the pelvis is less likely to tip backwards to produce outward curving (kyphosis) of the spine (2). Early studies of back muscle activity and intervertebral disc pressure revealed that unsupported seating with spinal kyphosis resulted in higher muscular loads and higher disc core pressures than when a backrest was used and that the loads on these tissues decreased as the backrest angle increased (3). Furthermore many people who suffer from back disorders find the normal flattening or kyphosis of the spine during seating to be very uncomfortable. It has been generally accepted that postures with spinal kyphosis should therefore be avoided.

The study described in this paper was undertaken to evaluate in real workplaces a new seatbase profile which had previously been tested in laboratory studies (4). The initial idea was to open the angle between the trunk and the thighs without causing the body to tip and slide forwards, a reported source of discomfort on forward sloping chairs (5). The seat profile under investigation was moulded such that the area underneath the ischial tuberosities remains either slightly backward sloping or parallel to the floor on a tiltable chair, whereas the front (from in

---

* We are grateful to the firm Giroflex Entwicklungs AG, Koblenz, for the technical support that made this study possible.

front of the ischial tuberosities) portion of the seat always slopes downwards (see Figure 1). Laboratory trials over one hour of seated assembly and VDU work showed that the test profile reduced the incidence of kyphotic seating postures and produced a more even distribution of upper body postures (forward/middle/backward). The open question was whether the changes in seating behaviour observed in the laboratory studies would be maintained over a longer period in a real workplace.

a) Chair with standard profile   b) Chair with test profile

Figure 1. The two chair profiles which were compared in the study.

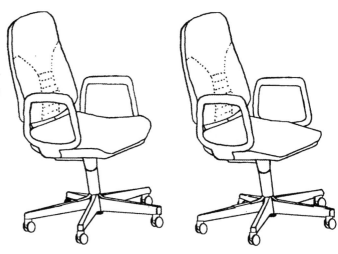

2. METHOD

2.1 Postural analysis

The work tasks in the investigation involved principally computer programming, word processing or data analysis (termed here VDU work). The workplaces were of generally very good standard, having been designed in collaboration with ergonomists. An initial investigation of seating behaviour was undertaken using the subjects' usual chairs for later comparison. These chairs were identical to the chairs on which the new profile was mounted. Six subjects (5 males and 1 female with no history of back disorder) were observed for one hour. Their postures were recorded each minute using a previously developed posture classification system (6). The procedure was repeated immediately following the introduction of the test profiles and then again one month later, still on the test profiles. The frequency of the various trunk, thigh and lower leg positions were compared between the two types of seat profile, as well as the frequency of marked kyphosis. The frequency of postural change was also compared for each body part. The maximum period that postures were held and the mean period that they were held were also calculated. Significance was tested using a sign test.

2.2 Comfort assessment

Additionally, the subjects were given a questionnaire (see Table 1) on each testing occasion. This contained specific items requiring yes/no answers and several general items relating to comfort and stability where the subjects had to rate their subjective impressions on a seven point scale. It also contained a body diagram where the subjects had to mark any areas of discomfort which they perceived.

3. RESULTS

3.1 Postural analysis

No statistically significant differences ($p<0.05$) were found in the frequencies of the various upper body positions (Figure 2). In both the first and second series the tendency was for the forward working posture to be the most common and the backwards posture the most infrequent. In the final series the middle posture tended to be the most frequent, increasing at the expense of both other positions.

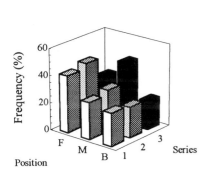

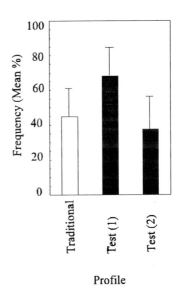

Figure 2. Relative frequency of body positions (F = leaning forwards, M = upright, B = leaning backwards). The new profile was in use for series 2 and 3. The frequency is calculated as a mean percent value.

Figure 3. Relative frequency of kyphotic postures. The bars indicate the standard error.

It can be seen in Figure 3 that the frequency of kyphotic postures appears to initially increase on the test profile but then to decrease to the level found on the traditional profiles after one month, however these differences are not statistically significant ($p= 0.11$). The same pattern of initial increase followed by decrease to below original levels was, however, also found for the maximum period and the mean period that a kyphotic posture was held (see Figure 4). The mean duration of the kyphotic posture on the second series (the first trial of the new profile) was significantly longer ($p=.04$) than for both other series. In Figures 5, 6 and 7 the postural analysis of the torso, thigh and lower leg positions can be seen. None of these differences reached statistical significance.

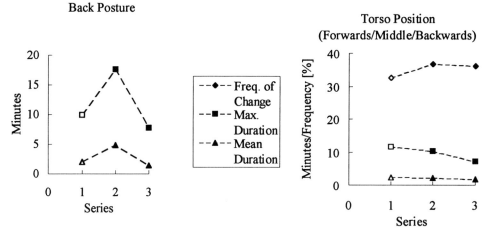

Figure 4. The results of the movement analysis for back posture (marked kyphosis).

Figure 5. The movement analysis of the torso positions. The frequency of position change is a mean percent value whereas the other two measures are mean time variables.

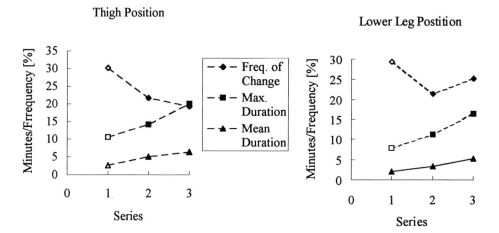

Figure 6. The movement analysis of the thigh postitions.

Figure 7. The movement analysis of the lower leg positions.

3.2 Comfort assessment

The questionnaires indicated good acceptance of the test profile (see Table 1). At the end of the study only one subject (with 46 years the oldest in the study) preferred the traditional profile. Reports of discomfort were minimal with both profiles so they were not analysed further. The general rating of the chair was poorest for the test profile on the last series, however the difference was small and not statistically significant.

Table 1.
The results of the questionnaire analysis.

Questions (Translation from German)	Standard Profile	Test Profile First day	Test After 1 month
The following questions required a yes/no answer.	*(Number of positive answers)*		
1. Do you understand in how your chair works?	6	5	6
2. Do you know how to set your chair height correctly?	3	3	3
3. Is the seat depth comfortable for you?	3	4	6
4. Is the seatbase angle comfortable for you?	4	5	5
5. Do you feel that you are slipping out of the chair?	1	0	1
6. Does the chair feel too hard or too soft?	4	4	5
7. Does the backrest feel comfortable?	4	5	6
8. Do you have enough leg room?	6	5	6
9. Is the table too high or too low?	6	6	6
10. Is the angle of the table right for you?	6	6	6
The following questions required a rating from 1 to 7. (the higher score is the most positive)			
11. How would you generally rate this chair?	5.7	5.7	5.5
12. How well supported did you feel?	4.8	6.0	5.7
13. How relaxed did you feel on the chair?	5.0	5.5	5.3
14. How easy did you find changing your position?	5.3	6.7	6.0
The following question was only given after test chair use		*(positive for test profile)*	
15. Which chair do you prefer?		4	5

4. DISCUSSION

Traditionally, but probably more for aesthetic reasons, people are taught as children to sit up straight, that is, to reduce the tendency of the body to slump into kyphosis. As mentioned in the introduction, early findings about back muscle activity and disc pressures also lent weight to the assumption that immobile upright postures were the most beneficial to health if not comfort. There is however be a confusion here between secondary causes of back pain and primary causes. Sitting up straight requires muscular effort which cannot be maintained indefinitely. The function of a backrest is therefore to reduce the effort that is needed to overcome the tendency of the pelvis to tip backwards when we sit, and thus to reduce the muscular load.

Sitting is however a very natural posture. It is more energy efficient than standing and does not compromise venous blood flow as much. Short term kyphotic postures are also not dangerous as such. The spine is very flexible and both muscles and intervertebral discs depend to a large extent on movement for their nutrition. But both the quality and quantity of body movements are important (7). Good seat design should be determined by the ease and quality of postural change that a chair allows. The reduction of lengthy kyphotic postures is an important but not definitive factor. Furthermore, studies of seated postures can only be valid if they take into account postural behaviour over time, as fatigue effects must logically be included. The effect of fatigue on posture may account for the disparities in findings from studies which have been done on forward sloping chairs (1, 4, 5, 8).

No chair can guarantee good seating postures as multiple factors affect postural behaviour. The chair can only have a positive or negative effect on that behaviour. The findings of this study, after one month of experience on the new seat profiles, support the conclusions from the laboratory studies only in so far that seating behaviour was not negatively effected. The magnitude of the differences which were found in the laboratory studies could not be replicated and an initial deterioration of postures may occur, using the frequency and duration of kyphosis as a standard. The significant changes to the postural range (more even spread of forward, middle and backward postures) which was found in the laboratory studies also could not be replicated. This may be due to the lower number of subjects in the field trials as a similar tendancy was found, however a significant change in postural behaviour, in the sense of meaningful change, would have been detected.

One effect of the tested seat profile, as for forward sloping chairs, is to raise the body by a few centimetres over the height of the front edge of the chair (the standard ergonomic recommendation for chair height). In the laboratory studies, where table height was fixed, increased muscle activity in the thoracic region was found, possibly due to the resulting mismatch between seat and table height. No complaints of shoulder or upper body pain or discomfort were however registered in these field trials wher the subjects were able to adjust the height of their tables to compensate for their increased sitting height.

The benefit of increased postural mobility would be particularly advantageous for work tasks where postural fixation likely contributes to the development of musculoskeletal disorders. Most likely the differences between these two types of profile are not great enough to produce any significant change in behaviour. Further studies are nevertheless underway to test the profile in industrial workplaces and for cashiering tasks. It is possibly however more profitable to seek improvements in postural behaviour by education and increased postural awareness rather than chair design.

REFERENCES

1. Mandal, A.C., 1976. Work-chair with Tilting Seat. Ergonomics, 19(2), 157-164.
2. Bridger, R.S., von Eisenhart-Rothe, C. and Henneberg, M., 1989. Effects of Seat Slope and Hip Flexion on Spinal Angles in Sitting. Human Factors, 31(6): 679-688.
3. Andersson, B.J.G , Örtengren, R., Nachemson, A. and Elfström, G., 1974. Lumbar disc pressure and myoelectric back muscle activity during sitting. I. Studies on an experimental chair. Scandinavian Journal of Rehabilitation Medicine, 3, 104-114.
4. Graf, M.C., Guggenbühl, U. and Krueger, H., 1993. Investigations on the effects of seat shape and slope on posture, comfort and back muscle activity. International Journal of Industrial Ergonomics, 12 (1-2), 91-103.
5. Drury, C.G. and Francher, M., 1985. Evaluation of a forward-sloping chair. Applied Ergonomics, 16(1), 41-47.
6. Graf, M.C., Guggenbühl, U. and Krueger, H., 1991. Movement dynamics of sitting behavior during different activities. In: Y. Quèinnec and F. Daniellou (Eds), Designing for Everyone; Proc. 11th Congress of the International Ergonomics Association. Taylor and Francis, London, pp. 15-17.
7. Grieco, A. 1986 . Sitting Posture: An old problem and a new one. Ergonomics, 29(3), 345-362.
8. Bendix, T., 1984. Seated Trunk Posture at Various Seat Inclinations, Seat Heights, and Table Heights. Human Factors, 26(6), 695-703.

Check list for studying VDU workplaces in order to observe where minimum levels, laid down by EEC Directive 270/90, are not being respected.

D. Colombini, E. Occhipinti, G. Bernazzani, G. Bocchi, A. Petri, A. Soccio, E. Tosatto, F. De Marco

Research Unit for the Ergonomics of Posture and Movement
CEMOC - AZIENDA USSL 41 - Via Riva Villasanta, 11 - 20145 Milano

1. OBJECTIVES

As the various countries adopt EEC directive 270/90, with reference to minimum safety and health levels for work activities involving VDUs, employers will be obliged to take measures to adapt both old and new workplaces, to within the established limits. The following check-list has been prepared and tested with the aim of providing an agile, flexible, yet standardised tool with which to analyse, in VDU workplaces, how closely the minimum levels required by the directive and its annexes are being adhered to. Such an analysis will also allow employers to evaluate the funds and time required for any investments needed to bring themselves in line with the contents of the directive.

2. METHODS

Due to space restrictions the check-list cannot be presented here in full. In figures 1a, 1b and 1c, only the check list sections regarding the analysis of natural and artificial lighting and office furnitures are represented. However, a version in English is available from the authors. The contents and application methods will be briefly described here.

a) <u>Contents</u>. These refer to points 1 and 2 of the Annex to the EEC Directive: equipment (screen, keyboard, work surface and seat) and environment (space, lighting, reflections, noise, micro-climate). Analysis of point 3, which deals with software, has been deliberately left out: this is actually more concerned with what the work contains and is not part of the analysis of the workplace, which is the aim of this check-list. The parameters used to evaluate how closely the minimum requirements are being met are described quite succinctly in Tables 1 and 2, together with the results of a first application in 4 different working set-ups. The first of these (A) is a public body sited in a skyscraper (897 VDU stations), the second (B) is another public body on a smaller scale (70 VDU stations). The third and fourth (C and D) are the two administration offices of a multinational chemical company (160 VDU stations) and a big pharmaceutical industry (120 VDU

stations), respectively.
b) <u>Application methods</u>. The check-list has been laid out in an easily understood and compiled form (limited-choice answers - drawings - judgements rendered objective by numeric parameters etc. ...). In this way it can be filled out by research staff or carried out through interviews, or even compiled directly by the workers themselves: the latter being indispensable in situations where there are a large number of workers.

3. RESULTS

The results of the check-list in the 4 situations are described in Tables 1 and 2. In companies A and B it was filled in by the workers themselves; in D it was filled in by research staff (and thus lacks the most subjective data), in C it was filled in both by research staff and the workers themselves (no differences emerged). To sum up the results: a) there are no particular problems with the technical characteristics of screens and keyboards: luminosity problems seem to derive from the incorrect positioning of the screen rather than intrinsic problems and the way the light is distributed on the screen. b) Dimensions and the possibility of adjusting work surfaces and seats, do not - to a great extent - meet the minimum requirements of the directive. The results obtained confirm the usefulness of the check-list as a screening tool. It was also noted that the main problems in adopting the directive concern the choice of furnishings (tables-chairs-accessories) and their correct positioning within the layout of the spaces.

Table 1
Results of the application of the check-list in four large offices: non-fulfilment of the minimum standards of EEC directive 270/90, with reference to the environmental parameters.

CEE 270/90

ENVIRONMENTAL PARAMETERS	A	B	C	D
HUMIDITY - air too dry	58.40	40	44	-
NOISE - bothered in own office	25	56.3	17	-
REFLECTIONS AND GLARE				
- incorrectly positioned with respect to the windows (in front and behind)	28	38	62	48
	13	26	22	18
- lack of suitable screening from the window	33	9.9	4.8	6
- lack of suitable screening from artificial light	0.3	0	15.4	0
- white walls				
LIGHTING - uncomfortable lighting	49	45	41	-
TOTAL NUMBER OF VDU WORKSTATIONS	897	70	166	120

Table 2
Results of the application of the check-list in four large offices: non-fulfilment of the minimum standards of EEC directive 270/90, with reference to equipment.

EQUIPMENT	270/90			
	A	B	C	D
SCREEN				
- brightness and/or contrast not adjustable	8	8.6	5.6	10
- screen not adjustable	24	9.9	23.9	28
- reflections on the surface of the screen	68	35	26	39
KEYBOARD				
- too thick and/or not separate from the screen	29	5.6	16	21
- space in front of the keyboard insufficient for resting hands and forearms (less than 15cm.)	32	10	35	24
WORK SURFACE				
- surface reflects (shiny)	22	1.4	8	9
- pure white or black surface	70	80	72	13
- inadequate surface dimensions (width less than 100cm.)	40	49.3	46.6	28
- inadequate leg room (not possible to cross legs)	50	50	40	52
- inflexibility (keyboard plain lowered/fixed)	26.6	4.2	61	24
- screen-to-eye distance of less than 50 cm.	15	22	23	11
- reading stand useful but not provided	25	35	23	-
CHAIR				
- seat not height-adjustable	29	79	13	24
- back-rest not adjustable	77	87	58	50
- footrest useful but not provided	48	66	35	-

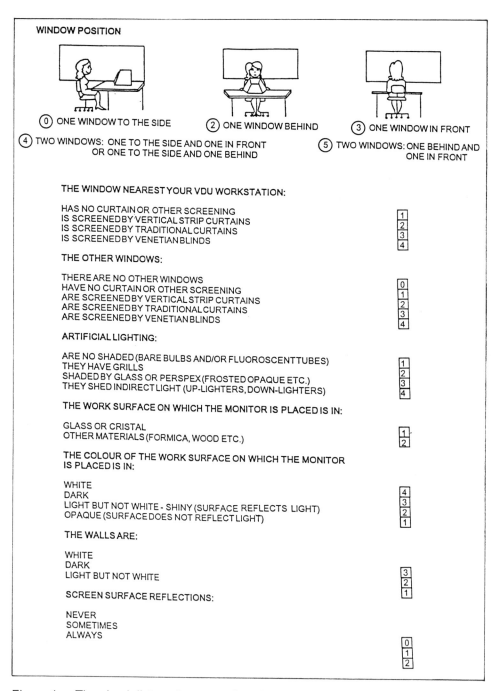

Figure 1a. The check list section regarding the analysis of natural and artificial lithing.

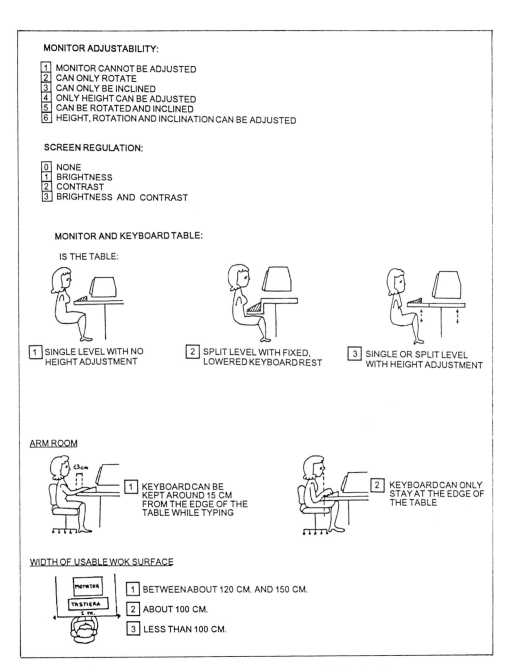

Figure 1b. The check list section regarding layout and office furnitures.

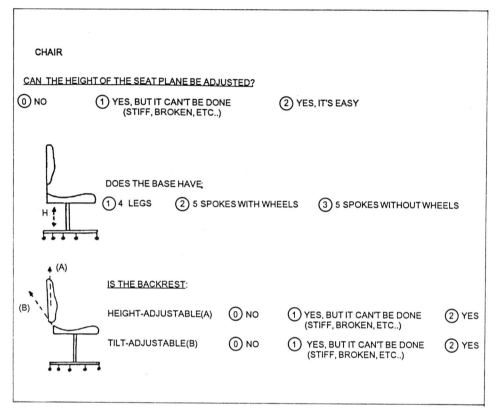

Figure 1c. The check list sections regarding office chair.

4. CONCLUSIONS

Even when filled out by the work-force themselves, the check-list prepared for studying VDU work-places has proved to be useful, easily applied and elaborated.

It was possible to use it as a means of supplying employers with data on how their environments and equipment shape up to EEC Directive 270/90, in a short time and at relative low cost.

The results showed that the greatest problems in VDU work stations are related to the choice of furnishing (tables - chairs - accessories) and their correct positioning within the layout.

Employers should direct their efforts and investments toward solving these problems if they are to get in line with the EEC's new directives.

New methods to evaluate VDU screen glare

I. C. Pasini[a], D. K. Tiller[b] and G. R. Newsham[b]

[a]Public Works and Government Services Canada, Sir Charles Tupper Bldg., Riverside Drive, Ottawa, Ontario, K1A0M2, Canada

[b]Institute for Research in Construction, National Research Council, Ottawa, Ontario, K1A0R6, Canada

1. INTRODUCTION

Public Works and Government Services Canada (PWGSC) is the common service agency of the Canadian Federal Government charged with the responsibility to design, construct and maintain building facilities needed by the federal government. With approximately 8 million square metres of office space across Canada, PWGSC represents the largest landlord in North America for this type of accommodation. The responsibility to provide and maintain a productive work environment for more than 210,000 employees is the principle motivation behind this work, which aims to identify and develop methods to efficiently measure the actual and perceived quality of the built environment. A successful realization of this project is expected to produce significant improvements in the environmental quality of office lighting, and a considerable reduction in commissioning and remedial costs associated with lighting systems. This report describes three new tools developed to facilitate the collection of enough *in situ* workplace data to establish more clearly the link between physical photometric data and subjective judgments of lighting conditions.

2. CURRENT TECHNOLOGY

Although illuminating engineering and lighting design are mature, technically sophisticated disciplines, the problem of ensuring that a work site provides adequate illumination remains a major challenge. At least in part, this is because collecting enough post-occupancy evaluation field survey data and on site photometric data, which are required to establish links between illuminated environments and occupant satisfaction, is time consuming and costly. Current methods assess the visual and luminous quality of workplaces primarily by surveying task and ambient luminance and illuminance distribution. The results are then analyzed and compared against a set of established professional, national or international criteria. However, luminance and illuminance photometry are often cumbersome when applied *in situ*, and rarely produce data that can be unambiguously related to occupant satisfaction. Similarly, post-occupancy evaluation field surveys involve labour intensive questionnaire administration, scoring and analysis, and in the end only provide a snapshot of occupant opinion at the time the questionnaire was administered. As a consequence of these limitations, experimenters are often forced to limit their efforts and collect relatively few data. This paucity of data can weaken conclusions reached by experimenters, and can also prevent meaningful cross-comparisons among different studies.

3. PROPOSED TECHNOLOGY

PWGSC has been at the leading edge of the development of innovative lighting diagnostic tools, aimed at improving our ability to collect and analyze vast and complex amounts of field data. The three tools described in this paper were originally developed independently of one another, but provide complementary information. The tools are: 1) Custom software, named 'NRCQ'[1], that is capable of building and administering an electronic questionnaire; 2) A second custom software tool, named 'Reflect'[1], which can be used by workers to interactively identify and give their subjective opinion about the severity of Video Display Unit (VDU) screen glare, and; 3) A new type of proprietary digital imaging photometer, known as 'IQCam™', which is used to describe the photometric characteristics of the same sources of VDU glare as identified by the worker. These new tools provide an economical, simple and yet comprehensive common basis for quick data collection, and easy subsequent comparison of field data collected by different investigators, at sites located anywhere in the world.

4. HOW THE THREE TOOLS WORK

'NRCQ', the questionnaire survey software package, has been designed to help investigators economically and effectively monitor occupant reactions

---

[1] These software tools were developed by IRC/NRC, with financial support from PWGSC. Both packages operate in a WINDOWS™ environment.

by automatically administering a post-occupancy evaluation questionnaire at predefined times, then record the questionnaire responses to a data file for subsequent collection and analysis. The software package can be installed on several hundred computers in a variety of buildings, representing different office layouts and lighting systems. The complete package consists of two parts: a *Form Builder,* software which is used to generate the questionnaire; and an *Administrator*, software which initiates the questionnaire at specified dates and times, and stores the responses to hard disk.

The *Form Builder* allows the experimenter to generate a questionnaire consisting of an unlimited number of questions, using three standard question formats. The first format is a numeric scale, where response options consist of a set of mutually exclusive and exhaustive response options; the second possible format is a check list from which more than one item may be selected by the subject as applicable; the third and final possible format is a graphic or 'thermometer' scale, in which the subject uses a sliding cursor to place a marker on the scale indicating their opinion.

The questionnaire *Administrator* program resides in the computer's memory and initiates each questionnaire session, based on a schedule of specific questions to be asked and specific times to ask these questions that has been previously created by the investigator. For example, it is possible to create a schedule that ensures questions are posed in random order at random intervals during the workday. When the *Administrator* detects that the time has arrived to initiate a questionnaire session, the following sequence occurs:

1. A warning banner appears, which indicates to the subject that a questionnaire session is scheduled. The subject has the option of allowing the questionnaire to appear, or canceling the session. If the session is canceled by the subject, the questions scheduled for that session are abandoned, and the *Administrator* waits until the next scheduled session.
2. If the subject agrees to answer questions, their current work is suspended, and the *Administrator* paints the questions for the session onto the VDU screen following the sequence specified by the schedule. The subject answers the questions using the mouse.
3. Once all questions have been answered, the *Administrator* writes the date and time the questionnaire session started and finished, along with the identifying file names for all questions presented during the session and their respective answers, to a hidden and encrypted data file on the computer hard disk. The data file is hidden and encrypted to prevent tampering.
4. At the completion of a session, the computer is returned to its previous state.

The 'Reflect' package allows for a more precise and in-depth characterization of the specific areas of VDU screens that are problematic. 'Reflect' is used by the computer operator to trace the outline of actual veiling reflections or glare sources as they appear on the VDU screen, and to rank order these sources in terms of severity. The resulting 'map' and rank ordering produced by the subject are then written to disk for later collection, analysis and comparison with photometric images of the same screen. All data are stored in a hidden and encrypted data file on the computer hard disk. The data file is hidden and encrypted to prevent tampering.

The panel to the right depicts 'Reflect's' main menu, outlining the operation and function of the software

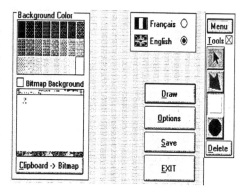

The toolbar (far right) controls the drawing functions, which are used by the subject to trace the outline of problematic veiling reflections in the VDU screen. It is possible to trace the outline of any shape: squares, circles and even irregular shaped polygons are allowed. The 'arrow' pointer at the top of the toolbar allows users to select shapes for further manipulation.

Images of veiling reflections can be traced against either a uniform background (a specific gray-scale value for the background can be selected by clicking on the desired item from the 'Background Colour' box at the top right of the menu). Alternatively, veiling reflection images can be traced using a bitmap image of an actual software screen (e.g., a WordPerfect or other word processing software screen). This is achieved using the 'Bitmap Background' and 'Clipboard --> Bitmap' menu items at the middle and bottom right of the menu. 'Reflect' supports multilingual operation; language choice is selected by clicking the button next to the desired language. The other four buttons control and regulate the actual drawing and data storage functions of the software.

Finally, the actual photometric characteristics of the VDU screen can be completely and precisely described using 'IQCam™'. 'IQCam™' is a video photometer that is used to take a calibrated image of the scene of interest (i.e. a VDU screen in this case) from the same vantage point as the observer (who has already described the VDU using 'NRCQ' and 'Reflect'). 'IQCam™' is comprised of a black and white or colour CCD camera, and a complementary software package that incorporates extensive image processing and analysis capabilities. The panel below depicts the 'IQCam™' main software menu. The image of the VDU screen that has been captured is made up of approximately 140,000 pixels. Different lenses are available that have fields of view ranging from 3.5° x 5°, up to 20° x 25°.

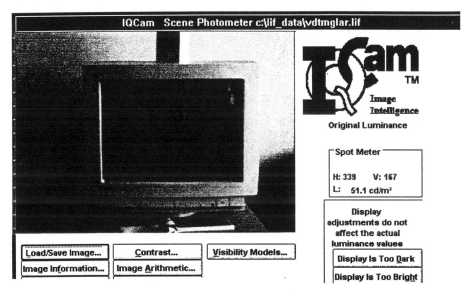

The software package offers a powerful suite of analysis capabilities. For example, the distribution of luminances in the whole image or any portion thereof can be determined and plotted as a histogram; visual target and background areas within the image can be defined, and contrasts between the visual target and any area in the image background can be computed; finally, the software incorporates calculation routines for several standard visibility models, which can be used to model and predict the effects of different scenes on human visual function.

Taken together, these three sources of data (subjective questionnaire rating, trace outline of problematic VDU veiling reflections, and photometric image of VDU screen), provide a complete and potentially dynamic picture of the worker's assessment of their luminous environment.

5. PRINCIPLE ADVANTAGES

These new tools, when used together, will enable the lighting professional to: electronically design and administer dynamic subjective evaluation surveys (i.e., ask different questions at different times); administer questions repeatedly at varying intervals to observe if responses change; collect more subjective reactions data than ever before possible, and; avoid keypunch data entry costs since all data are stored on computer disk at the time of response. Video photometry enables quick and accurate collection and analysis of the photometric quantities that are presumably responsible for the observed subjective ratings.

6. CONCLUSIONS

These three new tools offer unrivaled opportunities for data collection that will help bridge the gap between photometric measurements of lighting system performance, and the elusive subjective effects that lighting can have on office worker subjective reaction and productivity. The new tools can be used to systematically and economically collect large amounts of data, since they rely on automated methods.

The data collected with these tools can be used to compile lighting system 'subjective performance' databases, which would relate the physical photometric performance of different lighting systems and VDU treatments, to worker opinions. Such a comparison would provide a firm empirical basis for selecting among different lighting system alternatives that are otherwise comparable on cost and other physical features. Until now this has not been possible simply because it has been impractical to collect enough data to compile a requisite database. For example, before these software packages existed, it would have been impossible to administer a different questionnaire twice daily for a year, or allow users to record their opinions about their VDU on demand. Both are now a possibility.

This new approach can be extended to other features of work environments, when used in conjunction with the appropriate physical measurement devices (e.g., acoustics, thermal comfort, and air quality). Ultimately, this approach offers significant opportunities to improve the ability of the practitioner to measure and deliver better indoor environments.

Brightness: highest luminance or background luminance?

G.P.J. Spenkelink and J. Besuijen
Department of Ergonomics, University of Twente,
P.O. Box 217, 7500 AE Enschede, Netherlands

1. INTRODUCTION

There are two main reasons that a positive display polarity, i.e. dark characters on a light background, is recommended. The first reason is that the disturbing influence of reflections can be decreased by choosing a high luminance for the background area of the display. Reflections can affect the performance and comfort of working with displays. Since reflections add a constant value to the luminance output of the display, the contrast between foreground and background of the image is reduced. Therefore reflections of high luminance deteriorate the visibility of the image and may even wash out (part of) the image completely.

The second reason is that the ambient light determines the lightness of the keyboard or written documents that are frequently gazed at during display work. The lightness of these parts of the surround relative to the brightness of the display defines the luminance balance or display surround contrast. A luminance imbalance or high display surround contrast may result in ocular or visual problems. Apart from glare resulting from high levels of illumination, large differences in the (reflected) luminance of the display on the one hand and of the keyboard or document on the other hand may decrease comfort and increase visual complaints according to some authors. Others do not find any critical relationship, unless the contrast is very high, e.g. higher than 1:20 (for a discussion see Pawlak 1986). The above mentioned effects are often attributed to fast brightness adaptation processes (eg. Kokoschka & Haubner 1985) which are assumed to take place between gaze shifts. Adaptation influences visual acuity and contrast sensitivity, and visual fatigue may built up due to frequent re-adaptation. In order to achieve a good luminance balance, a positive display polarity is often recommended. This recommendation is based on the notion that the level of adaptation is a function of the average luminance or the luminance of the largest surface (which, for text displays, is the background area of the display). An adaptation experiment by Rupp and Taylor (1986) however, indicated that adaptation level is strongly biased in the direction of the highest luminance. In this case the polarity of the display is much less or even non-critical for the luminance balance. The display luminances used by Rupp and Taylor were much higher than are found under office work conditions, because they did not find any effects in a pilot study with lower luminances.

There is also one reason for *not* using the positive polarity but rather bright characters on a dark background. If flicker is perceived by the display user, which may be the case for refresh rates up to about 90Hz for flicker sensitive users, using a negative polarity is advantageous. The threshold for flicker increases with decreasing luminance and area. In most cases flicker goes unnoticed in the small character area, even at high luminance. In the background area flicker is noticed even at moderate luminance and becomes more disturbing with increasing luminance. In practical working conditions there often is a trade off between disturbance by reflection and flicker. Which is the most disturbing depends on the ideosyncracies of environment and user.

Through the processes of brightness perception and adaptation the display luminance and polarity have a great relevance with respect to flicker and reflection. The present experiment is aimed at assessing the relevance of display polarity for the luminance balance, which is often assumed, eg. (ISO, 1992), but denied by others (Rupp and Taylor, 1986). This experiment also tries to replicate the findings of Rupp and Taylor under office work conditions.

2. DESIGN AND PROCEDURE

The stimuli consisted of black on white (positive polarity) and white on black (negative polarity) screens of text, each consisting of 22 lines of text with 60 character positions. The text consisted of nonsense words. The stimuli were generated and displayed by a 486 Windows configuration with an EIZO Flexscan T560i 17-inch color display. This display has a pitch of .26 mm and a resolution of 1280*1024. The display was driven at 69 Hz. The reflection coefficient is .028. The display elements or DELs (simulated pixels) consisted of 2*2 display pixels. The 7*9 DEL characters were designed in a 8*18 DEL font matrix. Following the definition of the ISO (1992), this resulted in characters of 17 arcminutes high at the nominal viewing distance of 95 cm.

The dependent variables were ratings of foreground brightness, background brightness, global brightness, contrast and illumination level on a scale from 'too low' to 'too high' with an optimum in the middle, reflections on a scale from 'not at all' to 'much too much', and readability and overall quality with a scale from 'bad' to 'good'. The ratings were given on a quasi continuous 21-point response scale (Spenkelink et al. 1993). The scale items were presented in fixed order on a second display, the rating display. This was a 14" monochrome amber Hercules screen, with a luminance of 22 cd/m^2 (on pixels) and 0.8 cd/m^2 (off pixels).

Three independent variables were defined: the polarity of the *rating* display (positive or negative), the polarity of the *stimulus* display (positive or negative) and fixed combinations of higher and lower luminances on the stimulus display (7.0/1.0; 12.9/1.8; 23.7/3.4; 43.5/6.2 and 80.0/11.4 cd/m^2). These were actually measured values and thus incorporate the diffuse reflection component. The display luminance was defined as the highest of the two luminances and thus is identical for both polarities. The contrast is the same for each combination (M=.75). In total there were 2*2*5=20 experimental conditions. The subjects rated the stimuli under all experimental conditions. These were administered in two separate sessions (order balanced). The polarity of the rating display was blocked with session. Stimulus display polarity was blocked within session (order balanced) and luminance was balanced within stimulus display polarity. The ratings and stimulus presentation were self paced.

In advance of the first session the subjects read written instructions explaining the task and procedure as well as descriptions of the rating items. In both sessions, the subjects rated ten stimulus displays after practising.

3. RESULTS AND DISCUSSION

The inter-rater reliability (Guilford 1954) of all ratings was significantly high ($p<.001$). There was no significant effect of the polarity of the *rating* display on any of the ratings (all $p > .05$). Thus there was no advantage for equal polarities of both displays, in spite of frequent gaze shifts between the two displays which were necessary while rating.

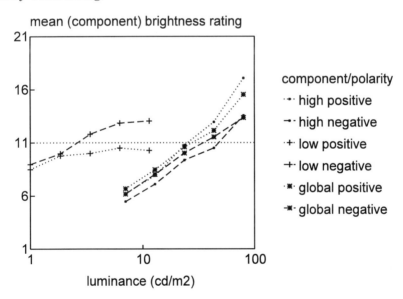

Figure 1 rating of luminance components for both display polarities

The relation between display luminance and brightness ratings is shown in figure 1. The ratings of foreground, background and global brightness are plotted separately. The dotted lines in figure 1 pertain to positive polarity displays and the dashed lines to negative polarity displays. The global brightness ratings correlated .81 with the high component and .38 with low component.

The global brightness ratings differed significantly between luminances (F 132.7;

p<.001). The stimulus polarity main effect, although small (.5 rating point), is also significant (F 18.12; p<.001). For positive polarity displays, the brightness rating strongly increased at the highest luminance. The polarity difference for the lower four luminance levels however, is still significant (F 6,70; p.010). Regression of global brightness ratings on the highest luminance gives 6.7*log(highest luminance) + .56 for negative polarity displays and 7.0*log(highest luminance) + .76 for positive polarity displays (disregarding the condition of 80 cd/m^2), with RSQ's of .998 and .996 respectively. In figure 2, for both polarities the mean global brightness rating is plotted against highest luminance and weighed luminance. The weighed luminance is the mean luminance output of the stimulus display in the text area and thus depends on the relative number of on-DELs. This was 25% in the present experiment. Weighed luminance is lower than highest luminance and thus the curves are shifted to the left in the figure. This effect is stronger for negative polarity displays than for positive polarity displays. If plotted against the highest luminance the curves for the two polarities are much closer than if plotted against the weighed luminance.

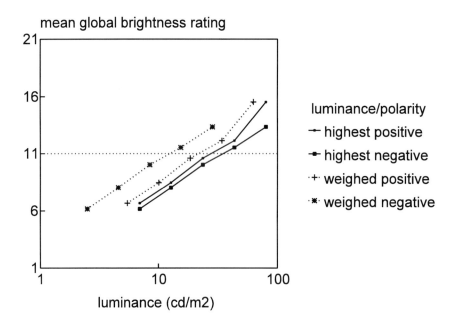

Figure 2 brightness rating by highest and weighed luminance

The main effects of polarity and luminance on the rating of contrast are significant (F 6.29; p .013 and F 35.61; p <.001 respectively). With increasing luminance the contrast was rated higher. The polarity effect is due to a much higher score in the condition with the highest luminance for the positive polarity display. For the lower four luminance levels the polarity effect is non-significant.

The rated brightness of the surroundings significantly differs for the two polarities of the stimulus displays (F 10.90; p.001) and between display luminances (F 3.16; p.015). The significant effect of display luminance is due to the highest luminance condition for the positive polarity display. Without this condition the effect in non-significant. The illumination level is rated higher for negative polarity displays than for positive polarity displays (this coincides with a slightly lower brightness rating for negative polarity displays). The range of the mean ratings is very small however. The largest difference between any of the conditions is only 3 rating points.

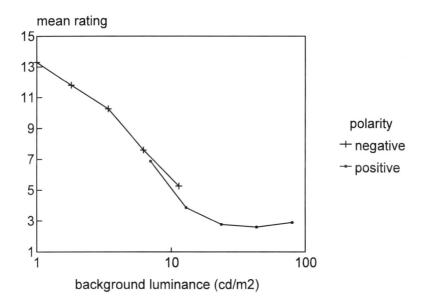

Figure 3 rated reflections as function of background luminance

Figure 3 shows the relation between rated reflections and the background luminance of the stimulus display. This DES item was formulated in a 'not at all-much too much' dimension and therefore has an absolute optimum at a score of 1. The ratings differ significantly between luminances (F 27.26; p<.001) and polarity of the stimulus display (F 193.57; p<.001). Furthermore the interaction between those factors is significant (F 6.52; p<.001). The curve in figure 3 flattens at the higher luminances, which are obtained with positive polarity. The linear regression of rated reflection on the logarithm of the background luminance for the negative polarity displays gives an RSQ of .98. The relation is given by: rating = 13.7 - 7.66 * log(background luminance).

The ratings of readability and the overall impression were highly correlated (r .96). Both were highly correlated with rated brightness (r .87 and .94 respectively)

and, within polarity, with rated reflections (-.90<r<-.72). Because display luminance and reflections were not independently varied in the experiment, the readability and overall impression data were not further analyzed.

4. CONCLUSIONS

Identical area weighted luminances were associated with large differences in global brightness scores. These results indicate that the brightness was strongly biased in the direction of the highest luminance. This also explains that no difference was found between rating display polarities: the ratio of highest luminances of the two displays is both small and identical in all polarity conditions. Therefore it is unlikely that readaptation due to shifts of gaze between rating display and stimulus display occurred.

If the brightness is predominantly determined by the highest luminance component in text displays, there are several options for the configuration of a display in actual working situations. The choice between positive and negative display polarity should be made contingent upon the problems of both reflection and flicker. If the brightness (adaptation) is determined by the highest luminance component, the polarity of the display has no effect on the luminance balance. Four situations can exist, in which flicker and/or reflections are or are not problematic. If both reflection and flicker cause problems or if both do not pose any problems, the user should be free to choose the polarity in order to minimize the problem he or she judges most severe or to effect the individual preference. If only flicker is problematic, a negative polarity should be used. If only reflections are problematic positive polarity should be preferred.

The ratings of readability and the overall impression were highly correlated (r .96), correlated high with rated brightness (r .87 and .94 respectively) and, within polarity, with rated reflections (-.90<r<-.72). This indicates that both aspects are (subjectively) important.

REFERENCES

1. Guilford, J.P., 1954, Psychometric methods, McGraw-Hill, New York, 395-398.
2. ISO, 1992, Ergonomic requirements for office work with visual display terminals (VDTs), part 3: visual display requirements, ISO 9241-3.
3. Kokoschka, S., Haubner, P., 1985, Luminance ratios at visual display work stations and visual performance, Lighting Res. and Technology, 17, 138-144.
4. Pawlak, U., 1986, Ergonomic aspects of image polarity, Behaviour and Information Technology, 5, 4, 335-348.
5. Rupp, B.A., Taylor, S.E., 1986, Retinal adaptation to non-uniform fields: average luminance or symbol luminance?, Beh.& Inf. Tech., 5, 4, 375-379.
6. Spenkelink, G.P.J., Besuijen, K., Brok, J., 1993, An instrument for the measurement of the visual quality of displays, Beh. & Inf. Tech., 12, 4, 249-260.

Daylighting Potentials in Display Office Workplaces: Japan, the US, and Sweden

G. Sweitzer*

Department of Architecture, Musashi Institute of Technology
1-28-1 Tamazutsumi, Setagaya-ku, Tokyo 158, Japan

Abstract
Daylighting potentials are compared for display users in standard perimeter office workplaces in Japan, the US, and Sweden. The means considered can aid user access to window view and daylight while limiting visual discomfort and demand for electric lighting: perimeter window glazings, integrated day- and electric-lighting controls, workplace layout, display hardware and software, and user knowledge. It is concluded that individual display users can be empowered to use their tacit knowledge to exploit daylighting potentials precluded by currently promulgated display user guidelines.

1. INTRODUCTION

Display users have reached every corner of the office workplace. Cost-effective advances in display hardware and software now enable more and more users to satisfactorily perform a wide range of tasks. Office layout and work organisation patterns are changing accordingly, but not without limitations. Daylighting is among these.

Daylighting is a limitation in part because it is widely promulgated as an anathema to display users. Although it is rightly considered as a potential source of visual discomfort in the direct- and screen-reflected-visual fields, there is no basis for indiscriminately locating display screens remote from and perpendicular to windows, especially windows that can be satisfactorily shaded (1). To do so diminishes vital access to window view and daylight in favour of uniform electric lighting, the basis for most current lighting guidelines for display workplaces. Accordingly, daylighting potentials in display office workplaces remain largely untapped.

2. DAYLIGHTING POTENTIALS

Daylighting potentials in perimeter office workplace are nevertheless of increasing interest for three reasons: 1) to enhance user well-being; 2) to limit electric-lighting and cooling loads; and 3) to save space. In addition, it is argued that means to achieve the above are not incompatible, but rather

---
* Fellow, Japan Society for the Promotion of Science / US National Science Foundation

2.1. Perimeter window glazing

Advanced insulating glazings can aid both goals, by limiting heat loss while admitting a higher fraction of visible light compared to solar heat gain. Accordingly, workplace users can sit closer to the window wall without experiencing additional thermal discomfort, in hot or cold climates (1). In addition, "window workplaces" promote visual access to the usually more informative and lower luminance (versus the sky) ground plane. At the same time, hand reach to window daylighting controls is improved.

2.2. Day- and electric-lighting controls

Window daylighting controls include those outside of, integral with, and inside of window glazing. Each may be fixed or adjustable, manually or automatically. Among the many systems introduced into office buildings in response to the energy crises of the 1970s, however, only a few survive. Many have been abandoned due to misuse, disuse, or even sabatoge – in part because these systems proved "unfamiliar" to their users (2). As an outcome, there are few - if any - exemplary daylighting control systems that satisfy the needs of display users in contemporary perimeter office workplaces.

In contrast, artifical office lighting is generally designed to be uniformly distributed, with task and ambient lighting components provided by the same sources. The standard is fixed, ceiling-mounted luminaires with fluorescent tube lamps, with or without baffles or parabolic louvers. Otherwise, luminaire control is usually limited to remote on/off switching, manually, or, automatically in response to motion- or light-sensors. An alternative automatic control that may prove both less annoying to users and more energy-efficient is continuous dimming. This control can automatically regulate the lighting output in response to available daylight. Sensor placement and control area are accordingly critical to user acceptance.

Differences in individual demand for lighting point to the benefits of local task lighting. Personally-adjustable task lighting, for example, can enable users to choose source direction and intensity for illuminating display screen and associated paper document and keyboard tasks. In addition, this lighting can be used to balance display screen/surround luminance ratios while proving more energy-efficient than fixed task/ambient ceiling lighting. Careful procurement of task luminaires and lamps can help avoid complaints of visual and/or thermal discomforts.

2.3. Workplace layout

Workplace layout meanwhile can extend window and daylighting benefits by providing for task and user mobility, including compensatory behaviors (3). The latter include, for example, use of the body to shade tasks that otherwise might prove annoying. Workplace layout can also aid work organization.

2.4. Display equipment

Procurement of display equipment can further aid users. Fundamental differences distinguish desktop cathode ray tube (CRT) units from the more portable and increasingly popular flat panel displays (FPDs). CRTs feature larger, curved glass-covered displays that reflect a larger visual field. Meanwhile, FPD screens are smaller and feature liquid crystal displays (LCD) that are sensitive to viewing angle. In addition, the smaller, fixed FPD keyboards limit adjustments for gaze angle (4), viewing distance, and hand and arm support. Meanwhile, both display types offer positive-polarity screens, dark symbols on a light background, now widely accepted as mandatory in daylighted workplaces.

For the future, software considerations will be increasingly important in daylighted workplaces. Users of larger CRT or FPD screens will undoubtedly require improved screen window markings.

2.5. User knowledge
All of the above provisions, moreover, will be appreciated by cognizant and participatory users. Although users of the first office workplaces also controlled their environments, including day- and artificial-lighting, contemporary users are commonly unable to do so. This limitation may explain some of the dissatisfaction among office workers toward their workplaces, especially that for lighting (5).

Opportunities to enhance user control of lighting in contemporary office workplaces could well be expanded if the initial designs were *less* specific. That is, personally-adjustable task lighting could be introduced when and where needed by users. Means to empower users to confidently make such decisions are being developed. One program provides a checklist for workers to evaluate their own workplace and then initiate the desired changes (6). In this way, workplace users can become more responsible for and, probably, more satisfied with their work environment.

At the same time, international lighting standards for office workplaces are being promulgated (7,8). These standards, however, discount local and regional differences in available daylight and lighting culture. As examples, prevailing lighting conditions are compared for users of standard perimeter office workplaces in Japan, the US, and Sweden. Differences are reflected in the use of window glazings, day- and electric-lighting controls, workplace layout, display hardware, and user knowledge.

3. COMPARISONS: JAPAN, the US, and SWEDEN

3.1. Perimeter window glazings
Similarly-appearing glass-clad office buildings can be found in each of the three countries compared. In each case, however, this external appearance belies significant differences in window performance and office use behind. While fixed single (tinted) glazing is most common in Japan, fixed, selectively-coated double-pane insulating glazings are now most common in the US, in hot and cold climates. Meanwhile, two, three, or even four-pane insulating glaz-ings, set in inward-opening frames, are the norm in Sweden. Each of these window configurations affects incoming daylight and solar heat gain as well as heat loss.

3.2. Day- and electric-lighting controls
Window daylighting controls vary in each country as well. While external shading controls are noticeably absent in Japan and the US, fixed and operable exterior window shading is common in Sweden. This can be used to limit incoming low-angle sunlight that may annoy display users.

Likewise, interior window roller blinds and drapes are more extensively used in Sweden, in part to control the light reflected by the window openings, set in thick insulating perimeter walls. Such controls support the (office white-collar union) requirement that each office user have access to window view and daylight. Meanwhile, adjustable venetian blinds, which can cast shadow patterns at spatial frequencies annoying to display users, are the norm in Japan and the US.

Office electric lighting controls vary as well. While remotely-controlled fixed ceiling-mounted luminaires commonly provide task and ambient lighting in Japan and the US, these components are commonly separated in Sweden. Here personally-adjustable task lights are the norm (availability required) and, in some cases, adjustable overhead hung ambient lighting as well. These choices enable users to "stretch" the benefits of available daylight.

3.3. Workplace layout
Justification for the above described window glazing and day- and electric-lighting controls may be further explained by the perimeter office workplace layouts in the three countries (see Figure 1).

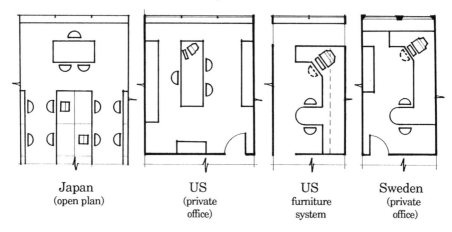

Japan
(open plan)

US
(private office)

US
furniture system

Sweden
(private office)

Figure 1. Floor plans of perimeter office workplaces

Perimeter office areas in Japan (mostly open plan) are occupied primarily by supervisors. Each is located, however, to face the interior, to oversee rows of office workers aligned perpendicular to the window wall. They are seated side-by-side and, often, face-to-face. While this layout enables supervisors to comfortably view the workers, each worker's view of the window is often diminished by a silhouetted supervisor. Another outcome of this configuration is that ceiling-mounted electric lighting, rather than daylighting, is of consequence to workers that use displays.

Daylighted perimeter areas in US offices meanwhile are commonly occupied by senior staff in one of two ways: 1) in comparatively large private offices linked by an interior corridor or 2) in open plan areas divided by partial-height furniture systems. In the first case, the user is typically seated behind a freestanding desk, removed from and oriented perpendicular to the window wall. This vantage affords a sidelighted overview of the window and room, including the door and visitor position(s) opposite the desk. Viewing of displays located to either side of the work surface, however, may be complicated by either direct or screen-reflected window views.

Users of office furniture, meanwhile, may or may not have control over daylighting. Those with storage cabinets above work surfaces, however, will likely have one or more integral task lamps afixed to the underside of the cabinet, in order to illuminate the horizontal work surface below. Display equipment is usually located on this surface.

In contrast, smaller (10-12m^2) and proportionally long and narrow private perimeter offices are found in Sweden. Each of these offices, by default, is divided into two zones: a semi-private area opening from the corridor, to receive guests; and a private work area near the window. Most often this arrangement dictates that the display unit be located in the workplace corner formed by the wall partition and the window wall. Accordingly, the reflected visual field, assuming a downward gaze angle, is toward upper wall and ceiling surfaces, those usually most protected from daylight penetration. The direct visual field, meanwhile, can be controlled with the window controls near at hand. Meanwhile, silhouette effects at the interior meeting area, remote from the window, can be mitigated by local tasklighting, usually located above the table.

3.4. Display equipment
CRTs are currently the most commonly used display type in each of the three countries, although FPD use is growing rapidly in each. Procurement of display equipment, however, differs among the three countries. In Japan and the US there is often a bias toward national products while this is less of an issue in Sweden. Here, more stringent procurement is in effect, again at the initiative of the white collar union. Their interests include screen, keyboard, and software characteristics.

3.5. User knowledge
Changes in the nature of office work have placed new demands on display users. Although task needs will continue to change, basic needs for human access to window view and daylight will not. Means to address these needs vary case-by-case, worldwide. The examples indicate that user knowledge is currently being exploited more in Sweden than in either the US or Japan.

4. CONCLUSIONS

1) *Daylighting potentials* for display users in perimeter office workplaces should first be considered on a local, even individual, basis rather than on an international level.

2) *Perimeter window glazings*, usually selected to endure a building lifetime, should not limit access to window view or daylight or compromise thermal comfort for office users located in perimeter areas.

3) *Day- and electric lighting controls* should be integrated for ambient lighting but segregated for task lighting; the outcome should limit visual discomfort as well as demand for electric lighting.

4) *Workplace layouts* should enhance user mobility; work surfaces should be easily adjustable in order to maintain access to window view and daylight and lighting controls;

5) *Display equipment* should be personally-adjustable in response to individual lighting needs and preferences;

6) *User knowledge* to exploit daylighting potentials for CRT and FPD users should be addressed in the respective ISO/TC159/SC4 working drafts now under development.

REFERENCES

1. Sweitzer, G, Arasteh, D, & Selkowitz, S, 1987, "Effects of Low-Emissivity Glazings on Energy-Use Patterns in Nonresidential Buildings", ASHRAE Transactions 93 (2)

2. Sweitzer, G, 1993, User-Adjustable Daylighting Controls for Perimeter VDU Office Workplaces, Doctoral Dissertation, Department of Architectural Lighting, The Royal Institute of Technology, Stockholm

3. Japan Institute of Architects, 1994, Architectural Design Data, 2nd (compact) Edition, Maruzen, Tokyo

4. Krueger, H, 1994, "Gaze Angle Potentials in Daylighted VDU Workplaces", presented at Work With Display Units,1994, Milan

5. Çakir, A, 1991, Light and Health: Influences of lighting on health and well-being of office and computer workers, Ergonomic Institute for Social and Occupational Sciences Research Co., Ltd., Berlin

6. Berndsen, M, 1994, "Daylighted VDU workplaces in the Netherlands", presented at Work With Display Units,1994, Milan

7. ISO/TC 159/SC4/WG2, 1994, "Ergonomic requirements for work with visual display units employing flat panel technology", ISO, Berlin

8. ISO/TC 159/SC4/WG3, 1993, "Ergonomic requirements for office work with visual display terminals (VDTs)". Part 6: BSI, London

Thermal environments in workplaces with video display terminals (VDTs): a draft standard*

G. Alfano and F.R. d'Ambrosio

D.E.TE.C. - University of Naples "Federico II" - P.le Tecchio, 80 - 80125 Naples

1. EXISTING STANDARDS FOR INDOOR THERMAL COMFORT

Many advances have been made over the past twenty years in the measurement of indoor thermal comfort, which then resulted in many international standards being produced. A list of such standards is provided in Table 1.

Undoubtedly, the most important and widespread standard is ISO 7730 (ISO, 1994). However, it must be pointed out that in order to assess any environment based on this standard, global discomfort conditions must be measured which depend on two subjective variables (activity, M, and clothing thermal insulation, I_{cl}) and on four environmental variables (air temperature t_a, air velocity v_a, air humidity ϕ, and mean radiant temperature, t_{mr}). Based on the values of these six quantities it is possible to determine an index, PMV, which provides a score of thermal sensations as perceived by an average person, and the relative percentage of dissatisfied, PPD. Measurements must also be made of local discomfort conditions, i.e. sensations confined to a specific area of the body, which are due to asymmetries in horizontal or vertical mean radiant temperatures, $\Delta t_{pr,h}$ and $\Delta t_{pr,v}$, to the high vertical difference of temperature, $\Delta t_{a)v}$, the excessively high or low floor temperature, t_p, or, yet, air draughts. The latter is the most important and hardest-to-assess cause of discomfort as it depends on the temperature, mean velocity and turbulence of air. A PPD is associated to each of such magnitudes. Table 2 shows the conditions set by ISO 7730, in winter, for standard winter clothing and sedentary activities. The related PPDs are also provided.

The ASHRAE-ANSI 55 Standard (ASHRAE, 1992) relies on a different model but, ultimately, gives the same results as ISO 7730.

ISO 7726 (ISO, 1985, ISO, 1933c) deals with the measurement of the physical parameters referred to both in ISO 7730 and in ASHRAE-ANSI 55.

ISO 10551 (ISO, 1933a) suggests, instead, a method for the evaluation of the thermal environment by means of a questionnaire based on subjective judgment scales, to be administered to the occupants.

Last, Working Group 6 of CEN TC 156 has worked out a draft standard which is currently being voted as prENV 1752 (CEN, 1994) and which applies ISO 7730 to its thermal

---

* The cost of this research work has been funded by MURST 40%.

requirements (in fact, this documents also deals with air quality and acoustic conditions). The draft standard also suggests that environments should be classified into three categories - A, B and C - with less restrictive prescriptions when switching from A to C, and with the prescriptions for category B virtually coinciding with those of ISO 7730 (as shown in Table 3).

Besides, CEN has already accepted ISO 7730 and ISO 7626 as EN standards, and the PQ[1] procedure for ISO 10551 is in progress.

Table 1
Standards referring to indoor thermal comfort.

Standard	year	title
ISO 7726[2]	1985	Thermal environments - Instruments and methods for measuring physical quantities
ANSI/ASHRAE 55	1992[3]	Thermal Environmental conditions for human occupancy
ISO 7730	1994[4]	Moderate thermal environments - Determination of the PMV and PPD indices and specification of the conditions for thermal comfort
ISO/DIS 10551	1993	Ergonomics of the thermal environment - Assessment of the influence of the thermal environment using subjective judgement scales
CEN prENV 1752	1994	Ventilation for buildings design for the indoor environment

Table 2
Conditions for thermal comfort in winter (I_{cl} = 1.0 clo) for sedentary or light activity (M ≤ 1.2 met) as provided by the standard ISO 7730 (ISO, 1994).

Quantity	Condition	PPD (%)
PMV	$-0.50 \div +0.50$	≤ 10
$\Delta t_{a)v}$	$(t_{a,1.1} - t_{a,0.1}) \leq 3°C$	≤ 5
$\Delta t_{pr,0.6)h}$	≤ 10°C	≤ 5°C
$\Delta t_{pr,0.6)v}$	≤ 5°C	≤ 5°C
draft	---	≤ 15
t_p	$19 < t_p \leq 26°C$[5]	≤ 10

---

[1] Primary Questionnaire procedure
[2] Being revised, see (ISO 1993c).
[3] The previous issue dates back to 1981.
[4] The first edition is (ISO, 1984).
[5] When floors are heated, the upper limit of the acceptability range becomes 29 °C.

Table 3
Conditions for thermal comfort in Class A, B and C environments, as proposed in the prENV 1752 (CEN, 1994).

Quantity	Class A		Class B		Class C	
	Condition	PPD(%)	Condition	PPD(%)	Condition	PPD(%)
PMV	$-0.20 \div 0.20$	<6	$-0.50 \div +0.50$	<10	$-0.70 \div +0.70$	<15
$t_{a,1.1}-t_{a,0.1}$	<2°C	<3	<3°C	<5	<4°C	<10
$\Delta t_{pr,0.6)h}$	<10°C	<5	<10°C	<5	<13°C	<10
$\Delta t_{pr,0.6)v}$	<5°C	<5	<5°C	<5	<7°C	<10
draft	---	<15	---	<20	---	<25
t_p	$19 \div 29°C$	<10	$19 \div 29°C$	<10	$17 \div 31 °C$	≤15

2. ISO/CD 9241-6.2 FOR ENVIRONMENTS WITH VDTS

A draft standard on the requirements of environments with VDTs is currently being designed, ISO 9241-6.2 (ISO, 1993b). Section 8 and Annex D of this draft, which deal with thermal conditions, only duplicate the prescriptions set out by both ISO 7730 in its earlier (ISO, 1984), not the revised, version and by ISO 7726. However, some inaccuracies can be observed:
1. for global discomfort:
    1.1 air, not operative, temperature is considered. Operative temperature is defined as the weighted average of air temperature and mean radiant temperature, where the weighting coefficients are given by the convective and radiative heat transfer coefficients. This means that, as far as global discomfort is concerned, the draft standard does not consider mean radiant temperature.
    1.2 for relative humidity, the extreme values of the range are assigned as a function of temperature, i.e. 40÷80%, while ISO 7730 indicates 30÷70%;
2. for local discomfort:
    2.1 as to the height at which measurements must be made, the Draft Standard sets out slightly different prescriptions than those provided by ISO 7726 (ISO, 1985, 1993c);
    2.2 the criterion to evaluate discomfort caused by air draughts is solely based on the mean velocity value, i.e. no account is taken of air temperature and turbulence intensity which are, indeed, involved in this type of discomfort (ISO, 1994). In other words, reference is only made to the first issue of ISO 7730;
    2.3 as to thermal radiation, plane radiant temperature is never mentioned; only "irradiance" is considered, which is not used in practice and which the document itself does not relate to any discomfort index whatsoever;
3. generally:
    3.1 it does not consider the comfort conditions in summer time;

3.2 the draft standard only briefly mentions the need of individual adjustments, but provides no specific indication.

3. PROPOSED CHANGES

In premises accomodating VDTs, the environment, notably the thermal environment, must be very accurately designed since the operator spends most of his working hours in performing activities which often demand high concentration.

Based on what indicated above and as a result of the experience gained in several field trials where experimental measurements were made, the authors feel that, insofar as the thermal requirements are concerned, ISO 9241-6.2 (ISO, 1993b) could refer to the standard ISO 7730 (ISO, 1994); however, the comfort conditions which are set out in the CEN prENV (CEN, 1994) for Class A environments should be used in order to obtain more favourable environmental conditions than those indicated by ISO 7730. Moreover, in the section which deals with measurements, the draft standard should make full reference to ISO 7726 (ISO, 1985; ISO, 1993). In particular, the ways of measuring thermal radiation as well as the heights at which measurements must be taken should be changed (even if, in the latter case, only minimal differences are observed).

Furthermore, given the specificity of the environments being considered, the draft standard should more clearly indicate the need for "individual adjustments", to allow for interpersonal differences. In fact, it should be recalled that the laboratory trials underpinning the theories of thermal comfort (Fanger, 1972; Nevins et al. 1966; Rohles, 1970) provided evidence that people dressed in the same way and performing the same activity in the same environment, do not, all, feel the same thermal sensations. For example, in trials made in Copenhagen (Fanger, 1972) out of 144 people placed in a climatic chamber at t_o = 25.6°C, $v_a \leq 0.10$ m/s and ϕ = 0.50, with I_{cl} = 0.60 clo and M = 1.0 met, the score was + 2 (warm) for 4 subjects, + 1 (slightly warm) for 27 subjects, O (thermally neutral) for 83 subjects, -1 (slightly cold) for 26 subjects, -2 (cold) for 3 subjects and, even, -3 (very cold) for one subject. This means that in indoor environments, because of interpersonal differences, a given percentage of people dissatisfied with the thermal environment is, indeed, physiological.

The last column of table 2 shows the maximum number of people who can be dissatisfied, PPD. Fortunately, such percentages do not add, and it is estimated that in an environment where all the conditions of Table 2 are simultaneously met, the number of dissatisfied does not exceed 20%. This estimate, however, is not rigorous given that very few trials are made under multiple concomitant discomfort causes (Melikov and Nielses, 1989). Consider, also, that the PPD values of Table 2 have been derived from laboratory tests whereas, in the real world, conditions may occur that are not found in laboratory trials (activities other than sedentary activities, occupational maladjustment, personal problems, acoustic discomfort, lighting discomfort, drowsiness, hunger, physical unfitness, non-steady-state thermal conditions) and which tend to further increase the percentage of dissatisfied (Alfano and d'Ambrosio, 1991). In sum, it is unthinkable to produce, in indoor environments, a thermal environment which satisfies all occupants. Of course, the effort of designers and maintainance engineers must be directed to minimizing the percentage of dissatisfied. This holds especially if VDTs are installed in the environments, in which case it is crucial to ensure comfort conditions to all occupants.

The authors, therefore, deem it appropriate to make the following proposals.

<u>Clothing</u>. Clothing can be a useful means to cancel out almost all interpersonal differences and the effects of the inevitable changes occurring in the various parameters affecting global

comfort (Alfano and d'Ambrosio, 1991). To a certain extent, this instrument is already being used: generally speaking, if one knows that in a given environment he/she has once felt cold (warm), he/she will wear heavier (lighter) clothes when returning to that environment. Educating workers to adopt this behavioural pattern is deemed most appropriate. In addition, they must be given the possibility of keeping some garments at their workplace, in lockers, so that they may change the clothing thermal insulation during their working day.

Manual Adjustment. There is also a psychological reason why some people are dissatisfied when occupying air-conditioned environments. It is the result of their inability to decide on the thermal environment characteristics of the space they live in, and of the need to accept conditions that are set by others. This dissatisfaction disappears if the person is able to adjust manually, by fine tuning, the conditions of the space that he/she generally occupies (Wyon, 1988; Kroner and Stark-Martin, 1994). Obviously, this adjustment (which can be obtained by fan coils, radiating panels, table air vents) also has the same advantages as clothes, i.e. it allows to make up for interpersonal differences and for the effects produced by different working activities. Clearly, manual adjustments must be studied so as not to cause localized discomfort or change the microclimate in adjacent spaces occupied by other people who are likely to express different thermal requirements. On this issue a Seminar on "Personally Controlled Environment: Today and Tomorrow" was held in January 1995 at the Chicago ASHRAE Winter Meeting.

Last, the standard draft could suggest periodical protocols for the thermal evaluation of environments, which could be based on objective, i.e. instrumental, and on subjective investigations, i.e. carried out via the administration of *ad hoc* questionnaires (ISO 1993a; Alfano et al., 1993). These latter are deemed of crucial importance, given the need to discriminate the effects of the thermal environment from many other psycho-physiological effects often observed in this type of indoor environments.

4. CONCLUSIONS

Due to the inherent characteristics of workplaces with VDTs, a high level of thermal comfort must be ensured to each occupant.

Therefore, the authors feel that, with respect to this, the proposed ISO standard must be amended both to allow for the more advanced standards available in this specific field, and to explicitly provide for the absolute need of using individual adjustment instruments.

REFERENCES

ASHRAE. 1992. Thermal environmental conditions for human occupancy. ANSI/ASHRAE Standard 55-1992. Atlanta: American Society of Heating, Refrigerating, and Air Conditioning Engineers Inc.

Alfano G. and d'Ambrosio F.R. 1991. Clothing: an essential individual adjustment factor for obtaining general thermal comfort. Environment International, 17(4), 205-209.

Alfano G., Cirillo E., d'Ambrosio F.R., Fanelli C., Fato I., Fattorini E., Leonardis C., Riccio G., Strambi F. and Valentini F. 1993. Proposta di questionario per la valutazione soggettiva del benessere termoigrometrico. Proc. V National Conference S.I.E., Palermo.

CEN. 1994. Ventilation for buildings. Design criteria for the indoor environment. CEN prENV 1752.

P.O. Fanger. 1972. Thermal Comfort. Malabar: R.E Krieger Pub. Company.

ISO. 1984. Moderate thermal environments. Determination of the PMV and PPD indices and specification of the conditions for thermal comfort. ISO 7730. Geneva: International Organization for Standardization.

ISO. 1985. Thermal environments. Instruments and methods for measuring physical quantities. ISO 7726. Geneva: International Organization for Standardization.

ISO. 1993a. Ergonomics of the thermal environments. Assessment of the influence of the thermal environment using subjective judgement scales. ISO/DIS 10551. Geneva: International Organization Standardization.

ISO. 1993b. Ergonomic requirements for office work with visual display terminals (VDTs) - Part 6: Enviromental requirements. ISO/CD 9241-6.2. Geneva: International Organization for Standardization, 1993.

ISO. 1993c. Thermal environments. Instruments and methods for measuring physical quantities. ISO/DIS 7726. Geneva: International Organization for Standardization, 1993.

ISO. 1994. Moderate thermal environments. Determination of the PMV and PPD indices nd specification of the conditions for thermal comfort. ISO 7730. Geneva: International Organization for Standardization.

Kroner W.M. and Stark-Martin J.A. 1994. Environmentally responsive workstations and office-worker productivity. ASHRAE Transactions, 100(2), paper OR-94-8-3.

Melikov A.K., and Nielsen J.B. 1989. Local thermal discomfort due to draft and vertical temperature difference in rooms with displacement ventilation. ASHRAE Transactions, 95(2), 1050-1057.

Nevins R.G., Rholes F.H., Springer W., and Feyerherm A.M. 1966. A temperature-humidity chart for thermal comfort of seated person. ASHRAE Journal, April, 55-61.

Rohles F.H. 1970 Thermal sensations of sedentary man in moderate temperatures. Special Report 1970. Manhattan: Institute for Environmetal Research, Kansas State University.

Wyon D. 1988. Buildings to live and work in. How do we get healthy buildings?. 14-16. Swedish Council for Building Research.

An application of "Adaptation Level theory" to experimental data concerning temperature judgment. -Quantification of the KANSEI (human sensitivity) attribute.

E. Masuyama

Faculty of Humanities and Social Sciences, Tokyo Metropolitan University, 1-1, Minamiosawa, Hachioji City, Tokyo

Introduction

It is known that Fechner's law (equation(1)) holds well between physical value X_i and psychological value J_i, while S_0 represents the stimulus threshold.

Fechner's law is defined as follows:

$$J_i = c \log X_i / S_0 \tag{1}$$

If you look at this equation more closely, then we realize that it lacks the following two variables: the background variable (Y_j) and the individual variable (T_k).

Even though S_0, in equation(1), represents the absolute reference point, that is, it doesn't move, in fact the reference point is influenced by both background and individual variables.

The eminent psychologist, H. Helson developed the theory of Adaptation Level (AL). Helson regards AL as the relative reference point rather than the absolute reference point.

Consequently, when a stimulus (X_i) is presented to subject, AL is the function of the background stimulus (Y_j) and the individual variable (T_k).

So, if we express AL A_{ijk}, then we derive equation(2):

$$A_{ijk} = f(X_i, Y_j, T_k) \tag{2}$$

But, if we always use the same stimulus set (X_i), the effect is regarded as negligible. In such cases, the above equation can be redefined as follows:

$$A_{jk} = f(Y_j, T_k) \tag{3}$$

Accordingly, Helson constructed his AL theory in the 1940's. Yet it is unfortunate that he only applied his theory to two areas: i.e. the color experiment and the weight lifting experiment[1].

Fig.1 shows the experimental result[2] for weight lifting with the same procedure as Helson used.

In Fig.1, we use that Adaptation Levels, A_{jk} is designated a crossing point where the zero category horizontal line intersects each regression line. After lifting a heavy weight (i.e. a heavy anchor), for example, $Y_j=130g$, then A_{jk} increases. Whereas when lifting a light weight, for example, $Y_j=10g$, A_{jk} decreases. When A_{jk} increases, we felt that the usual weight was comparatively

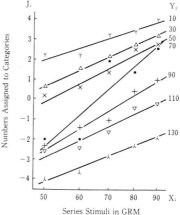

Fig. 1 Shifts in scale-value of stimuli for subject It in comparative rating methods with different anchors. Anchor (Y_j) : $10g=Y$, $30g=\triangle$, $50g=\times$, $70g=\bullet$, $90g=+$, $110g=\triangledown$, $130g=\lambda$.

lighter. In contrast, if A_{jk} decreases, we felt that the usual weigh was comparatively heavier. Accordingly Fig.1 effectively illustrates the mechanism of Helson's AL theory when applied to a weight lifting experiment.

After he published the results of his two experiments, many researchers recommended an application of his AL theory to other experimental situations, but it is a matter of regret that this does not occur.

I now wish to present the results of an application of AL theory to experimental data concerning temperature judgment[3].

Six tanks made of plastic were placed in our laboratory and into each of them the apparatus, which makes water temperature constant was inserted. The apparatus consists of a heater, an air pump and a thermometer. The experimenter turns the knob above and adjusts the temperature as previously decided and continuously observes the digital thermometer.

If the temperature remains below the decided value, then the heater operates and water temperature increases. In addition, the air pump works continuously and mixes the water.

An application of AL theory to hot-cold temperature judgment

For background stimuli, Y_j, we used five sets of heated water: $Y_1=26°C$, $Y_2=34$

℃, $Y_3=42℃$, $Y_4=48℃$, $Y_5=54℃$. Correspondingly, the stimuli presented to subjects, X_i were similarly five sets of varying temperature i.e.: $X_1=26℃$, $X_2=30℃$, $X_3=34℃$, $X_4=38℃$, $X_5=42℃$.

Experimental procedure

Firstly, each subject puts his right hand into a nominated sub-set (for example Y_4:48℃ hot water) for about 2 seconds and then removed his hand and places it in the stimulus water (for example X_2:30℃ hot water) for about 2 seconds.

Then, the subject rated his temperature impression of X_2 by using a 9 graded scale (see Fig.2) The reported value is designated as J_2. The subject then reported the procedure, for example, using Y_4 and X_3, Y_4 and X_1, Y_4 and X_5, lastly Y_4 and X_4, etc.

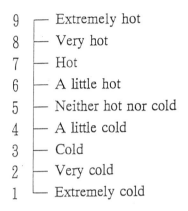

Fig.2 A nine-graded scale of hot or cold sensation

Subsequently, we can express equation(3) more specially as follows:

$$\log A_{jk} = q \log Y_j + r \log T_k \tag{4}$$

If $q+r=1$ (5)

then accordingly equation(4) can now be represented as follows:

$$\log A_{jk} = q \log Y_j + (1-q)\log T_k \tag{6}$$

Now, if we express $\log A_{jk}$ as z_{jk}, $\log Y_j$ as y_j and $\log T_k$ as t_k, then equation(6) changes accordingly:

$$z_{jk} = qy_j + (1-q)t_k \tag{7}$$

Equation(7) is a form of two-way analysis of variance in experimental design. As shown in Tab.1, the first term of the right-hand side (qy_j) expresses the background effect (row effect) and the second term ($(1-q)t_k$) express the individual effect (column effect).

Tab.1 Computation of five constants.

$Y_i(y_i)$	Subjects												$\bar{z}_i$
	1)As	2)Ik	3)Iz	4)On	5)Om	6)Kay	7)Kaw	8)Kom	9)Sa	10)Ta	11)Ma	12)Ya	
$Y_1 = 26°C (y_1 = 3.258)$	3.443	3.466	3.247	3.498	3.513	3.438	3.485	3.434	3.459	3.419	3.439	3.455	3.411
$Y_2 = 34°C (y_2 = 3.526)$	3.513	3.513	3.513	3.542	3.535	3.513	3.537	3.499	3.538	3.566	3.555	3.525	3.529
$Y_3 = 42°C (y_3 = 3.738)$	3.635	3.500	3.652	3.526	3.504	3.543	3.513	3.565	3.485	3.547	3.571	3.626	3.556
$Y_4 = 48°C (y_4 = 3.871)$	3.574	3.471	3.720	3.536	3.531	3.556	3.549	3.632	3.547	3.577	3.634	3.686	3.584
$Y_5 = 54°C (y_5 = 3.989)$	3.540	3.555	3.620	3.524	3.543	3.556	3.513	3.663	3.555	3.581	3.593	3.513	3.563
$\bar{z}_{.k}$	3.541	3.501	3.550	3.525	3.525	3.521	3.519	3.559	3.517	3.538	3.558	3.561	
$t_{me\cdot k}$	3.519	3.473	3.530	3.501	3.501	3.496	3.494	3.540	3.491	3.516	3.539	3.542	
$t_{md\cdot k}$	3.516	3.468	3.526	3.497	3.497	3.492	3.487	3.537	3.487	3.512	3.536	3.540	
T_k	33.75	32.23	34.12	33.15	33.15	32.98	32.92	34.47	32.82	33.65	34.43	34.54	Range = 2.31°C
$T_k{'}$	33.65	32.07	33.99	33.02	33.02	32.85	32.69	34.36	32.68	33.52	34.33	34.47	Range = 2.40°C

Note : Min., Max.

From equation(7), we can easily get the following equation:

$$q_{ij} = \frac{y_j - y_i}{z_j - z_i} \qquad (8)$$

If we put 'q' into equation(7) and rearrange the equation, then we can get the following equation:

$$t_k = \frac{z_k - qy_i}{1 - q} \qquad (9)$$

If the resulting value is 't_k', then we can obtain an individual constant as follows:

$$T_k = e^{t_k} \qquad (10)$$

An example of subject Kom is shown in Fig.3. From Fig.3, it can be seen that after the subject placed his right hand into hot water, for example $Y_4=48°C$, he rates J_i as relatively low. In contrast, he placed his hand into cold water, for example $Y_1=26°C$, he rates J_i as relatively high.

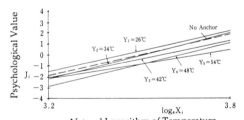

Fig.3 Shifts in scale-value of stimuli for subject Kom with different anchors.

This temperature sensation demonstration is the third application of Helson's AL theory.

A similar computation for any subject is evident in Tab.1. As the data for Tab.1 is tabulated for an analysis of variance, we can undertake a two-way analysis of variance. The result of this computation is shown in Tab.2. From Tab.2 we observe a 1% level significant difference between the background effect, but no significant difference between individual effect. Next, we calculates the coefficient q_{ij} by using equation(8). This expresses the background as shown above. And,

Tab.2 Two way analysis of variance.

Factor	S	ϕ	V	F_0
Individual	.021	11	.00191	.578
Background	.149	4	.0373	11.3**
Residual	.145	44	.00330	
Total	.315	59	.00534	

as there are five conditions in background, there are $_5C_2=10$ combinations.
Accordingly, we calculated the mean value $\overline{q}$ of 10 q_{ij} as follows:

$$\overline{q} = \frac{1}{10} \sum_i \sum_j q_{ij} \quad (i<j)$$

$$= \frac{1}{10} (.328+.240+.233+.167+.127-.157+.073+.211+.028-.178)$$

$$= .1388$$

Conversely, the individual coefficient r can be calculated by using equation(5)

$$\overline{r} = 1 - \overline{q}$$
$$= .8612$$

If we substitute these two values into equation(7), we can get a theoretical value $\dot{Z}_{jk}$, And plotting Z_{jk} and the corresponding $\dot{Z}_{jk}$, we derive a correlation diagram represented by Fig.4.

The correspondence between Z_{jk} and $\dot{Z}_{jk}$ is represented by r and the value of .6809 is quite good. Now, if we observe the background coefficient q_{ij} more precisely, we find that the distribution of q_{ij} is not symmetrical, but rather is a little skewed as shown in Fig.5.

In this case, the better measure may be 'median'. So, we calculated a median: $q_{med.} = .163$.

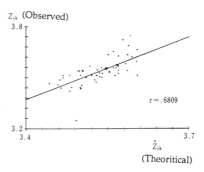

Fig.4 Correlation diagram between $\dot{z}_{jk}$ and z_{jk} is predicted from mean q value.

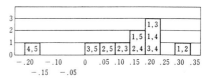

Fig.5 Histogram of q_{ij}.

By substituting this into equation(5), we derived: $r_{med.} = .837$.
Substituting these values into equation(7), we derived $\dot{Z}_{jk}$. By plotting Z_{jk}, and

the corresponding new $\dot{Z}_{jk}$, we derived a new correlation diagram as shown in Fig.6. The correspondence is better than in Fig.4.

Finally, we calculate the individual constant. In retrospect, from the time of Wundt (19c), the derivation of an individual constant has been the important issue for experimental psychology. And so, it is regrettable that psychologists have not succeeded in acquiring a correct and reliable

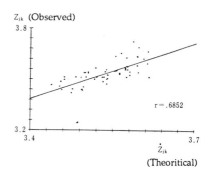

Fig.6 Correlation diagram between $\dot{z}_{jk}$ and z_{jk} is predicted from median q value.

value for the individual constant. If we scrutinize Tab.1 carefully, we observe T_k and T_k'. These constants should be designated as individual constants and can be calculated by using equation(9) and (10), successively.

From $\overline{q}$, we can derive $t_{me,k}$ and then T_k. Similarly, from q_{med}, we can get $t_{md,k}$ and then T_k'. Suffix 'k' designates the individual subject.

So, as T_k varies from 32.07℃ to 34.54℃, we observe the Range: R=2.31℃.

On the other hand, as T_k' varies from 32.07℃ to 34.47℃, we observe the Range: R=2.40℃. But as either T_k or T_k' represents the individual adapted temperature, we were surprised to find a narrowness in temperature range. A more interesting and important finding is that familiar 'physiological zero point' i.e. 32~33℃ is contained within both the T_k and T_k' range.

Conclusion

Following the successful application of AL theory to hot-cold water experimentation, we could also apply the theory to another two areas.The result of such applications may be reported in future. To summarize, the human attribute, known in Japanese as KANSEI, is translatable as 'human sensitivity'.

Reference

1) Appley, m. H.: Adaptation-Level Theory -A Symposium-, Academic Press, 1971.
2) Eitaro Masuyama: Application of "Adaptation-level theory" to Human Experiment on Temperature Sensation, Ningen Kogaku vol.30, no.4, 1994.
3) Eitaro Masuyama: An Application of 'Adaptation Level Theory' to Experimental Data Concerning Temperature Judgment.-Quantification of the KANSEI Attribute-, WWDU '94, Oral Contribution, Milan, Italy.

Biological and subjective responses to EMF exposure. A double-blind provocation study.

B. Andersson[a], B. Arnetz[b], M. Berg[c], L. Melin[a], I. Langlet[d] and S. Lidén[c] *

[a]Department of Clinical Psychology, University of Uppsala, Box 1225, S-751 42 Uppsala, Sweden

[b]Section for Occupational and Environmental Health and Stress Research Section, Karolinska Institute, Huddinge University Hospital - R64, S-141 86 Huddinge, Sweden

[c]Department of Dermatology, Karolinska Hospital, S-171 77 Stockholm, Sweden

[d]The Swedish National Institute of Radiation Protection, S-171 16 Stockholm, Sweden

1. INTRODUCTION

Epidemiological data suggest an association between EMF exposure and certain malignancies, primarily leukemia and brain tumors. There have also been a number of in vitro studies concerning possible biological effects of EMF. During the last decade there have been a growing number of people who purport that they suffer from hypersensitivity to electricity and video display units - VDUs. They report symptoms from the central nervous system, the skin and the gastro-intestinal system that they believe are elicited by EMF. We have previously reported the results of a psychophysiological study of electrically hypersensitive VDU employees, as compared to healthy controls, during work as well as leisure under electromagnetically similar conditions (1). In the following study we were interested to assess whether EMF exposure under double-blind controlled conditions is associated with any measurable symptoms.
The objective of the study was thus to assess possible biological and subjective reactions in humans purported to be sensitive to electromagnetic fields in a controlled double-blind laboratory setting.

2. SUBJECTS AND METHODS

Out of a total of 35 patients purported to suffer from sensitivity to electricity and VDUs, 17 (12 women and 5 men) fulfilled the inclusion criteria. These were that a person should experience a clear connection between being in an "electrical environment" and the induction of symptoms typical of "electric hypersensitivity". The duration of the problem should have

---

*This research was supported by a grant from the Swedish Work Environment Fund. A modified version has been submitted to The Journal of Occupational Medicine for consideration to be published.

been at least 6 months, the disorder should have a major impact on the patient's social life and occupational capacity, there should be no immediate concomitant need for medical or psychiatric treatment, and symptoms should appear within 30 minutes following the initiation of electromagnetic exposure.

Each participant filled out a comprehensive questionnaire concerning sociodemographics, work, health and well-being, as well as impact of the disorder on quality of life. The limitation the hypersensitivity to electricity placed on the patients in their daily living was also recorded. A number of the assessments were done using Visual Analogue Scales (VAS) 100 mm in length with the two anchoring points 'not at all' and 'maximum'.

Blood samples were taken prior to and immediately following the provocation session. Blood was either used fresh or frozen for later analysis for electrolytes, fibronogen, cholesterol, apolipoproteins, prolactin, testosterone, dehydroepiandrosterone, and cortisol.

2.1. The provocation procedure

Each person was scheduled for the electromagnetic provocation test at either eight o'clock or ten o'clock in the morning. Following a 15 minutes' rest period, subjects filled out a present symptoms check-list. Blood was sampled. Then the 30 minute provocation period started. Either the source was on or off for the entire 30 minute period. The provocation was double-blind and regulated by a remote computer software program. Following the provocation, subjects once again rated their symptoms and blood was sampled.

The electromagnetic provocation apparatus was set out in a specially designated house in such a way that there were no electric cables or water pipes close by. The patients were seated in front of the apparatus, which was actually an old VDU. Neither the patient nor the researcher was aware whether the apparatus was turned on or off. The screen had been darkened even though it was bombarded by electrons when turned on. The patients were seated 50-60 cm away from the screen.

The magnetic fields in the "on"-conditions were 245 nT (5Hz-2kHz) and 19 nT (2 kHz-400 kHz), respectively. In the "off"-conditions the equivalent fields were less than background level (< 2 nT). The electric fields in the 'on'-conditions were 7 V/m and 10 V/m, respectively. When "off", the electric fields were at the background noise levels.

2.2. Statistics

χ-square and ANOVA tests were used to study possible differences between the "on" and "off" conditions with regard to biological and subjective responses.

The study had been approved by the Karolinska Institute's Ethics Committee and participants were free to withdraw at any point in time.

3. RESULTS

Sixteen of the 17 patients completed 4 provocation tests or more. One of the patients did not go through the required test series due to technical problems. Thus, the results are based on 16 patients. Table 1 depicts the results of the provocation tests.

Table 1
Individual results of the provocation tests. Number of correct judgements and mean and range for certainty ratings.

Object no	No of correct judgements /total no of judgements	Certainty* (0-100 mm) mean	range
1	4/8	56.7	10-95
2	3/8	17.3	0-80
3	3/6	45.8	10-91
4	2/4	9.0	0-19
5	3/4	45.0	6-67
6	3/4	74.5	44-91
7	2/6	53.5	5-84
8	2/4	29.3	19-50
9	2/4	29.0	0-49
10	2/4	24.3	5-47
11	1/4	47.8	0-100
12	2/6	89.8	71-100
13	2/6	61.7	44-79
14	3/4	41.8	8-71
15	*4/4*	*63.5*	*46-87*
16	3/4	53.3	20-96
Total	41/80	46.4	0-100

* How certain a patient was about the correctness of his/her judgement as to whether the apparatus was "on" or "off".

The participants did not guess correctly significantly more often that would have been expected by chance (χ-square = 5.75, n.s.). They were no more certain in their guess when they actually were right than wrong with regard to the exposure condition. There were no statistically significant differences in subjective symptoms when the fields were on, as compared to off. However, when participants judged the fields to be on, regardless of the actual situation, participants rated their symptoms as significantly stronger.
There were no associations between objective measures and the on/off-condition.

4. DISCUSSION

In the present study we looked at possible biological and subjective effects of a double-blind elektromagnetic provocation test. The conditions were identical to those found in the working proximity to a regular VDU. We could not detect any significant biological nor subjective changes related to the actual provocation situation. However, if a person believed the fields to be "on" they signaled with more intense symptoms. Out of a total of 16 subjects tested, one was able to rate the exposure conditions correctly 4 times out of 4. For all other subjects, there were no results that deviated from those expected by chance alone. Some of the hormones tested, such as cortisol, are rather slow and would not be expected to show any significant changes in secretion within the aloted 30 minute period. However, prolactin is a fast-reacting hormone and would have been expected to respond, would there have been a direct exposure effect.

We are currently studying under double-blind controlled laboratory conditions whether combined environmental stress load may induce sensitivity to electromagnetic fields. We are combining electromagnetic and mental stress. Results from these latter studies are expected within a year. Total environmental load to the human body might facilitate enhanced susceptibility in some individuals to various specific environmental factors, such as electromagnetic fields (2). It is therefore important to apply a multidisciplinary approach when "sensitivity" to VDUs are being investigated.

REFERENCES

1. M. Berg, B.B. Arnetz, S. Lidén, P. Eneroth and A. Kallner, J. Occup. Med., 34 (1992) 698.
2. B. Arnetz, J. Occup. Med., in press (1995).

Whatever happened to MPR3 ?

D. Sawdon [1]

IBM United Kingdom Ltd

1.0 Introduction

In common with all electrical devices, Visual Display Units (VDUs) produce magnetic and electric emissions. Market pressure is convincing most VDU manufacturers to add "low-emission" displays to their product range and, despite the absence of any evidence of adverse health effects, these "low-emission" VDUs are quickly becoming the normal offering. Since the introduction of *MPR2*, IBM (in common with other major companies) has made a public statement that all new designs will fully meet the *MPR2* emission guidelines.

It is clear that there is still confusion and concern about the possibility of health hazards from low-frequency electromagnetic fields. In the absence of a *formal* standard for low-frequency VDU emissions some manufacturers are using the confusion to play on the safety theme to sell their products. Some organisations (ECMA, IEEE, JEIDA) are developing their own requirements. Many employees are probably confused by the multiplicity of sensationalised press articles on this topic. What is needed -by industry and users alike- is a single, formal, worldwide, pragmatic standard against which VDUs can be assessed.

As there is no generally accepted medical or scientific evidence which can be used to derive emission limits, any standard must initially be based on the premise that VDUs should not add appreciably to the pre-existing electromagnetic ambient levels. We already have a widely accepted de-facto standard (for both test methods and emission limits) in the Swedish *MPR2* guideline documents. These are based on achievable levels rather than scientific, medical or epidemiological research and can be used as the basis of such a standard until irrefutable evidence justifies a review.

The purpose of this paper is to report the progress of attempts to update *MPR2* and develop it into a formal, pragmatic, worldwide standard. At the time of writing, the work is incomplete and the proposals listed may be incomplete.

---

[1] Dave Sawdon is an EMC Consultant with IBM UK Ltd at Hursley Park, Winchester, Hampshire and is the IBM Corporate Standards Project Authority for Near Field Phenomena.

1.1 Existing guidelines

Largely in response to pressure from work unions, the Swedish government took the lead in the early 1980s by instructing their agency for technical accreditation (now called SWEDAC but then called MPR) to establish a system of voluntary product testing for all aspects of VDU design. Such a system naturally requires that voluntary emission limits (and therefore measurement methods) be produced but there was no sound scientific evidence on which to base such limits. The guideline levels were therefore developed on the basis that emissions from VDUs should not add appreciably to the electromagnetic background in which we all live. This is a perfectly laudable step, we obviously shouldn't add to pollution of any kind if we can prevent it, but it is important to realise at the outset that any recommended limits are **NOT** "safety limits" and are **NOT** based on biological research. These voluntary emission limits are "technically achievable" levels (although this term causes some of us who have to achieve them to wince) which do not add appreciably to the ambient electromagnetic levels.

The various National Radiological Protection Boards have since published exposure guidelines based on the accepted acute, or short term, effects but these are more than a thousand times higher than VDU emission levels. The International Radiation Protection Association (IRPA) and the World Health Organisation have stated that available epidemiological data does not provide any basis for health risk assessment and that nor is it useful for developing exposure limits.

The SWEDAC working group published a document early in 1987 called MPR-P 1987-2 *Testing VDUs - test methods* that is now universally known as MPR1.

1.1.1 MPR2

In 1990 SWEDAC re-formed the committee and initiated a review of the MPR1 measurement experience and of new research. The consensus was that there were difficulties in performing the "peak" measurement required in MPR1 and that this could best be overcome by replacing them with RMS measurements. MPR1 also required that measurements be made around a sphere but this was complex and unnecessary and was replaced by measurements around a cylinder. The research debate had moved away from inductive effects but, in its place, there was a new discussion on the possibility of adverse health effects being caused by lower frequency electric and magnetic fields. As a result of this review, new documents called MPR 1990:8 *Test Methods for VDUs* and MPR 1990:10 *Users Handbook for evaluating VDUs* were published in 1991 **and MPR1 was withdrawn**. These new documents are universally known as *MPR2* and, as with MPR1, are largely devoted to visual ergonomics.

The *MPR2* measurement protocol measures the magnetic field at 48 points on a 600 mm high cylinder, with a diameter equal to the length of the VDU plus 1 metre, which is centred on the optical axis of the VDU. The lower frequency electric field is measured at only 1 point on the cylinder, on the optical axis, whereas the higher frequency electric field is measured at the 4 cardinal points on a horizontal plane through the centre of the VDU.

The equivalent surface potential is measured at a distance of 100 mm along the optical axis of the CRT, at a prescribed temperature and relative humidity.

The *MPR2* guideline levels are generally known, wrongly, as *limits* and are shown in the box below.

┌─ MPR2 Guidelines ───┐
Magnetic field strength (RMS):
    5Hz to 2kHz   250nT
    2kHz to 400kHz 25nT
Electric field strength (RMS):
    5Hz to 2kHz   25V/m
    2kHz to 400kHz 2.5V/m
Equivalent surface potential:
    500 volts, 20 minutes after switch-on.
└───┘

1.1.2 Guidance from other Bodies

The Swedish TCO union were part of the *MPR2* review group but disagreed with the recommendations. Because of this they published their own recommendations (shown below) in a booklet called *Screen Facts*. The TCO measurement points are as described earlier for *MPR2* but with an additional point at 300 mm from the screen centre (along the optical axis) for all except the higher frequency magnetic measurement. No test method is provided and this is a problem since the maximum recommended levels for all except the higher frequency magnetic fields are at the lower limit of the published validity range of the *MPR2* method. Because of this the TCO recommendations cannot include measurement uncertainty.

┌─ TCO Guidelines ──┐
Magnetic field strength (RMS):
    5Hz to 2kHz   200nT
    2kHz to 400kHz 25nT
Electric field strength (RMS):
    5Hz to 2kHz   10V/m
    2kHz to 400kHz 1.0V/m
Equivalent surface potential:
    500 volts, 20 minutes after switch-on.
└───┘

The European Display Screen Directive (90/270) stipulates that emissions should be "reduced to negligible levels from (a health and safety) viewpoint" but offers no further help or suggestions. The UK Health and Safety Executive (HSE) have stated that "so little radiation is emitted from current designs of (VDUs) that no special action by users is necessary to meet (the requirements of the Directive)."

Both the European Computer Manufacturers Association (ECMA-TC20) and the Institute of Electrical and Electronic Engineers (IEEE-P1140) have wrestled with the topic. Unfortunately, for many reasons, neither would accept the concept of recommended limits or guideline levels. The P1140 committee spent several months debating whether some "achievable" levels should be quoted in an annex because there is "insufficient information to define safe or unsafe levels"; the final version has had this section removed.

The draft document published recently by JEIDA (Japan Electronic Industries Development Association) stipulates the levels shown in the box below for Japanese domestic products; when finalised it will come into force in 1998.

┌── **JEIDA VDU Emission requirements** ────────────────────────────┐
Magnetic field strength (RMS):
    5Hz to 2kHz   200nT
    2kHz to 400kHz 25nT
Electric field strength (RMS):
    5Hz to 2kHz   Grounded: 50V/m, Ungrounded: 250V/m
    2kHz to 400kHz Grounded: 10V/m, Ungrounded: 10V/m
└──┘

1.2 The new standard

When SWEDAC were approached about the need to update *MPR2* they stated that they had no wish to work on this as such work is outside their remit as an accreditation agency. SEK (the Swedish National Committee of the IEC) have since formed a working group to develop a formal Swedish standard; members include manufacturers, labour unions, measurement laboratories and scientists.

CENELEC have been formally notified of this work and have assigned a formal working group number, as a result of this step the membership of the WG is expanding. ECMA, IEEE, JEIDA and IEC have all been notified of the work and have received copies of working drafts.

1.2.1 Detailed proposals

Visual Ergonomics
    This section of *MPR2* has been overtaken by ISO 9241/3 and will be removed.

X-ray Radiation
    This is already covered by EN60950 (to which all office electrical equipment must conform) and will be removed to avoid duplication.

Electrostatic Discharge (keyboard)
    The requirement for a keyboard to provide an operator with an electrostatic discharge path to ground may or may not be valid in conditions of very low humidity. It most certainly is not valid to include this requirement in a VDU emission standard and it will be removed.

Electrostatic Potential, Alternating Electric and Magnetic Fields
    There are several detailed aspects of the *MPR2* test method which need clarifying and updating but the experience of the last four years has shown the method to be basically good. The number of magnetic measurement points around the VDU will be reduced to 8 per plane rather than the 16 required by *MPR2*. Clarification of the testing of multi-mode and multi-sync displays will be added, as will the testing of non-CRT products.

Emission categories
    3 emission categories (class A, B and C) will be introduced. These are approximately equivalent to the existing TCO (class A), *MPR2* (class B) and JEIDA/IEEE (class C) guideline levels. This should allow all interested parties to accept the new standard, rather than developing their own.

Label
    A non-text label will be introduced. This will indicate whether the VDU has been tested by an accredited test house and assessed as emission class A, B or C. Currently manufacturers are inventing their own (occasionally sensational) labels.

In-situ measurements
    We recognise that there is a need for measurements to be made outside a laboratory and will include a suitable standard test method. In-situ measurements will necessarily be far

less accurate than those made in a laboratory so a simple calculator will be provided to enable measurement uncertainty to be assessed.

Measurement Uncertainty

The laboratories that are accredited to perform measurements using the *MPR2* method (IBM UK and Semko) are required to report a value which includes the calculated measurement uncertainty. The measurement uncertainty will be reported separately from the measured value (in line with normal practise) and the detailed statistical method will be included to ensure that all labs report comparable uncertainty data.

1.3 Summary

It is clear that the markets and manufacturers around the world need a single formal standard, against which to assess and design VDUs. The difficulty is that the only solid scientific data that can be used to derive emission limits are the national exposure guidelines and the markets have indicated that these are not acceptable. In the absence of solid data some groups are developing their own limits or are marketing low emission products as "ultra-safe," both of these actions can lead to a heightened concern amongst VDU users that can not be justified.

I recognise that the concept of a pragmatic standard based on what can be achieved, rather than what must be achieved, is unusual but I believe that the circumstances surrounding this issue are such as to justify the proposal. A formal standard for VDU emissions will allow users and manufacturers to compare the emission performance of different products and will hopefully be adopted internationally.

If you wish to support this work you should lobby your national standards organisation to send a delegate to the WG. Please contact the author for further details.

Hypersensitivity to electricity - a Round Table discussion

Ulf Bergqvist

Department of Neuromedicine, National Institute of Occupational Health, S-171 82 Solna, Sweden

1. INTRODUCTION

The term "hypersensitivity to electricity" is used below to indicate a phenomenon, where an individual experiences one or several adverse health reaction symptoms, together with the attribution of the onset of these symptoms to an "exposure to electricity", often conceptualized as an exposure to an electric or magnetic field emanating from an electrical appliance. The inclusion of "hypersensitivity" in the term stems from the observations that such adverse reactions are not perceived by all, but apparently only by a subset of those exposed - these being in some way "hypersensitive". The quotation marks are used to indicate that the general causal attribution of the reaction to "electricity" is not taken for granted, but remains one of the hypotheses to be tested by ongoing research.

The appearance of these individuals' reactions have been noted in several countries, but in somewhat different settings where the first reactions were noted. For example, most cases in Sweden described as "hypersensitive to electricity" perceived their first reactions when working in front of a Visual Display Unit (VDU), and sometimes also in the vicinity of fluorescent lighting. In Austria, a common setting was the vicinity of a power line. In the USA, some individuals who reported themselves to be Multiple Chemical Sensitive (MCS), have also reported reactions to various electrical appliances such as VDUs, fluorescent lights and various electrical household appliances.

The structure of this discussion centers on a number of rather basic issues:
- Can we give a distinct description of "hypersensitivity to electricity", for example in terms of symptoms? Can this lead to a definition - diagnosis if you so will - of the problem? If we do manage this, have we then managed to define the extent of the problems, i.e. how many are afflicted?
- What may be causes of the problems? We may need to focus on electric and magnetic fields, on other physical factors, on other external factors such as stressful conditions, and on individual traits. What has been investigated, and what is known?
- Finally, we need to take a look at intervention. What has been tried in order to improve the situation for an afflicted individual - or to prevent new cases? What has worked?

This topic was discussed at a Round Table at the WWDU´94 conference in Milano. Participants were Dr Bengt Arnetz from the National Institute for Psychosocial Factors and Health in Sweden, Dr Ulf Bergqvist from the National Institute of Occupational Health in Sweden, Dr Yngve Hamnerius from the Chalmers University of Technology in Sweden, Dr Lena Hillert from the Huddinge Hospital in Sweden, Dr William Rea from the Environmental Health Center in Dallas, USA, and Professor Arne Wennberg from the National Institute of Occupational Health in Sweden. Dr Bergqvist chaired the session. This summary paper has been written by Dr Bergqvist - and represent at least one attempt to give a coherent structure to this phenomenon.

2. CASE DESCRIPTIONS

2.1 A case description

A 38 year old married woman (2 adult children), nonsmoker, she began working with a VDU in the seventies. When she began work with a new VDU in 1985, she experienced heat sensations in the face after about a week. At the same time, she suffered from (left-sided) sinusitis and excessive thirst. In 1986, she began work with yet another VDU, and promptly developed pronounced reactions; aches and rashes on the left side of the forehead and chin, with blisters appearing in these areas. Pain from the left eye, with milder symptoms also from the right. Symptoms appeared in the mouth, and later also as numbness and tingling in the left foot. Other symptoms included dizziness and asthma-like troubles.

Symptoms appeared with a new VDU, and with the VDU placed to the left of the subject. A grounded filter did not alleviate the problems. Later on, the VDU was removed, but she noticed that problems now appeared due to electric typewriters and fluorescent lighting, and subsequently also due to any electrical appliance. With time a pronounced sensitivity developed in response to various light sources, including daylight and white surfaces.

The subject can now only work in candlelight with a manual typewriter. She has problems with transportation and daylight. She is on long-term sickleave - and has also suffered major social consequences of the disease (description from (1)).

2.2 Symptoms of cases

The first topic at the Round Table was that of symptoms involved in this phenomenon of "hypersensitivity to electricity". Case descriptions from both Sweden and the US were presented by Prof Arne Wennberg, Dr Lena Hillert and Dr William Rea.

Both Prof Wennberg and Dr Hillert described symptoms of cases of "hypersensitivity to electricity" as found in Sweden. By and large, these symptoms center on either symptoms from the skin or symptoms which can be described as coming from the nervous system. A non-comprehensive list of such symptoms could be; redness, blushing, heat or burning sensations, tinglings and aches among skin symptoms, and dizziness, tinglings, tiredness and headaches among nervous system symptoms. (A description - referred to by Prof Wennberg - can be found in (1)). In the discussions, the relative emphasis of skin versus nervous system symptoms varied somewhat - Dr Hillert and coworkers as well as some other investigators did emphasize primarily the skin symptoms, and regarded nervous system symptoms (or "generalized symptoms") as something more apt to describe a person who has had this problem for quite some time, and where the symptomatology has become less well defined - or perhaps an individual with an entirely different symptomatology.

Dr William Rea presented a somewhat different description of his patients, in that principal signs and symptoms were neurological (tingling, sleepiness, headache, dizziness and unconsciousness), followed by some patients with also musculoskeletal, cardiovascular or respiratory symptoms. Skin symptoms did occur, but were less common. (See a description in (2).)

Thus the Round Table was not able to present a common description of symptoms involved in "hypersensitivity to electricity", due to the large variability across individuals, and perhaps also between case series from Sweden and the US. In consequences, studies (epidemiological, provocational etc) into the phenomenon have not - at present - been able to fall back on a clear definition of the ailment - but has generally relied upon a self-declaration by the individual as to "hypersensitivity to electricity".

2.3 Extent of the problem

Both Dr Yngve Hamnerius and Dr Ulf Bergqvist commented on the possible extent of the problem of "hypersensitivity to electricity" in Sweden. While the number of individuals claiming this problem has grown in recent years, the above-mentioned inability to give a more stringent case definition has made it virtually impossible to arrive at a definite statement as to the extent of the problem.

Dr Bergqvist gave one example. The inclusion of various - but often mild - skin reactions among VDU users could, judging by certain cohort studies, bring the number up to perhaps a few percent of the population. However, several investigations have suggested that this fairly large group appear at least partially explainable by factors such as stress, indoor air climate etc, and often with a good prognosis, see e.g. (3-5). It may be that the term "hypersensitivity to electricity" should either be reserved for individuals with more emphasis on symptoms from the nervous system, or as a small(er) subgroup of individuals with skin symptoms and with less good prognosis. Regardless of this distinction, and arguments have been presented both ways, it appears as if the group of "hypersensitive to electricity" represent a growing but still small subgroup of Swedish workers.

In for example a survey made by the Swedish Foundation for Occupational Health and Safety for State Employees ("Statshälsan") in 1990 at 118 health care centres, 1650 patients with skin symptoms reminescent of those experienced in "hypersensitivity to electricity" were revealed (6). 60 (3.6%) of these were severely affected in that their life style and fitness for work were affected.

3. SUGGESTED CAUSE OF HYPERSENSITIVITY TO ELECTRICITY

3.1 Some general remarks

It is well known that the etiology of diseases most often is multi-factorial, i.e. a disease is very seldom caused by one single factors - several factors are needed. There is no reason to suppose that "hypersensitivity to electricity" should be an exception to this. Based primarily on the experiences of those afflicted, it is at present not possible to exclude the possibility that exposure to very weak electric or magnetic fields could constitute some of these causal factors. On the other hand, it is not possible to refrain from considering a number of other factors, both external and related to individual traits.

From the observations of the afflicted individuals, a number of factor have been suggested in connection with "hypersensitivity to electricity". Some of these are "external" in the sence that they describe the situation in which the "hypersensitive" person reacts, prime examples being:
- Electric and/or magnetic field. This suggestion is primarily based on the description of the cases as to where their reactions occur.
- Some characteristics of light. Likewise, the description of the cases support this suggestion.
- Humidity and/or room temperature. This appear a reasonably well established factor for (at least) certain mild skin reactions.
- Workplace conditions conducive to stress. Again, a reasonably well established factor for VDU-skin reactions.
- Work or non-work traumatic experiences. This appear to be a fairly common description among several cases as to the situation when symptoms of "hypersensitivity to electricity" first appeared.

It should be noted that these observations, being reported by afflicted individuals, still need to be confirmed by scientific investigations. In terms of "hypersensitivity to electricity", few such confirmations have as yet been obtained, see further below.

3.2 Exposure to electric or magnetic fields

Implied in the name "hypersensitivity to electricity" is the suggestion that the reactions are caused by "electricity", viz exposure to electric and/or magnetic fields. One avenue of investigations utilized have been that of controlled provocation studies.

One such study was described by Dr William Rea. In this study, a single challenge using a situation with a magnetic field exposure with varying frequency (0.1 Hz to 5 MHz) was given to 100 patients and 25 controls. Responses were either in terms of reported symptoms, or by changes in the pupil size. In the first phase, 100 patients were challenged, whereby 25 (25%) reacted. In the second experiment, these 25 positive patients were tested together with 25 controls, whereby none of the controls but 16 of the patients (64%) reacted. The conclusion of the authors was that "electromagnetic field sensitivity" had been demonstrated (2).

In another provocation study by Dr Hamnerius and coworkers (7), simulated VDU electric and magnetic fields at various VDU-relevant frequencies were used to expose 30 patients (defined primarily on their skin symptoms). The design utilized both exposures and sham exposures of 1 hour each (repeated). Ability to detect fields from sham exposures, symptoms and certain measurements of the skin (e.g. temperature) were all used as responses. In none of the 30 tested patients could any measure reproducibly separate real and sham exposures. Dr Hamnerius reported details from another study (8), where 7 individuals were tested with "real" VDUs, and where differences in magnetic field exposures were introduced by various forms of shielding or compensation coils. Again, fields from sham exposures, symptoms and skin measurements were used as responses. There was no secure demonstration of differences between exposures and sham, although a tendency in that direction could be seen. The limited size of the study precluded any definite conclusions.

Prof Arne Wennberg reported from a provocation study with simulated VDU electric and magnetic fields at ELF and VLF frequencies in short and recurring exposures. Field detection, skin temperature recordings and symptom were used as responses, utilizing 25 cases of "hypersensitivity to electricity" and 13 controls. There were no relationships between symptom or skin temperature and fields. Three individuals did manage to detect the fields at one occassion, but two of them failed an attempt to replicate this (the third was not tested) (9).

Dr Bergqvist reported the results of two epidemiological studies where exposure to electric and magnetic fields around VDUs were investigated in relation to various skin symptoms (5, 10-11). None of the studies found any association between the fields at the VDU position and skin problems, although in one of them (5, 10), there was an association between the electric 50 Hz field in other parts of the room and skin problems.

Some studies have, however, investigated associations between certain non-skin symptoms (predominantly depression and headaches) and vicinity to power lines among members of the general public or working people. In some of these, the results did indicate such relations, while other studies generally failed to do so (12-14).

Although there are suggestions in some studies of effects of electric and magnetic fields on various symptoms possibly related to "hypersensitivity to electricity", the overall impression by the Round Table discussion was that such effects had not been clearly demonstrated. In part, the lingering uncertainty about this may also be due to our difficulty in clearly defining "hypersensitive to electricity" individuals - it makes it rather difficult to compare different studies. For example, most Swedish provocation studies (possibly excluding the one by Prof Wennberg) had defined individuals based on their skin symptoms - but this had not been a primary symptom in the study by Rea and coworkers. The observations among VDU users may or may not have included individuals with "hypersensitivity to electricity", in at least one of them there were probably very few who had declared themselves so.

3.3 Other physicochemical factors

Both Dr Bergqvist, Dr Rea and Dr Hillert gave short accounts of other possible physical or chemical factors. Specifically, little evidence have been accrued on "hypersensitive" individuals' reactions to light under controlled conditions, although provocation experiments are currently being carried out. Some cases have reported a temporal sequence between eye discomforts and subsequent skin rashes. Thus, vasodilatory reactions due to ocular muscle fatigue - presumably due to adverse vision ergonomic situations - should perhaps be looked for in these individuals.

Among chemical factors, case reports have testified to the presence of contact sensitivity to various substances in the office environment among some afflicted individuals. Another chemical factor alluded to by some of the cases is amalgam fillings. These and similar factors were briefly discussed by Dr Hillert and Dr Rea.

Despite a general awareness of several such factors as important for health and well-being, there were - in conclusion - rather limited data specifically on those with "hypersensitivity to electricity".

3.4 Psychosocial factors and stress

In contrast to this paucity of findings on physical factors, there was a general agreement that various types of psychosocial factors often appear to be involved. Dr Bengt Arnetz gave a description of what could be called a "vicious circle", where initial problems of perhaps a more modest or even trivial nature are attributed to a specific agent ("electricity"). Subsequently, the (initially) mild symptoms are reinforced by the body´s reaction to anxiety and fear caused by this perceived source of problems. Reinforcing such theories are findings of more pronounced stress levels among cases with skin symptoms (15) when working with VDUs, also when their exposure to electric or magnetic fields were unaffected. In addition, the VDU work by itself could, by many, be experienced as stressful and underutilization of skills.

Dr Bergqvist also gave an account of stress factors and skin problems in the two epidemiological studies already mentioned (3, 5, 10), where indications of stress involvement with skin symptoms at VDU work were seen.

3.5 Final remarks on factors

Prof Arne Wennberg gave an account of the various types of factors that could be involved in "hypersensitivity to electricity" - or for which at least there is a need for further studies. It is clearly implicated by the above, that investigations into "hypersensitivity to electricity" should not be carried out under the hypothesis of a single factor being responsible, it should - as actually most diseases - be considered to have a multifactorial origin. Electric or magnetic fields have not at present been identified as part of such an etiology, but the possibility has - in general - not been excluded. In contrast, it was rather clearly expressed by most of the Round Table participants, that stress or other descriptions of psychosocial factors have been identified as at least a part - and an important part - of the etiology of "hypersensitivity to electricity".

4. INTERVENTION AND PREVENTION

While research is ongoing, the individuals afflicted - and in cases of workplace reactions also their employers - need advice on how to handle situations. With the uncertainty described above as to what (combination) of causal factors may be responsible, it appears difficult to formulate in full detail a general system of intervention for those afflicted by "hypersensitivity to electricity".

Nevertheless, examples of intervention and prevention strategies were presented and discussed by most of the participants. These have often showed to be rather effective - especially if they were resorted to at an early stage. The emphasis of physical vs psychosocial factors varied, however. It was remarked that of two reasonably well documented programs in Sweden, one included extensive reduction of electric and magnetic fields, while the other did not. Both programmes included actions taken to reduce stress or adverse organizational situations. The end result of both programs were fairly similar - the large majority of cases were able to return to their normal work. It was argued that programs involving psychosocial measures were at least as effective as programs that involved both psycholosocial and physical remedial methods.

In summary, an effective program could be constructed with the following components:
- A person afflicted by reactions attributed to "hypersensitivity to electricity" should be taken seriously - and whatever preventive or curative actions taken should be taken as soon as possible.
- A first step is to have a competent medical examination. In several cases, a diagnosable and treatable illness may be found. Sick leave should be avoided where possible.
- A thorough review of the situation(s) in which the reactions first occurred should be undertaken. Based on this, a number of measures may be undertaken. Such measures could encompass measures to alleviate both physical and organizational adverse conditions. (The extent and balance between different types of measures varies, both between individual applications, and between different programs, however.)

REFERENCES

1. Knave B, Bergqvist U, Wibom R. Symptom och subjektiva besvär vid "överkänslighet mot elektricitet" (Symptoms and subjective discomforts at "hypersensitivity to electricity", in Swedish). 1989 (National Institute of Occupational Health, Solna, Sweden). Report U1989:4.
2. Rea WJ, Pan Y, Fenyves EJ, Sujisawa I, Samadi N, Ross GH. Electromagnetic field sensitivity. J Bioelectr 10 (1991) 241-256.
3. Bergqvist U, Wahlberg J. Skin symptoms and disease during work with visual display terminals. Cont Derm 30 (1994) 197-204.
4. Norbäck D, Edling C. Environmental, occupational, and personal factors related to the prevalence of sick building syndrome in the general population. Br J Ind Med 48 (1991) 451-462.
5. Stenberg B, Office Illness. The Worker, the Work and the Workplace. 1994 (Umeå University, Umeå, Sweden) New Series Report 399.
6. Blomkvist A-C, Boivie PE, Hamnerius Y, Mild KH, Klittervall T, Östberg O. Electrical and magnetic sanitation of the office. In H. Luczak, A. Çakir, and G. Çakir (Eds). Work with Display Units '92 - Selected Proceedings of the 3rd International Conference WWDU '92, Berlin, Germany, 1-4 September 1992. (Elsevier Science Publ, B.V, Amsterdam) (1993) 77-84.
7. Hamnerius Y, Agrup G, Galt S, Nilsson R, Sandblom J, Lindgren R. Double-blind provocation study of hypersensitivity reactions associated with exposure to electromagnetic fields from VDUs. Preliminary short version. In C. Ramel (Ed). Seminarium om elöverkänslighet (Symposium on hypersensitivity to electricity). KVA report 1993:2. (Royal Swedish Academy of Science, Stockholm, Sweden) (1993) 67-72.
8. Hamnerius Y, Sjöberg P. Study of provoked hypersensitivity reactions from the electric and magnetic fields of a video display unit. In Proceedings of BEMS 1994, Copenhagen. The Bioelectromagnetic Society, p 21.
9. Wennberg A, Franzén O, Paulsson, L.E. Reaktioner vid exponering för elektriska och magnetiska fält. Provokationer av personer med och utan "elöverkänslighet". (Reactions to exposure to electric and magnetic fields - provocations of subjects with "electrical sensitivity", in Swedish). 1994 (National Institute of Occupational Health, Solna, Sweden). Report U1994:9
9. Sandström M, Mild HK, Lönnberg G, Stenberg B, Wall S. Inomhusmiljö och hälsa bland kontorsarbetare i Västerbotten. Elektriska och magnetiska fält: en fall - referentstudie bland bildskärmsarbetare (The Office Illness Project in Northern Sweden. Electric and magnetic fields: a case referent study among VDT workers, in Swedish). 1991 (National Institute of Occupational Health, Solna, Sweden). Report U1991:12
10. Bergqvist U, Wahlberg JE, Skin diseases, symptoms and complaints at VDU work - investigating the impact of electric and magnetic fields. In H. Luczak, A. Çakir, and G. Çakir (Eds). Work with Display Units '92 - Selected Proceedings of the 3rd International Conference WWDU '92, Berlin, Germany, 1-4 September 1992. (Elsevier Science Publ, B.V, Amsterdam) (1993) 64-69.
11. Dowson DI, Lewith GT, Campbell M, Mullee MA, Brewster LA. Overhead high-voltage cables and recurrent headache and depressions. The Practitioner 323 (1988) 435-436.
12. Poole C, Kavet R, Funch DP, Donelan K, Cherry JM, Dreyer N. Depressive symptoms and headaches in relation to proximity of residence to an alternating-current transmission line right-of-way. Am J Epidemiol 137 (1993) 318-330.
13. Savitz DA, Boyle CA, Holmgreen P. Prevalence of depression among electrical workers. Am J Ind Med 25 (1994) 165-176.
14. Berg M, Arnetz B, Lidén S, Eneroth P, Kallner A. Techno-Stress. A Psychophysiological Study of Employees with VDU-Associated Skin Complaints. J Occup Med 34 (1992) 698-701.

Hypersensitivity to electricity and preferred remedial measures

A.C. Blomkvist and S. Almgren

Department of Human Work Science, Luleå University, S-97187 Luleå

There will always be an element of concern connecting electromagnetism with health issues. As one expression for this concern, hypersensitivity to electricity has been debated in Sweden for ten years. The present debate stems from symptoms such as reactions from the nervous system, skin irritations and general symptoms of disease, and causes are often attributed to VDUs and/or other electric equipment and high voltage transmission [1]. The National Board of Health and Welfare refers to the lack of explaining mechanisms and nonappearance of effects in provocation studies, while possible psychological and psychosomatic mechanisms are described at length [2].

A study of 32 afflicted persons, conducted in spring 1988 [3] listed the following main classes of symptoms, presented here with approximate percentages in parentheses: Complexion (98), nervous system (62), eyes (54), stomach (25) pain (25) - and eliciting factors given were VDU work (91), fluorescent lights (9), light bulbs and sun (50), electric equipment (38) and amalgam (13). At the time of the interviews as much as 53 percent claimed that they then were sensitive to fluorescent lights. The authors stated that interviewees differed according to how they were recruited, that complexion or skin symptoms have more positive prognoses than symptoms from the nervous system, and that the most successful therapy for skin problems reported was to avoid the VDU, something that was also confirmed in a study in 1992 [4].

A correspondence between skin problems and relatively high electric fields in offices was noted in a study in northern Sweden in 1991 [5]. Two Swedish companies have documented their rehabilitation efforts [6, 7], which include general improvement of the physical environment, lowering electric and magnetic fields, for example with shielding and protective earthing, i.e. 'electrical sanitation', improvement of the psychosocial environment, and 'taking the afflicted person seriously'. One company [6] reported some success with acupuncture.

In spring 1992, a project, 'Elkontoro'* was initiated by departments at six government offices, with the aim of designing a common rehabilitation program for employees suffering from hypersensitivity to electricity. The project includes mapping of the work environment, measures for rehabilitation, and follow up studies. Themes addressed in this report are symptoms and rehabilitation measures as described by afflicted persons themselves in tree studies for mapping. Follow up interviews will be reported later.

To begin with, five hypersensitive veterans were interviewed in a Mapping Study 1. Then, in Mapping Study 2, telephone interviews were carried out with 29 persons contacted via various local branches of the 'Swedish Work Life Foundation' through which their employers had received financial support for rehabilitation measures - disregarding private or governmental employment. In connection with these interviews, people involved with rehabilitation measures were interviewed as well. Last, in Mapping Study 3, 23 persons were interviewed at work after their departments had joined the Elkontoro-project, which the interviewees had approved of. The results of the Mapping Studies are discussed with reference to discussions in three recent Swedish dissertations on environmental problems [8] and treatments [9, 10].

All afflicted persons in this study have classified themselves as hypersensitive; we know of no other way to select them. There may be other ongoing studies on hypersensitivity to electricity where subjects have been selected on the bases of symptoms, for instance skin problems.

---

* Sponsored by the Swedish Work Life Foundation [Arbetslivsfonden], Nacka, Sweden

1. MAPPING STUDY 1

The veterans were interviewed at the start of the project so that they could advise us concerning questions to ask in the interviews to follow. The veterans were members of FEB, a Swedish organisation for persons with symptoms from electricity and VDUs. Three were interviewed by phone, one in his own home, and the fifth in the home of one of the interviewers. From this small group we learnt that there was no direct correspondence between source and symptom; the symptoms may be immediate or delayed after exposure, and different sources do not cause different symptoms in the same person, although there may be symptoms of varying intensity. It was further seen that these persons had periodic symptoms and after the onset of a period of more severe illness, the persons were sensitive to a wider range of stimuli. We thus state that there are sources of primary and secondary kind, the latter coming into effect when a period has started. Merging of these descriptions of periods gives a picture illustrated in Fig.1.

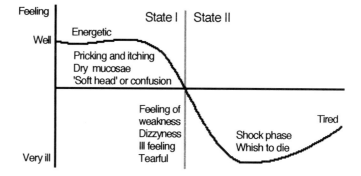

Figure 1.
A picture of qualitative descriptions of a period of hypersensitivity by five 'veterans' with severe symptoms.

State I and II refer to descriptions of change in sensitivity to environmental stimuli.

1.1. Reflections on Mapping Study 1

The periodicity of severe symptoms is of importance, we think, because the repeated onsets stimulate the search for eliciting factors, and because it is always difficult to find the correct match. The veterans reported having been active or in a good mood when the symptoms interrupted them. The dynamic development of a period could be compared to attacks of migraine, involving, for instance, prodromal symptoms, as described for classification [11, 12, 13]. Further, the periodicity may cause an optimistic response [14]; so that people report that they feel better, independent of actual change. In Figure 1 we indicate that there is a change in sensitivity to environmental stimuli by drawing a line between State I, with relative tolerance, and State II, where persons report being sensitive to stimulations from several sources. The sensitizing effect after onset causes the disease to seem more based on multi-factors than showing multi-symptoms. The lengths of the periods vary.

2. MAPPING STUDY 2

Twenty-nine hypersensitive office workers, 9 men and 20 women were interviewed [15]. The telephone interviews were conducted according to a prepared questionnaire, with open questions, were the subjects freely described their experiences. They were asked about symptoms, remedial measures taken at their work sites, measures taken in private life, and improvement. The interviews took place from autumn 1992 till early spring 1993. Interviews lasted from 30 to 60 minutes and were recorded. Also, 28 company employees, 'helpful representatives', who had tried to assist the afflicted persons, were interviewed.

2.1. Summary of results

Results are listed in Tables 1-4. Answers were categorized, and their frequency counted. As seen from Table 1, more women than men reported skin irritations. Complexion problems are dominant within the responses from the women. More women also have lighter measures taken; a filter for the VDU, fluorescent lighting turned off, and stop working with VDU. Protective earthing of lamps, cables, and equipment are frequent measures as well. Measures are seen in Table 2. Table 3 shows answers to the question about the cause of hypersensitivity. The interviewees were hesitant about number the of actions taken at home, so no frequency counts are presented, but Table 4 shows some of the actions recalled. Among the answers there was also concern about what would happen if they would have to go to the hospital, where there are fluorescent tubes, and regrets at being unable to see the children's teachers at school meetings, go to a pharmacy, a supermarket, or a library etc.

Table 1.
Number of reported symptoms by men (M) and women (F) in a telephone interview with workers in rehabilitation

Most frequently reported subjective symptoms:	M (9)	F (20)	All (29)
Pricking sensation in face	5	12	17
Burning sensations	4	12	16
Facial skin rashes	4	11	15
Extreme tiredness	5	7	12
Itching face	4	4	8
Headaches	3	4	7
Palpitations	2	4	6
Pimples	1	4	5
Dizziness	1	4	5
Listlessness	2	1	3
Smarting eye pain	2	-	2

Table 2.
Number of reported measures for men (M) and women (F) in a telephone interview with workers in rehabilitation

Most frequently reported measures at work site:	M (9)	F (20)	All (29)
Filter for VDU	4	12	16
Fluorescent lights off	4	11	15
Stop working at VDU	3	11	14
Fluorescent lights to earth	6	7	13
Shielding cables	6	5	11
Shielded cables to earth	5	5	10
Battery calculator	5	4	9
Incandescent lamp at table	3	6	9
Lamp on table to earth	3	5	8
Cabling to earth	4	4	8

Table 3.
Sources reported by men (M) and women (F) in a telephone interview with workers in rehabilitation

Sources suspected at start:	M (9)	F (20)	All (29)
Work place	4	3	7
Allergy	-	3	3
Lighting	1	1	2
Computer	2	6	8
Computer & other el. eq.	-	4	4
Amalgam	-	1	1
TV	1	1	2
No idea	1	1	2

Table 4.
Number of reported measures at home reported in a telephone interview with workers in rehabilitation

Most frequently reported measures at home:

Electrical sanitation
El. turned off at night
Move clock radio away
Do more housework manually
Exchange fluorescent lamps for bulbs
Watch TV at distance
Lower indoor temperature

All, except 2 men and 2 women, felt better after the remedial measures had been taken, even though all not programs were completed. All interviewed persons felt that their colleagues and families had been supportive. Some of the hypersensitive persons had their homes electrically sanitized, but most of them modified their routines and recreation behavior instead. 15 of the 29 persons had had, or were undergoing, amalgam sanitation of their teeth. In Table 5 remedial measures remembered by 'helpful' representatives in corresponding companies are listed.

Table 5
Number of remedial measures at work places supported by 'helpful representatives' according to a telephone interview

Most frequent measures at work site reported by 'helpful representatives':	All (28)	(cont.)	
Filter for VDU	14	Battery calculator	8
Shielding cables	12	Lamp on table to earth	7
Fluorescent lights to earth	12	Incandescent lamp at table	3
Buy LCDs	10	Fluorescent lights off	3
Shielded cables to earth	10	Stop working at VDU	-

2.2. Reflections on Mapping Study 2

From this study it seems as if facial skin problems were the subjective criterion for electrical hypersensitivity. Further, most symptoms improved; an outcome similar to other studies in this area [6,7]. It is not possible to know what role is played by spontaneous healing. Some of the afflicted persons have had symptoms for a long time. Despite the fact that they came to our knowledge because they wanted measures for electrical hypersensitivity, not all of them attributed the cause of their symptoms to electrical equipment. Measures reported by 'helpful representatives' at the work confirm those reported by afflicted persons; various degrees of electrical sanitation were the main steps taken. 'Stop working at VDU' as reported by afflicted persons, was not mentioned in by 'helpful representatives', who have been involved in physical measures, rather than organizational measures.

3. MAPPING STUDY 3

The 23 persons interviewed at work in the last mapping study were interviewed about symptoms and about their work environment. At the same time, electric and magnetic fields were measured at and around their work places, and ergonomic factors were observed.

3.1. Summary of symptoms

A structured form was used for the interview covering skin problems, nervous system symptoms and questions on psycho social matters. Frequency of symptoms are shown in Table 6.

There were complaints about the organization, or psychosocial issues, but very few demands for changes, apart from wishes to have electrical sanitation done and getting low emission VDUs.

Half of the persons agreed very strongly on diarrhoea. As further can be seen in Table 6, there is no single symptom which is shared by more than half of the persons, despite our effort to put structured questions corresponding with arising conventional ideas on the matter.

No interviewees thought that mood could have an effect on the complexion. However, one man said that he wondered wether he would not 'be able to think away' the pricking sensations, and one woman said that she got red spots on her face when angry.

Table 6.
Number of reported symptoms by men (M) and women (W) interviewed at work

Most frequently reported subjective symptoms:	M (8)	F (15)	All (23)
Pricking sensation in face	4	10	14
Headaches	4	9	13
Diarrhoea	3	9	12
Flushed face	2	10	12
Extreme tiredness	2	8	10
Sun sensitive skin	1	8	9
Light sensitive eyes	1	8	9
Heavy limbs	1	7	8
Pimples	0	8	8
Skin feels stretched tight	3	5	8
Forgetful	2	6	8

All interviewees but four had already received some amount of electrical sanitation. One way or another they manage to get help. Three men had taken the sanitation measures themselves. One person had a medical diagnosis, rosacea, but felt that protective earthing of the electric equipment was comforting anyway. Two persons came to the work place for the interview despite sick leave. They both experimented with amalgam sanitation of their teeth and electrical sanitation in their homes.

Symptoms varied among persons. Their thoughts on electrical sanitation varied less. LCDs, filters and protective earthing were desired measures. Six of them spoke spontaneously of anti-oxidants in the form of pills to strengthen their immune defense, not as an alternative to electrical sanitation but as a complementary measure.

3.2. Reflections on Mapping Study 3

The symptoms varied and do not inspire to any grouping of the hyper sensitive persons, nor to any differentiation with respect to measures to take. Conventional medical care seemed to have had nothing to offer. Afflicted persons had either received no medical care at all or turned to alternative medicines, with the exception of the worker with rosacea. As they were employed in organisations prepared to meet their demands, they represent people eager to manage continuing work. The two persons staying away both felt that their symptoms were rather unpleasant.

4. DISCUSSION AND CONCLUSION

Persons hypersensitive to electricity form no apparent subgroups, and there is no obvious way to select means for rehabilitation for them. Some people have periods of recurrent symptoms, with onsets which are hard to predict, and it is understandable if they look for eliciting factors all around them. We think that periodicity and increased sensitivity during periods cause a spread in attribution to new stimuli. Persons only sensing complexion irritations which grow during the work spell form a larger group and could be sensitive to various irritants for various reasons. It is understandable that they restrict their suspicions to their nearest environment. Moreover, research on the effects of electromagnetic fields do still not rule out the possibility of an influence of these fields on humans.

In comparison to the findings from 1988 [3], it is uncertain wether the VDUs play the same dominant role here in eliciting the disease. Another remark is that in the 1988 study and in Mapping Study 3 stomach problems were mentioned, but in Mapping Study 2, where persons describe the symptoms in their own words, stomach problems were not among the main symptoms.

"Do you believe this is a physical or a psychosomatic disease?", some interviewed started their counter-fire. This is difficult to respond to, but it seems to mean that their problems are not psychosomatic because they have not made them up voluntarily, and further, if the problems were psychosomatic, it should be as easy to think them away, as it had been to think them up - and it is not so. Psychosomatic hypotheses put the blame on the victim. Some hyper-sensitive people seem to prefer to deny psychic reactions totally, which could be a defence reaction? The only really common feature of the persons described here is that they want electrical sanitation. That is a message to us not to interfere with their integrity.

4.1. Measures to be taken

The affiliation of EMF afflicted persons in Sweden and other organizations or experts recommend immediate measures [1, 4]. Many afflicted persons avoid or restrict the use of VDUs, get rid of fluorescent lighting at work and at home and take long walks in the outdoors. Often they take an evening walk instead of watching television. Lower room temperature and better cleaning is said to minimize the risk for skin problems, and the overlaps between skin problems in general, headaches and atopic reactions should be born in mind. With reference to Fig. 1, we should try to diminish disturbing factors in State II, but remember to accept and understand the person's search for eliciting factors relevant to State I. As mentioned above, so called multi-factorial explanations might come up too easy by confusion of State I with State II.

The increase in use of electric equipment puts authorities in a difficult situation. It is too late to forbid electricity. From a historical perspective we realize that the 'technicalization' of the diffuse symptoms make them acceptable for men [8]. It is pointed out by the National Board of Health and Welfare that *psyche and soma* do interact. However, it is not pointed out that changes in the environment could be a mean to influence the psyche. Furthermore, in 'Refusing to be ill: A longitudinal study of patients' relationships with their asthma/allergy' [9] we are reminded that persons do want their own degree of health, strive for their own image of health, and interpret prescriptions and use medicine to fit their image, generally without deteriorative effects to their health. One drawback, which has been discussed in the context of recurrent panic attacks, is that they do not try other means than those preferred [10]. Our interpretation of Mapping Studies 2 and 3 and the company programs mentioned [6,7], is that electrical sanitation is preferred and carried out, also by afflicted persons themselves. When there is no decidedly better remedy at hand, which is also accepted by the afflicted, there is no real argument against sanitation.

REFERENCES

1. Blomkvist, A.C., Boivie, P-E., Hamnerius, Y., Hansson Mild,K., Klittervall,T., & Östberg, O. Electric and Magnetic sanitation of the office. In H. Luczak, A. Cakir, G. Cakir (Ed.) Work With Display Units '92-Selected proceedings of the Third International Conference WWDU'92, Berlin, Germany, 1-4 September 1992. Amsterdam: Elsevier, 1993. Pp 77-83.
2. Electric and Magnetic Fields and Wellfare. Report from a working group at The National Board of Health and Welfare, 1995-01-17. [In Swedish]. Stockholm: Socialstyrelsen, 1995.
3. Knave, B., Bergqvist, U., & Wibom, R. Symptom and subjective difficulties at 'hypersensitivity to electricity'. Investigation report 1989:4. [In Swedish]. Stockholm: National Institute of Occupational Health, 1989.
4. Gustavsson,P.,& Ekenwall, L. With shorter work spells at the VDU, symptoms of hyper-sensitivity to electricity can diminish. [In Swedish]. Läkartidningen, 1992,89, 4141-4142.
5. Sandström, M. Hansson Mild, K. Lönnberg, G. Stenberg B.,& Wall S. The Office Illness Project in Northern Sweden. [In Swedish]. Umeå: National Institute of Occupational Health, 1991. Investigation Report 1992:2.
6. Sandell, K.(Ed.) Hypersensitivity in the work environment. [In Swedish]. Stockholm: Ellemtel, 1993.
7. Johansson, K. I. Background to the results of Swedish telecommunications' action programme for hypersensitivity to electricity. [In Swedish]. In C. Ramel (Ed.) A Seminar on Hypersensitivity to Electricity, 6-7 October 1992. Stockholm: Swedish Royal Science Academy/IVA, KVA report, nr 2, 1993.
8. Hillmo, T. The Arsenic Process. A hazardous substances Debate in Sweden 1850-1919. [In Swedish]. Ph.D. theses, Linköping Studies in Arts and Science. Report 102. Linköping University, 1994.
9. Hansson Sherman, M. Refusing to be ill: A longitudinal study of patients' relationships with their asthma/allergy. [In Swedish]. Göteborg Studies in Educational Sciences. Report 95. Göteborg University, 1994.
10. Westling, B.E. A Cognitive-Behavioural approach to Panic Disorder. Comprehensive summary of Uppsala dissertations from the Faculty of Social Sciences 43. Uppsala University, 1994.
11. Dahlöf, C.,& Schenkmanis, U. Migraine. What is it? [In Swedish]. Malmö: Carlsons, 1992.
12. Silberstein,S.O., Lipton, R.B., Solomon, S.,& Mathew, N.T. Classification of daily and near-daily headaches: Proposed revisions to the IHS criteria. Headache, 1994,34(1),1-7.
13. Martin,P.M., Milech,D.,& Natan,P.R. Towards a functional model of chronic headaches: Investigation of antecedents and consequences. Headache, 1993, 33(9),461-470.
14. Foster, D.A. &, Caplan, R. D. Cognitive Influences on Perceived Change in Social Support, Motivation, and Symptoms of Depression. Applied Cognitive Psychology, 1994, 8, 123-129.
15. Hjortsberg-Almgren, S. Actions against hypersensitivity to electricity by and for afflicted employees. [In Swedish]. Research Report, TULEA 1993:18, Luleå University, 1993.

Facial Skin Symptoms in Office Workers. A five year follow-up study.

Nils Eriksson[a], Jonas Höög[a], Berndt Stenberg[b], Monica Sandström[c]

[a]Department of Sociology, University of Umeå, S-901 87 Umeå, Sweden
[b]Department of Dermatology, University of Umeå, S-901 85 Umeå, Sweden
[c]National Institute of Occupational Health, Department of Medicine, S-907 16 Umeå, Sweden

1. INTRODUCTION

During the last 10-15 years facial skin problems related to VDT work have been reported from Sweden (1, 2, 3) as well as from other countries. It has been found that selfreported skin symptoms are more prevalent among VDT workers than among other office workers (1, 2, 3). Many possible explanations of the symptoms have been presented. In conducted studies electrostatic fields, alternating electro magnetic fields, work conditions and personal factors have been pointed out as potential risk-factors. Results from recently performed studies indicates that the causes of reported symptoms are of multifactorial origin (3).

Most studies of skin problems have so far been case-studies or cross-sectional ones, whereas longitudinal studies are rare and changes in reported symptoms have generally not been focused (4). The implication of this is that our knowledge is limited concerning the permanency and the variability in skin complaints among VDT-users.

During the last years there has been a debate in media, at least in Sweden, concerning the effects of different measures that have been taken due to symptoms. In addition, we do not know how common these kinds of actions are. Do affected workers change employer, work tasks, reduce their VDT-work, intervene in the electric environment etc?

2. AIMS OF THE STUDY

The main objectives of this study are to discuss facial skin symptoms among VDT-workers in the long term. The following questions will be focused:

How do facial skin symptoms turn out over time? Have they increased, decreased or ceased after five years?

What are the consequences for affected persons? Have they reduced their VDT-work, changed work tasks, reduced their work time, been absent from work due to their problems, have they quit their jobs etc?

Have any measures been taken at the workplace as a consequense of complaints? Have affected persons changed monitors, computers and other electric equipment? Have any interventions in the other electric environment taken place?

Are there any differences in personal, social or work-related factors between individuals with positive and negative changes in symptom-status?

3. MATERIAL AND METHODS

As a part of the *Office Illness Project in Northern Sweden* a case-referent study of facial skin symptoms in 163 subjects was conducted (5). The data acquisition, which included two questionnaires, assessments at the workplaces, interviews with representatives of the employers and a clinical examination lasted from late 1988 to spring 1989 (3, 5, 6, 7, 8). A case was defined as an employee reporting itching, stinging, tight or burning sensations in facial skin *and* facial skin erythema or dry facial skin every week during the preceeding three months. Office workers, not fullfilling the symptom criteria, constituted referents. All cases and referents had at least one hour of daily VDT work.

With the intention to get a picture of changes that have occurred during the past five years a questionnaire was mailed in January 1994 to all cases and referents that participated in the clinical examination in the 1988 data collection. The return rate was 86 percent (140/163). Ten formulas had to be excluded as they were not completely filled out. By using a panel, we got a possibility to find answers to questions concerning symptom-duration and changes and the relations between symptoms and changes in the work environment during the period.

The questionnaire contained detailed questions on the following subjects: symptom prevalences during the preceeding three months, changes in symptom patterns, sick-leave due to symptoms, measures taken at work due to symptoms, if accomplished changes have had any effect on symptoms.

4. RESULTS

Using the same criteria for the definition of a case as in the 1988 case/referent-study the distribution of respondents five years later is shown in figure 1 below.

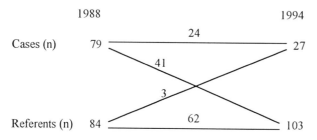

Figure 1. Distribution (n) of cases and referents 1988 and 1994.

Less then one third (30.4%) of the cases 1988 could still be defined as cases five years later, whereas for a little more than one half (51.9%) of them, the symptoms had decreased to such an extent that they no longer could be defined as cases. The 'recovery rate' could therefore be estimated to 0.52. The rest (17.7%) of the cases 1988 were dropouts.

Only three of the referents (3.6%) 1988 did report skin symptoms five years later, whereas the majority (73.8%) still could be defined as referents. The rest of the referents 1988 (22.6%) were dropouts. If we treat the individuals constituting referents 1988 as a separate cohort, and regard them as a risk population, the cumulative incidence rate for the five year period will be as low as 0.036.

Thus, we are dealing with four subpopulations: case 88/case 94, case 88/referent 94, referent 88/case 94 and referent 88/referent 94. In the following we will focus the two former, with the intention to find out why the symptoms have remained for some but not for others.

Persons defined as cases 1988 as well as 1994 more frequently reported other symptoms like headache, difficulties concentrating and mucosal symptoms 1994. In addition they reported more frequently that these other symptoms had increased during the five-year period. So in the case 88/case 94-group not only did the skin symptoms remain; other symptoms were added as well, whereas in the case 88/ref 94-group not only had the skin symptoms decreased; nor did other symptoms occur. Thus, the original 1988 case category was split into two categories (figure 2 below).

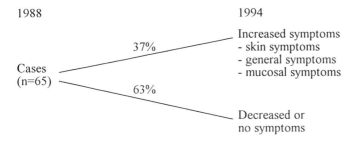

Figure 2: Changes in symptoms between 1988 and 1994 among cases 1988.

In 1988 a little more than half of the cases reported that they had symptoms independent of season. Five years later this figure have decreased to 29 percent, whereas those reporting that the symptoms are most prominent during the winter had increased from 24 to 41 percent. A minor group (11 %, 7/62) reported that they had been on sick leave at least ones a year during the period due to skin symptoms. No differences was found between those for whom the symptoms remained or increased and those with decreased or no symptoms 1994.

It is reasonable to assume that people perceiving facial skin symptoms have taken different measures due to their symptoms. Therefore some questions on this topic were put (table 1).

Table 1
Actions that have been taken during the period 1988-1994 due to symptoms among cases 1988. Percent (n=65).

Action	Symptoms 1994		
	Yes (n=24)	No (n=41)	Total (n=65)
Changed employer	4	-	2
Changed department	25	20	22
Changed building	25	22	23
Changed workroom	42	29	34
Changed work tasks	33	37	35
Reduced work hours	12	7	9
Reduced VDT-work	18	7	11

As shown in table 1 the majority have not taken any measures of this kind and there are no important differences between the two groups. Worth to take notice of is the small portion that have reduced their VDT-work.

Almost one half (46%) reported interventions in the electric environment (including the VDT) because of their facial skin symptoms (Table 2 below).

Table 2
Changes in the electric environment (including the VDT) between 1988 and 1994 due to facial skin symptoms 1988. Percent (n=30)

Changes	Symptoms 1994		
	Yes (n=12)	No (n=18)	Total (n=30)
VDT-filter	42	33	37
Monitor	67	44	53
Computer	42	50	47
Electric sanitation	67	56	60

Also concerning changes in the electric environment no clear differences between the two groups were found. An interesting issue in this context is what effects the respondents report that all the taken measures have had on skin symptoms. A little more than one half (57%) of the respondents answered the questions concerning the effects of measures taken (Table 3).

Table 3
Reported effects of measures (listed in table 1 and table 2 above) taken on facial skin symptoms. Percent (n=37).

Reported effects on symptom changes	Symptoms 1994		
	Yes (n=13)	No (n=24)	Total (n=37)
Yes	62	54	37
No	38	46	53

As shown in table 3 above, only marginal differences between the two groups were found.

In previous analyses in *The Office Illness Project in Northern Sweden* a number of exogenous factors were found to be related to an excessed risk of having skin symptoms; atopic dermatitis, amount of VDT-work, background electric fields (E_ELF), VDT-related magnetic field (B_ELF) and psychosocial factors (low support from co-workers, the combination of high demands and low support from supervisors) were factors that seemed to play a significant role in the etiology of facial skin symptoms among VDT-workers (5, 9).

If we regard these factors as long-term risk indicators, we can analyze if there are any connections between excessed risks 1988 and symptoms five years later.

Initial bivariate analyses shows that there seem to be no important differences between the 'symptomfree'- and symptom-group 1994 concerning social background, health status and employment situation. They do not differ according to age, sex, atopy, smoking, education, marital status or parenthood. An often vulnerable group, singles with small children, is not at all represented in the case88/case94-group. Nor do region, problems in the building they live/ work in, type of heating system at home, private or public employer, work time, length of employment, work tasks in general or hierachical position separate the two groups.

The case 88/case 94-group had a similar physical work environment as the case 88/ref 94-group concerning amount and type of VDT-work, exposure to different paper (including self-copying paper), fluorescent tubes, perceived static electricity and cleaning frequency in the office. The case 88/ref 94-group were more concentrated to the medium exposure group when it comes to the background electric fields in the working room (E_ELF). 41 percent of the case 88/case 94-group belonged to the high exposure group compared to 30 percent among the former. The VDT-related magnetic field (B-ELF) was slightly higher on average in the case 88/case 94-group, though the difference was not significant.

Among the psychosocial factors we found those that seem to be most important to discriminate between the groups. Satisfaction with the work-situation, relation to work-mates and to supervisors, workload and work control, all seemed to be factors that affect the probability to get better during the period. There are on average a 25 percent higher proportion of respondents in the case 88/case 94-group that belong to the psychosocial risk-groups. Due to the small number of respondents some of the covariations are not statistically significant on the 5 percent level (Chi-square) but for factors like workload/support from supervisors and job satisfaction we find a quit strong relation to the risk of still being a case 1994 when tested in a logistic regression. The lack of space in this article forces us to exclude any further discussion based on multivariat analysis.

5. DISCUSSION

The main objectives of this part of *The Office Illness Project in Northern Sweden* were to study the long term changes of facial skin symptoms among VDT-workers. So far, we have found that a majority of those defined as cases 1988, five years later had recovered; i.e. could no longer be defined as cases, whereas for a minority the symptoms had rather increased. Thus, there seem to be a relatively good prognosis for many VDT-workers with this kind of self-reported symptoms. However, as this prognosis doesn't include all, we might be dealing with different symptom-patterns and/or different risks-groups.

Different actions like change of department, building, work room and work tasks taken due to symptoms were quite usual among the respondents, but no differences were found between the 'recovery-group' and the 'symptom-group'. Interestingly, most respondents reported that they had *not* reduced amount of VDT-work, especially in the 'recovery-group'. Almost one half of the respondents reported interventions in the electric environment (including the VDT), but no differences between the two groups were found.

Bivariate analyses of the connection between factors associated with excessed risks and facial skin symptoms five years later shows that the most important factors seem to originate from the psychosocial work environment.

The conclusions are: (1) there is a relatively good prognosis for the majority of office workers with self-reported facial skin symptoms, (2) with the exception of a minority group for whom the symptoms tend to aggravate and expand, (3) concerning measures taken due to symptoms there are no difference between those with increased symptoms and those with decreased symptoms and (4) factors that promote a decrease in symptoms seem firstly to be of psychosocial character.

REFERENCES

1. Knave, B et al. Work with video display terminals among office employees. I. Subjective symptoms and discomfort. *Scand J Env Health*, vol 11, 457-466, 1985.
2. Berg, M. Facial Skin Complaints and Work at Video Display Units. Epidemiological, clinical and histopathological studies. *Acta Derm Venerol*, suppl 150, 1989.
3. Stenberg, B et al. A Prevalence Study of the Sick Building Syndrome (SBS) and Facial Skin Symptoms in Office Workers. *Indoor Air*, vol 3, p 71-81, 1993.
4. Bergqvist, U et al.. A Longitudinal Study of VDT Work and Health. *Int J Human-Computer Interaction*, vol 4 (2), p 197-219, 1992.
5. Stenberg et al. Facial Skin Symptoms in Visual Display Terminal (VDT) Workers. A case referent study of personal, psychosocial, building- and VDT-related risk indicators. Submitted.
6. Eriksson, N and Höög, J. *Inomhusmiljö och hälsa bland kontorsarbetare i Västerbotten. Psykosociala faktorers betydelse för förekomst av "sjukahus-sjuka" och för hudbesvär bland bildskärmsarbetare.* Undersökningsrapport 1991:13, Arbetsmiljöinstitutet, Solna. (Summary in English)
7. Sundell, J et al. Sick Building Syndrome (SBS) in Office Workers and Facial Skin Symptoms among VDT Workers in Relation to Building and Room Characteristics. Two case referent studies. Submitted.
8. Sandtröm, M et al. A Survey of Electric and Magnetic Fields Among VDT Operators in Offices. *IEEE Transactions on Electromagnetic Compatibility*, vol 35, no 3, 1993.
9. Höög, J and Eriksson, N. The Office Illness Project in Northern Sweden. The significance of psychosocial factors for the prevalence of skin symptoms among VDT workers. A case referent study. *Proceedings WWDU 92*, Berlin, Germany. North-Holland, Netherlands, 1993.

Measurements of some physical factors in the office environment of employees who consider themselves hypersensitive to electricity

Ö. Medhage, C. Wadman, G. Linder, U. Bergqvist, B. Knave

National Institute of Occupational Health, Solna, Sweden

1. INTRODUCTION

About 20 years ago the first "electric hypersensitive" cases appeared. They were mostly VDU workers reporting skin symptoms and symptoms from the nervous system. However, symptom descriptions were often vague and not homogenous within the "electric hypersensitivity" group. Several studies have tried to investigate causes of these symptoms. Concerning physical factors, attempts have been made by provocation studies of electric and magnetic fields [1-3]. Few studies have been made in real work situations [4], although there are some studies (for example [5, 6]) concerning discomforts of VDU workers in general that should be applicable to discomforts also reported by "electric hypersensitive" individuals.

We are presently engaged in a large case-control study of individuals claiming "electric hypersensitivity", of which current exposure situations among cases constitute a part (see also the discussion). Physical parameters investigated in this study may be divided into three groups; 'Climate', 'Lighting' and 'Electric and Magnetic Fields'. Choices of parameters were based on the general environmental situation [7, 8], VDU work [5, 8-10] and reported triggering factors for cases [4]

The objectives of this paper are to describe lighting parameters, electric and magnetic fields in the work situation of individuals considering themselves to be "hypersensitive to electricity" and to investigate associations between electric and magnetic fields of different frequency ranges.

2. SUBJECTS AND METHODS

2.1. Subjects

Four Swedish companies (in different working fields) with existing problems of "electric hypersensitivity" were investigated. Out of 868 mailed questionnaires, 731 (84%) were returned. The reported frequency of "electric hypersensitivity" were 111 individuals (15%) out of 731. Subjects worked in office environments, both single rooms and landscapes. Most of the workers used VDUs (67%). Measurements have been performed on 92 of the 111 subjects, although some factors can only be measured on part of the subjects. For example it is only possible to measure screen flicker on individuals working with VDUs.

2.2. Lighting factors

The following lighting factors have been investigated further in the study: High visual luminance, low luminance level, screen flicker and fluorescent light modulation.

High luminances were measured using a Hagner instrument (model S2) with a visual angel of 1°. A work place with a manuscript luminance of less than 50 cd/m^2, a surrounding mean luminance of less than 30 cd/m^2, and a peripheral mean luminance of less than 100 cd/m^2 was considered a low luminance work place. Mean luminances have been measured by connecting the Hagner instrument to an external illuminance probe, limited by a cone with an incident visual angel of 30°. The system was calibrated using different patterns of known luminances.

Screen flicker was measured according to [10], i.e. taking into account vertical refresh rate, phosphorous duration time, mean luminance on screen, screen size, distance from screen and pupillary size. To resolve light variations on the VDU, an optic fibre detector was connected to the Hagner instrument and the signal output was displayed on an oscilloscope. Since it is not known whether the individuals can be influenced by non-visual flicker, a floating variable has been created from e_{obs}/e_{pred}. This means that when $e_{obs}/e_{pred}<1$ there is no visual flicker and when $e_{obs}/e_{pred} \geq 1$ there is visual flicker. The floating variable also has the advantage of being analysable as quartiles. The set-up used to measure VDU flicker was also used when measuring fluorescent tube modulation. The amplitude modulation was calculated as $(X_{max} - X_{min}) / (X_{max} + X_{min})$ [11], where X_{max} is the maximum amplitude and X_{min} the minimum amplitude.

2.3. Electric and magnetic field

Electric and magnetic fields were measured in two different frequency ranges, ELF (for the purpose of detecting VDU image frequency related fields and fields due also to the power supply) and VLF (for the purpose of detecting VDU line frequency related fields).

The electric and magnetic fields were measured in three directions with an extremely low frequency (ELF) and a very low frequency (VLF) "Holaday HI-3600" field strength meter. (Table 1 shows the frequency ranges). The device was not grounded. All readings of the electric fields were done via an optic fibre, with an external device about three metres from the field meter (i.e. the fields were measured in a situation where subjects and investigators were absent). Measurements were taken at a standard position (50 cm from screen) and in the subjects normal working position. For the extremely low frequency range, measurements were also taken at four different positions surrounding the working position. These four positions were selected in the same way for all workplaces and were designed to give information on the background field level in which the subjects moved when not at the work station.

Table 1. Frequency ranges for different field settings

Type of field	Frequency range	
	ELF	VLF
Electric field	20 Hz - 2500 Hz	1 kHz - 500 kHz
Magnetic field	20 Hz - 300 Hz	6 kHz - 400 kHz

2.4. Analysing methods

All analyses were made using the SAS system (computer software for data analysis), giving descriptive data as mean values and standard deviations. All correlation calculations have been made using the Pearson product-moment correlation. Probability values (p) are presented with the correlations. For detailed descriptions of the statistical methods see [12]. We have chosen a significance level of correlations to be less than 0.001 in order to reject the null hypothesis of no correlation [13]. When correlating magnetic (B) and electric fields with distance (d) from VDU screens the following assumptions were used:

$$B = const * d^{-k} \qquad (eq.1)$$

Using these expressions for two different situations (STD=Standard Position, WP=Working Position) involving the standard distance (50 cm) and the working distance (d_{WP}) the expressions yield:

$$B_{WP}/B_{STD} = (d_{WP}/d_{STD})^{-k} = (d_{WP}/50)^{-k} \qquad (eq.2)$$

Plotting $log(B_{WP}/B_{STD})$ by $log(d_{WP})$ will result in a straight line if the field decreases with distance from screen as proposed by (eq.1). Corresponding plot for the electric field should give similar results. Linear regression has been used to derive k.

3. RESULTS

3.1. Lighting factors

The variables high visual luminance and screen flicker were logarithmic normal distributed, while fluorescent light modulation was normal distributed. The logarithmic distribution was also suggested by the standard deviations being higher than the mean values. Mean values and standard deviations are shown in table 2 below. Concerning screen flicker the measurements suggested that 30 % of the individuals (i.e. 17 out of 58 individuals) should be able to see screen flicker. All fluorescent tubes showed a 100 Hz variation. Eleven tubes also showed a 50 Hz variation but the amplitude variation was always less than 5% of the 100 Hz variation. This 50 Hz variation will therefore not be investigated further. No mean value, standard deviation or distribution can be presented of the "Low Luminance Level" since it is a dichotomic variable. However, each of the parameters used to form the variables are logarithmic normal distributions. Out of 64 workplaces, 17 met with the low luminance level criteria.

Table 2. Averages and standard deviations of high visual luminance, fluorescent light modulation and screen flicker (see methods)

Light factor	Mean	Standard deviation
High visual luminance	5000 cd/m^2	11000 cd/m^2
Fluorescent light modulation	33 %	17 %
Screen flicker	0.95	1.30

3.2. Electric and magnetic field

Table 3 and 4 below show averages and standard deviations of the field resultants at standard position (50 cm from screen), at working position, and for the background. All electric and magnetic field parameters are logarithmic normal distributed.

Table 3. Averages of extremely low frequency and very low frequency electric field strengths at different positions

Field and position	Mean	Standard deviation
ELF, Standard position	11 V/m	10 V/m
ELF, Working position	11 V/m	9 V/m
ELF, Background	15 V/m	19 V/m
VLF, Standard position	1.0 V/m	1.0 V/m
VLF, Working position	0.5 V/m	0.4 V/m

Table 4. Averages of extremely low frequency and very low frequency magnetic field strengths at different positions

Field and position	Mean	Standard deviation
ELF, Standard position	0.28 µT	0.20 µT
ELF, Working position	0.21 µT	0.19 µT
ELF, Background	0.23 µT	0.18 µT
VLF, Standard position	8.7 nT	14 nT
VLF, Working position	2.2 nT	3.9 nT

Data shows that the electric and the magnetic VLF fields are well correlated with distance, while the electric and magnetic ELF fields are less well correlated with distance (Table 5), see also figure 1.

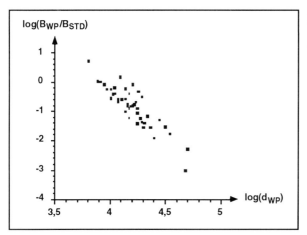

Figure 1. Plot of the magnetic VLF field (working position relative to standard position) by distance in a log-log sheet. Linear regression resulted in k=3.

Table 5. Correlation factors for VLF and ELF, electric and magnetic fields by distance from screen

Field	Correlation with distance			
	ELF		VLF	
Electric field	-0.47	(p<0.0001)	-0.71	(p<0.0001)
Magnetic field	-0.56	(p<0.0001)	-0.89	(p<0.0001)

The ELF magnetic fields at different positions are highly correlated to each other (table 6). The VLF magnetic fields at the standard and working positions are also correlated with one another (table 7). Concerning the ELF electric fields only the standard and working positions were correlated while the background field was somewhat less correlated to the others (table 8). The VLF electric fields for the two positions were correlated to each other (table 9).

Table 6. Correlation factors for ELF magnetic fields between different positions (ST = 50 cm from screen, WP = working position, B = background)

ELF, magnetic field	ST	WP	B
ST	1.0	0.9 (p<0.0001)	0.9 (p<0.0001)
WP	0.9 (p<0.0001)	1.0	0.9 (p<0.0001)
B	0.9 (p<0.0001)	0.9 (p<0.0001)	1.0

Table 7. Correlation factors for VLF magnetic fields between different positions (ST = 50 cm from screen, WP = working position)

VLF, magnetic field	ST	WP
ST	1.0	0.8 (p<0.0001)
WP	0.8 (p<0.0001)	1.0

Table 8. Correlation factors for ELF electric fields between different positions (ST = 50 cm from screen, WP = working position, B = background)

ELF, electric field	ST	WP	B
ST	1.0	0.9 (p<0.0001)	0.4 (p<0.003)
WP	0.9 (p<0.0001)	1.0	0.4 (p<0.0001)
B	0.4 (p<0.003)	0.4 (p<0.0001)	1.0

Table 9. Correlation factors for VLF electric fields between different positions (ST = 50 cm from screen, WP = working position)

VLF, electric field	ST	WP
ST	1.0	0.7 (p<0.0001)
WP	0.7 (p<0.0001)	1.0

4. DISCUSSION

The ongoing work will be directed to investigations of whether the physical parameters are related to current discomforts. This will also include a confounding analysis concerning other physical factors. At the same time personality factors and psychosocial environment will be investigated. Finally, these different aspects - physical, personality and psychosocial - will be combined in an overall analysis.

That the ELF fields are not so highly correlated with the distance from screen indicates that there are other sources than computers involved. This situation was taken care of by measurements of the background. The VLF fields obviously being more strongly dependent on the distance from the VDU when near it, suggest the VDU as a source of VLF fields. Still there is a theoretical possibility that other equipment on the writing-table may be VLF field sources.

In the ongoing analysis, dichotomised variables and quartiles will be used. This will sometimes make it hard to distinguish highly correlated parameters from each other, thus we will, in advance, have to decide upon which parameters that are to be analysed with respect to discomforts.

Only the current situation has been discussed in this paper. The reason for this is that the acute response pattern shown by the individuals, points to some triggering factor(s) which need to be evaluated. However, when it comes to factors that may have caused "electric hypersensitivity", we have to look back a couple of years and study the environment also when the cases were "initiated". An attempt has been made to reconstruct the electric and magnetic fields as they were by the time the symptoms were manifested for the first time. These data will be analysed later on. Physical factors other than the electric and magnetic fields will not be investigated in this "historical" analysis, since conditions, for these factors, change more rapidly, and it would not, for example, be realistic to try to recreate lighting factors as they were some years ago.

REFERENCES

1. Hamnerius, Y. and P. Sjöberg. *Study of provoked hypersensitivity reactions from the electric and magnetic fields of a video display unit.* in *BEMS.* 1994. Copenhagen: The Bioelectromagnetic Society.
2. Wennberg, A., O. Franzén, and L.E. Paulsson, *Reaktioner vid exponering för elektriska och magnetiska fält. Provokationer av personer med och utan "elöverkänslighet". (Reactions to exposure to electric and magnetic fields - provocations of subjects with "electrical sensitivity", in Swedish).* Arbete och Hälsa, 1994. (9): p. 1-19.
3. Rea, W.J., et al., *Electromagnetic field sensitivity.* J Bioelectr, 1991. **10**(1-2): p. 241-256.
4. Knave, B. *"Hypersensitivity to Electricity" - A Workplace Phenomenon Related to Low Frequency Electric and Magnetic Fields.* in *IRPA8.* 1992. Montreal:
5. Bergqvist, U. and J. Wahlberg, *Skin symptoms and disease during work with visual display terminals.* Contact Dermatitis, 1994. **30**: p. 197-204.
6. Bergqvist, U. and R. Wibom, *Work with visual display terminals, visual ergonomics and eye discomfort.* Human Factors, submitted. **xx**: p. xx-xx.
7. Skov, P., O. Valbjørn, and B.V. Pedersen, *Influence of Indoor Climate on the Sick Building Syndrome in an Office Environment.* Scand J Work Environ Health, 1990. **16**: p. 363-371.
8. Bergqvist, U., *Video display terminals and health.* Scand J Work Environ Health, 1984. **10**(Suppl 2): p. 1-87.
9. Knave, B., et al., *Work with video display terminals among office employees. II. Physical exposure factors.* Scand J Work Environ Health, 1985. **11**: p. 467-474.
10. ISO, *Visual Display Terminals (VDTs) Used for Office Tasks - Ergonomic Requirements - Part 3: Visual Displays.* 1992, International Organization for Standardization:
11. Wilkins, A.J. and C. Clark, *Modulation of Light from Fluorescent Lamps.* Light Res Technol, 1990. **22**(2): p. 103-109.
12. SAS Users Guide, *Statistics, 5th edition.* 1985, Cary, NC: SAS Institute Inc.
13. Zolman, J.F., *Biostatistics, Experimental Design and Statistical Inference.* 1993, New York: Oxford University Press, Inc. 343.

Overview of the special session on Melatonin and VDU work and personal results*

B. Piccoli*[a], R. Assini*[a], F. Fraschini[b]

[a]Institute of Occupational Health, University of Milan,
Via San Barnaba 8, 20122 Milano, Italy

[b]Department of Chemotherapy, University of Milan
Via Vanvitelli 32, 20129 Milano, Italy

1. Introduction

Professional activities, both industrial and "office", are almost exclusively conducted in indoor environments where the illumination is mainly artificial.

For some specific populations of workers the last hundred years has seen a progressive reduction in the already limited exposure to natural light due to technological changes. The enormous diffusion of computer based technology has caused, in the last twenty years, a further reduction. At present in almost all work situations the illuminance is ranging from 50 to 200 lux with spectral emissions which, regardless of the type of light sources (incandescent filament lamps, fluoriscent lamps, halogen lamps, etc.), are always much different from that emitted from the sun. It is now well known the effect that visually perceived light can produce via a retinal pathway on the pineal gland. This endocrine organ in the brain symthesizes a specific hormone, melatonin, which is present in the blood with high/low levels according to the dark/light cycle (3, 4, 6).

Melatonin is considered an internal "zeitgeber" translating the photoperiodic information from the environment (16) and the circadian melatonin signal is decoded by high affinity binding sites in the central nervous system (22). The exact role of melatonin in humans is not clear, but recent research demonstrates the presence of melatonin receptors in the human circadian clock (18), as well as the ability of humans to respond to the melatonin signal with a well-defined circadian phase-response curve (9). Changes in the melatonin rhythm and/or peripheral blood levels now seem to be implicated in a number of patho/physiological conditions, such as the seasonal affective disorder (27), regulation of the sleep-wake cycles (25), puberty (24), jet-lag (11) and reproduction (23).

Most circadian rhythms, including that of melatonin production, are driven by an endogenous circadian pacemaker located in the suprachiasmatic nuclei (SCN) of the hypothalamus. Starting perinatally and continuing until death, the SCN generates an approximately 24-hour rhythm in most, if not in all, bodily processes. In humans who are kept experimentally away from time cues (zeitgebers), their so called free-running circadian rhythms have an intrinsic period slightly longer than 24 hours. The SCN is reset earlier each day so that the entrained (syncronised) periodicity is that of the 24 hour light-dark cycle.

Apparently, humans require somewhat brighter light than other species (9). Perhaps this is because humans have adapted to ordinary-intensity indoor light. Sunlight, which is usually 20 to 200 times as intense as ordinary indoor light (except at twilight), appears to be the main "zeitgeber" for entrainment circadian rhythms.

Light arriving via the retinohypothalamic tract from the retina modulates SCN activity and both entrains and suppresses melatonin production. Exposure to light at night suppresses the synthesis of melatonin. Pineal sensitivity to light treatments of varying intensity, duration, and wavelength varies according to species studied (14). In humans high intensity light (seems like 2500 lux) is required to suppress its night-time production completely (9). Appropriately time dim light (300 lux) also suppresses nocturnal melatonin, but to a lesser extent (2). Inter-individual differences in that amount of light needed to suppress melatonin have also been noted (1). The degree of suppression thus depends on light intensity, exposure duration, exposure time, light wavelength (maximum suppression 509 nm) and the individuals' susceptibility (21), which plays a fundamental role in Occupational Health.

Bright light suitably timed can induce phase shifts in endogenous circadian rhythm including melatonin (5, 20). Volunteers receiving a skeleton spring photoperiod (bright light 8.00-9.00 and 19.30-20.30h) during an Antartic winter showed a phase advanced melatonin rhythm similar to that observed in summer (5). Urban populations in the U.K. (1) and Czechoslovakia (8) also showed phase advanced melatonin rhythms in summer. If subjects are kept in a strict light/dark cycle of 8h light and 16 h darkness (winter) an increased duration of melatonin secretion occurs compared with a summer photoperiod (10 h light, 14 h darkness) (25). So far Occupational Health investigations have been carried out on shift workers which, according to the most recent European estimates, are about 20% of the entire working population.

Night work is a well-known stressful condition, which interfers with the normal synchronization of the body functions as well as with the social habits. Desynchronization of internal circadian rhythms is considered one of the major causes of discomfort and health problems, as the adjustment of the body rhythms to the inversion of the normal routine is always only partial, even in case of prolonged periods of night shift work (6).

A new topic for research is represented by low and extremely low frequency electromagnetic fields which can reduce melatonin production and its protective effect against DNA damage made by carcinogens (16, 26, 28).

Besides shift work and electromagnetic fields exposure an opportune consideration should be given also to those operators who spend their work days with a non physiological exposure to only low intensity and limited spectrum artificial light. In the long term this could result in negative consequences both on operators' health and efficiency. Melatonin levels constantly higher than those normally present during day hours could reduce work performance and decisional ability with catastrophic consequences for those operators involved in some specific complex tasks, such as air traffic control, rail and underground traffic control, thermonuclear power station control and other similar professional activities.

The aim of the present study is the quantification of natural and artificial light exposure during a standard work-day in clerks operating in indoor environments.

2. Materials and methods

The study has been carried out on 17 clerks (11 male and 6 female) with an average age of 30 yrs, employed as VDU operators in "open-spaces" (group A) and traditional offices (group B),of two firms located in Milan metropolitan area. Each subject underwent a specific interview aimed at describing analytically his/her standard work-day. In the interview the characteristics of light during work-hours (task duration, outdoor work-time, out office phases, etc.) and extra work hours (type and time of travel, lunch off the premises, etc.) have been investigated in order to single out every possible moment of exposure to natural light. In addition lighting measurements by an Hagner S2 photometer at each single workstation (10-20 measurements) have been carried out, for a few days during May. The photometric analyses have been done by measurements of luminances (mainly in the "occupational visual field") and by illuminances on the working-planes, according to a methodology that we have devoloped and applied for many years, during on site investigations (7).

3. Results

Data concerning the light exposure pattern during the standard work-day of the two groups are reported in table 1.

Figures 1 and 2 show the exposure to natural and artificial light profile in subject 1 (the less exposed) and subject 17 (the most exposed) during a standard work day. The lamps used for group A environment were Osram L58W/20 and for group B environment were Osram L36W/20, both with a prevalent emission between 550-650 nm.

Table 1. Light exposure pattern of each operator during the standard work-day

Subject (group)	Waking uptime (h. a.m.)	Leaving home time (h. a.m.)	Hours worked a.m. - p.m.	Average illuminance (lux) *	Average luminance (cd/m^2) *	Commuting time	Arrival home time (h. p.m.)
1 (A)	7.00	7.50	8.30 - 5.20	60	10	60'/70'	6.00
2 (A)	7.00	7.20	8.00 - 5.30	60	10	80'	5.30
3 (A)	6.55	7.20	8.30 - 5.10	60	10	110'	6.30
4 (A)	6.45	8.20	8.45 - 5.30	170	--	60'/65'	6.10
5 (A)**	7.00	7.30	8.10 - 5.10	150	--	60'/80'	6.00
6 (A)	8.30	8.55	9.00 - 5.30	170	--	10'	5.35
7 (A)	6.30	7.00	8.30 - 4.40	150	20	100'+ 40'^	6.00
8 (A)	8.00	8.40	8.45 - 5.30	170	20	10'	5.35
9 (A)	7.15	7.35	8.25 - 4.40	150	18	60'/80'	5.20
10 (A)	6.30	7.15	8.00 - 4.40	160	18	80'/100'	5.40
11 (A)**	7.00	7.40	8.00 - 5.00	160	26	45'	5.30
12 (A)	7.00	8.20	8.30 - 5.30	160	16	20'	5.40
13 (B)	7.15	8.20	9.30 - 4.00	510	73	40'+ 45'^	4.50
14 (B)	8.00	9.00	9.30 - 8.15	380	38	45'	8.30
15 (B)	7.20	8.10	8.45 - 5.30	200	45	70'	6.10
16 (B)	7.00	8.15	9.45 - 4.00	450	52	105'	5.00
17 (B)	6.30	8.00	8.30 - 6.30	550	148	10'+ 20'^	7.00

* At the workstation (natural light only)   ^ By underground railway
** These operators spend respectively 15' and 30' outdoor during spring and summertime at lunch.

Fig. 1 Light exposure during a standard work day (subject 1)

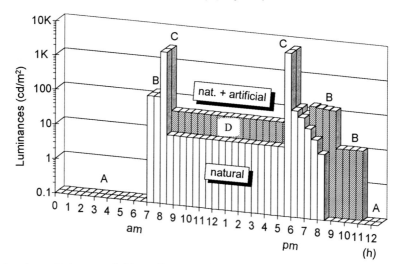

A: sleeping time - B: home activities - C: commuting time - D: working time

Fig. 2 Light exposure during a standard work day (subject 17)

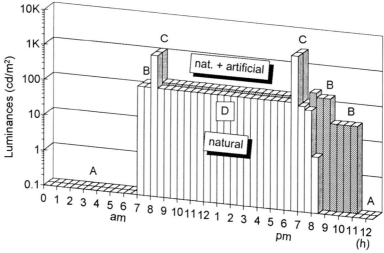

A: sleeping time - B: home activities - C: commuting time - D: working time

4. Conclusions

The photometric measurements have shown a low level of natural light at the workstation in both groups of workers, more accentuated in group A (open-space operators). These lighting conditions are, in our experience (over 50 firms investigated), very common among offices equipped with VDUs (a few million only in our region, Lombardy).

It should be pointed out that the two main methods for light measurements commonly used to evaluate the dose/response relationship in studies on melatonin, i.e. spectroradiometer (watts per unit area) and illuminance meter (lux) do not seem to be the most appropriate for this purpose. The first in fact, though very precise in terms of quantification, is very complicated to use and requires an analytic evaluation for limited bands of spectrum, therefore making it impractical for Occupational Health investigations. The other, developed mainly to measure the quantity of light present on the work surfaces, can not measure the actual amount of light that penetrates the subject's eyes, which is the parameter melatonin levels depend on. The illuminance meter, in fact, does not take into proper account, as the eye does, the reflection of light falling on the different "mediums" surrounding the operator (wall, ceiling, floors, tables, windows, etc.). For these purposes, and particularly in field studies, it seems much more appropriate to use a luminance meter.

To conclude it is evident that the exposure to dim-light during diurnal hours is today very common among office operators and particularly VDU operators. We believe that the consequences, both in terms of health and efficiency, of these working situations represent an interesting subject for pineal researchers and Occupational Health doctors and constitute an excellent occasion for developing interdisciplinary researches in this field.

REFERENCES

1. C.J. Bojkowski, J. Arendt, Annual changes in 6 sulphatoxymelatonin excretion in man, Acta Endocrinol., 117, 470-476 (1988).
2. C.J. Bojkowski, M. Aldhous, J. English, C. Franey, A.L. Poulton, D. Skene, J. Arendt Suppression of nocturnal plasma melatonin and 6-sulphatoxymelatonin by bright and dim light in mail, Horm. Metabol. Res., 19, 437-440 (1987).
3. G.C. Brainard, A.L. Lewy, M. Menaker, R.H. Fredrickson, L.S. Miller, R.G. Weleber, V. Cassone, D. Hudson.,Effect of light wavelength on the suppression of nocturnal plasma melatonin in human volunteers, Ann. N. Y. Acad. Sci.,452, 376-378 (1985).
4. G.C. Brainard, A.J. Lewy, M. Menaker, R.H. Fredrickson, L.S. Miller,R.G. Weleber, V. Cassone, D. Hudson, Dose-response relationship between light irradiance and the suppression of plasma melatonin in human volunteers, Brain Research, 454, 212-218 (1988).
5. J. Broadway, J. Arendt, S. Folkard, Bright light phase shifts the human melatonin rhythm during Antartic winter, Neurosc. Lett., 79, 185-189 (1987).
6. G. Costa, G. Ghirlanda, D.S. Minors, J. M., Effect of bright light tolerance to night work, Scand. J. Work Environ. Health, 19, 14-20 (1993).
7. A. Grieco, B. Piccoli, Visione e lavoro. Nota I: metodo per la valutazione del carico visivo e delle condizioni illuminotecniche nei luoghi di lavoro, Med. Lav., 73, 496-514 (1982).
8. Illnerova, P. Zvolski, J. Vanecek, The circadian rhythm in plasma melatonin concentration of the urbanized man: the effect of summer and winter time, Brain. Res. 328, 186-189 (1985).
9. A.J. Lewy, T. A. Wehr, F.K. Goodwin, D.A. Newsome, S.P Markey, Light suppresses melatonin secretion in humans, Science, 210, 1267-1269 (1980).

10. A.J. Lewy, R.L. Sack, M. Blood, V.K. Bauer, N. L. Cutler, Melatonin and the light-dark cycle. A. Grieco, G. Molteni, E. Occhipinti, B. Piccoli (eds), Book of short papers vol 3. Work with Display Units 1994, E 18.
11. K. Petrie, J.V. Conaglen, L. Thompson, K. Chamberlain, Effect of melatonin on jet-lag after long haul flights, Br. Med. J.,298, 705 (1989).
12. B. Piccoli, I. Gratton, R. Perris, A. Grieco, L'indagine ergoftalmologica sul campo: esempio di intervento su un gruppo di operatori video addetti a lavori di contabilità amministrativa, Med. Lav., 79,288-297 (1988).
13. B. Piccoli, R. Maltoni, P.L. Zambelli, A. Grieco, Lo studio delle luminanze al posto di lavoro: metodo e risultati di una esperienza sul campo. Proceedings from 8° National Congress of A.I.D.I.I., Como, Italy, 68-71 (1988).
14. R.J. Reiter, Action spectra, dose-response relationships, and temporal aspects of light effects on the pineal gland, Ann. N. Y. Acad. Sci., 215-230 (1985).
15. R.J. Reiter, F. Fraschini, Advance in pineal research: 2. R.J. Reiter, F. Fraschini (eds.) John Libbey London-Paris.
16. R.J. Reiter, Pineal melatonin: cell biology of its synthesis and of its pathological interactions, Endocr. Rev., 12, 151 (1991).
17. R.J. Reiter, Electromagnetic fields and melatonin: interactions and potential association with work at a video display unit, A. Grieco, G. Molteni, E. Occhipinti, B. Piccoli (eds), Book of short papers vol 3 . Work with Display Units 1994 E 12.
18. S.M. Reppert, D.R. Weaver, S.A. Rivkees, E.G. Stopa, Putative melatonin receptors in human biological clock, Science 242,78 (1988).
19. R.L Sack, M.L Blood, A.J. Lewy, Melatonin rhythms and shift workers, Sleep, 15 (2), 434-441 (1992).
20. T.L. Shanahan, C.A. Czeisler, Light exposure induces equivalent phase shifts of the endogenous circadian rhythms of circulating plasma melatonin and core body temperature in men, J. Clin. Endocrinol. Metab., 73, 227-235 (1991).
21. D. J. Skene, S. Deacon, J. Arendt, Light and melatonin responses in humans, A. Grieco, G. Molteni, E. Occhipinti, B. Piccoli (eds), Book of short papers vol 3. Work with Disply Units 1994 E 4.
22. B. Stankov, F. Fraschini, R. J. Reiter, The melatonin receptor: distribution, biochemistry and pharmacology. H-S. Yu, R.J. Reiter (eds), CRC Press, Boca Raton, chapter 7, 155-186 (1993).
23. B.C.G. Voordouw, R. Euser, R.E.R. Verdok, B.Th. Alberda,F.H. de Jong, A.C. Drogendijk, B.C.J.M. Fauser, M. Cohen, Melatonin and melatonin-progestin combinations alter pituitary-ovarian function in women and can inhibit ovulation, J. Clin. Endocrinol. Metab.,74, 108 (1992).
24. F. Waldahauser, H. Steger, Changes in melatonin secretion with age and pubescence, J. Neural. Transm. Suppl. 21, 183 (1986).
25. T. A. Wehr, The durations of human melatonin secretion and sleep respond to changes in daylength (photoperiod), J. Clin. Endocrinol. Metab. 73, 1276 (1991)
26. H. A. Welker, P. Semm, R. P. Willing, J. C. Commentz, W Wiltschko, L. Vollrath, Effects of artificial magnetic field on serotonin N-acetyltransferase activity and melatonin content of the rat pineal gland,Exp. Brain Res., 50, 426-432 (1983).
27. B.W. Wilson, L.E. Anderson, D.I. Hilton, R.D. Phillips, Chronic exposure to 60 Hz electric field: effects on pineal function in the rat, Bioelectromagnetic, 2, 371-380 (1981).
28. L. Wetterberg, J. Beck-Friis, B.F. Kiellman, Melatonin as a marker of a subgroup of depression in adults. M. Shafii, S.L. Shafii (eds), American Psychiatric Press, Washington, 69 (1990).

Mouse Input Devices and Work-Related Upper Limb Disorders

T. J. Armstrong[a]; B. J. Martin[a]; A. Franzblau[a], D. M. Rempel[b], P. W. Johnson[b]

[a]The Center for Ergonomics, The University of Michigan, Ann Arbor, MI 48109-2117

[b]The University of California Ergonomics Laboratory, Richmond, CA 94804

1. INTRODUCTION

There is general acceptance of the association between upper limb musculoskeletal disorders and work that entails repeated and sustained exertions — particularly in combination with high force, certain postures and localized contact stress [1]. This paper examines emerging evidence that these disorders and factors are associated with use of a mouse as an input device. Biomechanical arguments are used to examine the relationship between mouse and task design parameters and force exertion patterns and to develop recommendations for mouse design and use.

2. HEALTH AND MOUSE USE PATTERNS

Franzblau et al. [2] examined the incidence of carpal tunnel syndrome and the pattern of mouse usage in a medical illustration department. Three cases of carpal tunnel syndrome were identified from existing medical information among seven (4 female and 3 male) of the "graphic artists," while no cases were found among 39 (24 females and 15 males) "other" office workers. This trend was significant ($p<0.01$ Fisher's exact test) and was confirmed via an independent survey of symptoms and electrodiagnosis. The average age of the "graphic artists," 37 years, was not significantly different than "others," 38 years; both were significantly less than the mid-fifty range reported for "classic" carpal tunnel syndrome patients [3]. All three of the initial cases were among female "graphic artists," which suggests an association with gender. Findings of symptoms among male workers in the follow up survey, however, show that this is not a problem unique to female workers. Patterns of mouse usage were evaluated via a work sampling technique in which workers were observed at fixed intervals throughout their work shift to determine the percent time occupied by selected work tasks. Significant differences were found between "graphic artists" and "others" for "total mouse use" and "cut and paste " and paste with the mouse, 32% versus 13% and 13.5% versus <1% respectively. Although a small pilot study, these data suggest an association between mouse usage and upper limb disorders.

Johnson et al. [4], using video analysis of ten computer operators, found that mouse usage accounted for 30%, 40% and 65% of the time spent performing word processing, database/spreadsheet and graphics/drawing tasks. This finding is consistent with that reported by Franzblau; however, it does not mean that persons performing word processing and spreadsheet tasks do not do other things which would make them at risk of upper limb disorder, e.g., keyboard work or file handling. It does mean that mouse design is likely to have a greater effect on those performing the graphics/drawing tasks than those performing other tasks. A simple biomechanical analysis provides a vehicle for investigating the relationship between patterns of mouse usage and factors of upper limb musculoskeletal disorders and develop recommendations for mouse design and further research.

2.1. Force

The mouse is used to select commands for control of the computer and to move objects from one location to another. Some control commands require the user to position the cursor over a selected location on the screen and push the control button. These actions are characterized as "point and click." Other commands and certain editing commands require the user to hold the mouse button down while moving the mouse. These actions are characterized as "dragging." In either case, movements of the mouse are limited by the available work space or the range of joint motion. Therefore movements with the mouse tend to occur in a cyclical manner in which the mouse is slid in one direction and then lifted and moved in the opposite direction to the starting point.

Use of a mouse requires exertion of force with the fingers and palm to overcome the button, gravity, inertia and friction forces. The button and gravity forces are static, i.e., independent of velocity and acceleration, whereas the friction and inertial forces are dynamic. A simplified free body diagram of the mouse shown in Figure 1 illustrates the spatial relationship between the static forces. The gravity force and button force both act downward in the negative z direction. For simplicity, it is assumed that the center of pinch passes through the center of mouse gravity. This means that the mouse would balance between the two fingers when it is held without applying force on the button, F_b. The relationship between pinch force, F_p, weight of the mouse, W, and the coefficient of friction, μ, can be expressed with the following inequality:

$$F_p \geq W/2\mu \tag{1}$$

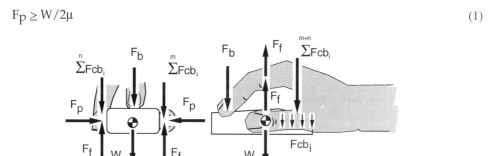

Figure 1. Free body diagram shows static forces on mouse while pressing button and holding mouse. (W, weight; F_b, finger-button force; F_p, pinch force, F_f, finger-mouse friction; Fcb_i counter-balance force on thumb, fingers and palm)

This expression is written as an inequality because F_p is a minimum and may be exceeded without dropping the mouse. Coefficient of friction, μ, data have not yet been reported for specific mouse materials. Buchholz et al. [5] reported that the coefficient of friction is highly variable; they reported values of 0.51±0.15 for vinyl-skin. It can be calculated that the average minimum force required to hold a widely used mouse weighing 1.3N would be 1.3N. Using a specially instrumented mouse, Johnson et al. [4] measured an average 1.4±1.1N pinch force for ten subjects lifting a 1.3N mouse. The average measured value exceeds the calculated value by a factor of only 1.1; but the measured force varied greatly from subject to subject and was skewed toward the higher values.

When force is applied to the button, the mouse tends to rotate out of the user's hand. This requires a counter balance force, ΣF_{cbj}, to prevent it from rotating. The counter balance force is written as a summation because the forces maybe distributed over the palm, thumb, or fingers. Thus additional force must be exerted to overcome F_b and ΣF_{cbj}. If it is assumed that the location of F_b and ΣF_{cbj} are equal distances from the center of pinch, then they will be equal and the total downward force will be double that of the button. Johnson et al. [4] measured 1.6±.4N and 2.0±1.0N respectively on the button requiring 0.7N for a single click to select a menu item and a sustained exertion required to drag. The average measured button force exceeds the minimum required force by a factor 2.3 to 2.8.

It can be calculated that a minimum of 2.6N is required to hold the 1.3N mouse and to activate the 0.7N button described by Johnson et al. 1994 . They measured 4.0±2.8N pinch forces to hold the mouse while dragging. The average measured force exceeds the predicted minimum by a factor of 1.5.

Johansson and Westling [6] referred to the force exerted above the minimum required as the "safety margin." They reported that the safety margin for subjects lifting 2-8N weights decreased from a factor exceeding 2 in the first second and stabilized at a factor of approximately 1.2 in the following ten seconds. Armstrong et al. [7] reported that forces exerted in keyboard use typically exceed the minimum required force by a factor of 2.5 to 3.9. Keystrokes typically required less than 50ms. The magnitude of the safety factors might be influenced by operator experience, style and anxiety. Taking into consideration the safety margin for the button, $F_{bsafety}$, the safety margin for holding the mouse, F_{safety}, pinch force can be estimated:

$$F_p = (W + (F_b + F_{bsafety}) + \Sigma F_{cbi})/2\mu + F_{safety} \qquad (2)$$

Figure 1 illustrates the case where the mouse is supported by the hand against the downward force of gravity. Pressing the mouse down on a work surface would produce a vertical force component upward that could exceed that of gravity. The weight of the hand should provide sufficient downward force in most cases; however, excess force may be exerted if the cursor does not respond properly.

Movement of the mouse over a work surface produces horizontal drag forces opposite the direction of motion. Movements side to side (perpendicular to the long axis of the forearm) produce drag that acts directly on the thumb or opposing fingers. Movements in and out (parallel to the long axis of the forearm) produce drag forces perpendicular to the fingers and thumb, which require increased pinch force. Friction forces are related to the downward contact force between the mouse and the work surface and to the coefficient of dynamic friction [8]. The coefficient of dynamic friction and the downward force should be low if the mouse is maintained properly.

The inertial force on the mouse is equal to mass x acceleration. As a practical matter, the inertial force on a 1N mouse will be small with respect to a 10N hand. The side to side hand acceleration could be as high as 2g's, which would increase the pinch force by two times the weight of the mouse or 2N for a 1N mouse [9]. High inertial forces cannot be sustained due to the limited range of joint motion. Also, it is unlikely that computer operations would require repetitive high mouse accelerations. Taking into consideration drag, F_{drag}, and inertial forces, $F_{inertial}$, Pinch force can be estimated:

$$F_p = (W + (F_b + F_{bsafety}) + \Sigma F_{cbi})/2\mu + F_{drag} + F_{inertial} + F_{safety} \qquad (3)$$

By convention, force is normalized as a percentage of maximum voluntary contraction (%MVC) as an index of physiological burden. For design purposes, it is common practice to consider the "worst case scenario," which would correspond the tasks with the highest force requirements performed by the weakest subjects. Dragging was identified as a possible risk factor by Franzblau et al. [2] and as the mouse tasks with the highest force requirements by [4]. An average button force of 2N would result in an exertion of 6%MVC for an average female with a second digit strength of 36N; however, 50% of the exertions were greater than 2N and 50% of the females were weaker than 36N [10]. Similarly the average pinch strength of 4N would result in an average button force of 8%MVC, but could be much higher for some exertions and some individuals. While relative workloads associated with mouse use are low for most people in comparison with industrial work in the industrial sector, studies show that prolonged exertions at low force levels may lead to adverse health effects [1]. Such problems might be associated with abnormal work schedules that result in high work loads and prolonged work shifts. All tasks, including mouse work should be designed so that there are conspicuous recovery periods at regular intervals. The force required to hold and use the mouse and the risk of upper limb disorders can be minimized by:
- minimizing mouse weight
- minimizing button force
- maximizing mouse-finger friction
    - selection of surface texture [8]
    - provide mechanical interference, e.g., indentations on sides of mouse
- orient button to reduce the vertical force component
- maintain mouse so that it tracks properly
- provide force feedback to users
- train users to minimize force of exertion and to relax between exertions

2.2. Contact Stress

Not only is the magnitude of the force important, but also so is the force location and the area of contact. Forces may be transferred through the surface of the skin and cause elevated pressure on underlying nerve and tendon tissues [11]. Although contact stress has not been specifically studied in the context of mouse use and upper limb disorders, it has been a suggested factor of disorders associated with certain hand tools [12, 13, 14].

Contact stress is related to the magnitude of the force divided by the area of contact. Some areas of the body are more vulnerable to adverse effects of contact stress than others. These include the sides of the fingers, the base of the palm and the elbow where contact stresses will be transmitted to underlying nerves. The pulps of the fingers and the fleshy areas at the base of the thumb and little finger should tolerate the stresses associated with mouse usage well as long as the user does not exert extremely high forces and the edges of the mouse are well rounded. The greatest stress concentrations

may come from the edges of the work surface or chair as the mouse is used. Contact stresses can be minimized by:
- minimizing force (see above)
- providing rounded edges on mouse
- providing rounded edges on work surfaces and chair
- locating mouse so as to avoid contact between wrist and work surface

2.3. Stressful postures

Stressful postures include radial and ulnar deviation of the wrist, flexion and extreme extension, inward rotation of the forearm and extended forward and sideward reaches [11,15,16,17]. Responding to musculoskeletal reports, Karlquist et al. [16] compared upper limb postures and movements in mouse users with those of non-mouse users. They found >15° ulnar wrist deviation and >30° outward shoulder rotation 64% and 81% of work time respectively for mouse users versus only 4% and 0% of work time for non-mouse users. These "non-neutral" postures and pinch forces both are associated with upper limb musculoskeletal disorders.

Radial and ulnar deviation is associated with side to side motions of the mouse. The required movement is related to the sensitivity of cursor to mouse movement and to the distance moved on the screen. There is a trade-off between the sensitivity required to maximize accuracy versus that required to minimize distance of movements. Each operator should be trained to adjust this sensitivity as needed. Deviations of the wrist may be minimized by using the entire forearm; however, there might be an energy penalty associated with the added mass of the forearm. Use of shorter motions could reduce deviations, but this would be slower and result in additional movements.

Flexion and extension of the wrist are related to the elevation of the mouse with respect to the elbow. Neither should be excessive if the mouse is located near elbow height. Inward rotation of the forearm is necessary to position the hand over the mouse. It might be reduced somewhat by an asymmetric mouse. This would required right and left handed mouse designs. Reaching for the mouse is related to where the mouse is located with respect to the user. It is desirable that the mouse be located directly in front of the user so that the user can keep the elbow close to the side of their torso. The work station should include room near the near keyboard so that both the keyboard and mouse can be adjusted for each operator as needed.

2.4. Frequency and Duration

In addition to the magnitude of the posture and force, the frequency and duration of exposure are also important factors of upper limb disorders [17, 18, 19]. The frequency of mouse operations are dictated by the task requirements. The force and time advantage between the keyboard and mouse will vary from task to task. In some cases tasks can be executed more quickly and with less force through a combination of keys than with a mouse and a pull down menu that require drag operations. In other cases it may be faster to point at a command than to type instructions. Theoretically, use of the fastest input device could free up some work time for recovery; however, in most cases that time is likely to be used to perform additional work. The choice of the mouse or keyboard input device most likely will be dictated by the work content, production quota, software, and user experience. If the mouse is used, then steps should be taken to minimize the magnitude of force and posture stresses. Further studies are required to determine acceptable work schedules for given tasks and equipment. In some cases it may be possible to optimize schedule tasks so that work is distributed among parts of the body according to each's capacity and no single part is overloaded.

3. SUMMARY

Use of a mouse input device exposes users to stresses associated with upper limb musculoskeletal disorders. Acceptable limits for these stresses have not yet been determined. In most cases, choice of a mouse or other input device will be based on other task and user factors. Whatever device is used, steps should be taken to minimize the magnitude of force and posture. Additional research is necessary for optimal mouse and work station designs that minimize force, contact and posture stresses. Further studies are also necessary to determine acceptable exposure regimes based on comfort, fatigue and risk of upper limb disorders.

REFERENCES

1. T. Armstrong, P. Buckle, L. Fine, M. Hagberg, B. Jonsson, A. Kilbom, I. Kuorinka, B. Silverstein, G. Sjogaard and E. Viikari-Juntura, Scand. J. Work Env. Hlth., 19 (1993) 73-84.
2. A. Franzblau, D. Flaschner, J. Albers, S. Blitz, R. Werner and T. Armstrong, Arch. Env. Hlth., 48 (1993) 164-170.
3. G. Franklin, J. Haug, N. Heyer, H. Checkoway, N. Peck. Occupational carpal tunnel syndrome in Washington State, 1984-1988. Am. J. Pub. Hlth., 81 (1991) 741-746.
4. P. Johnson, W. Smutz, R. Tal and D. Rempel, Proceedings of the 1994 International Ergonomics Association Conference, Toronto, Canada, 2 (1994) 208-210.
5. B. Buchholz, L. Frederick and T. Armstrong, Ergonomics, 31 (1988) 317-325.
6. R. Johansson and G. Westling, Exp. Brain Res., 56 (1984) 550-564.
7. T. Armstrong, J. Foulke, B. Martin, J. Gerson, and D. Rempel, Am. Indust. Hyg. Assoc. J. 55 (1994) 30-35.
8. O. Bobjer, S. Johansson and S. Piguet, Appl. Ergo., 24 (1993) 190-202.
9. D. Hoffman and P. Strick, II EMG Analysis. J. Neurosci., 10 (1990) 142-152.
10. A. Swanson, I. Matev and G. Groot. Bull. Pros. Res., 10 (1970) 145.
11. R. Gelberman, P. Hergenroeder, A. Hargens, G. Lundborg and W. Akeson, J. Bone Joint Surg., 63A (1981) 380-383.
12. J. Dobyns, E. O'Brien, R. Linscheid and G. Farrow, J. Bone Joint Surg., 54A (1972) 751-755.
13. J. Hoffman and P. Hoffman, J. Occ. Med., 27 (1985) 848-849.
14. S. Sauter, L. Chapman, S. Knutson and H. Anderson, Appl. Ergo., 18 (1987) 183-186.
15. T. Armstrong, in N. Corlett, J., J. Wilson, and I. Manenica (eds.), The Ergonomics of Working Postures, London: Taylor and Francis, (1986) 59-73.
16. L. Karlquist, M. Hagberg and K. Selin, Ergonomics, 37 (1994) 1261-1268.
17. R. Szabo and L. Chidgey, J. Hand Surg., 14A (1989) 624-627.
18. K. Maeda, Sumitomo Sangyo Eisei, 10 (1974)135-143.
19. M. Oxenburgh, Proceedings of the 21st Annual Conference of the Ergonomics Society of Australia and New Zealand, Sydney, Australia (1984) 137-143.

The "mouse-arm syndrome" - concurrence of musculoskeletal symptoms and possible pathogenesis among VDU operators

M. Hagberg

National Institute of Occupational Health, Division of Work and Environmental Physiology, S-17184 Solna, Sweden

1. INTRODUCTION

Symptoms in the neck, shoulder, forearm and wrist have been related to the introduction of to the use of the non-keyboard computer input device such as the computer mouse in case histories from occupational health care personnel in Sweden.

The symptoms among mouse users in Sweden have been termed "mouse-syndrome" or "mouse-arm syndrome" by the patients and occupational health care personnel. Whether there exist a specific syndrome is obscure. In the scientific literature there are neither reports describing the specific health outcomes of non-keyboard computer input devices nor reports on exposure-effect relationships.

1.1. Aim

The aim of this presentation is to evaluate the concurrence of musculoskeletal symptoms among computer mouse users. That means to answer the question whether the different symptoms exist simultaneous in the same operator. Furthermore to review possible pathogenic mechanisms and the implication in prevention of symptoms associated to non-keyboard computer input devices.

2. SUBJECTS AND METHODS

2.1. Operators.

Our study group consisted of 751 computer operators using a computer mouse. There were 570 men and 181 women. Both groups had a mean age of 39 years. They reported computer mouse use of mean 7 hours a week with a upper quartile at 10 hours a week and lower quartile at roughly 2 hours a week.

2.2. Questionnaire

A questionnaire with a mannequin was used (Figure 1). The operators answered whether they had symptoms "right now" in the following body regions; neck, shoulder -scapular, shoulder joint - upper arm, elbow - forearm ,wrist and hand - fingers. The intensity of symptoms were rated on a digital visual analogue scale (VAS).

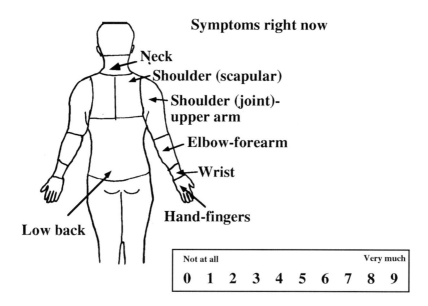

Figure 1. Mannequin used in the questionnaire for location of symptoms.

2.3. Alpha-coefficient

The association between symptoms in different body parts were examined by computation of the alpha coefficient. The alpha coefficient is a measure of the amount of internal consistency among a set of different symptoms that are combined to into a single outcome or index REF. The alpha coefficient (Cronbach´s alpha) measure the extent to which the symptoms reflect the same underlying construct ("condition"). Thus the alpha coefficient is one measure whether grouping of symptoms is a reliable measure.

An alpha coefficient below 0.4 is considered as poor, between 0.4 to 0.6 the reliability is said to be fair and between 0.6-0.8 the alpha coefficient is good and between 0.8-1.0 the alpha is excellent.

2.4. Analysis

The analysis was to determine which combination of symptoms reflect the same underlying condition among mouse users. We started out by only studying the 93% right handed operators of the study group and right sided symptoms. We compared the alpha coefficient among intense mouse users which we defined as operators reporting mouse use for at least 10 hours a week with non-intense mouse users defined as users using the mouse less then 2 hours a week. This division was based on the quartiles of the study group. The analysis was done using the factor procedure in SAS (1).

3 RESULTS AND DISCUSSION

3.1. Alpha coefficient and combination of symptoms

There was a good internal consistency for symptoms in neck, shoulder-scapular region, shoulder joint region, elbow - forearm, wrist and hand-fingers. With alpha coefficient in both group of mouse users above 0.60. However there was no major difference between intense and non-intense mouse users since the alpha coefficient was 0,71 for the intense mouse users and 0,69 for the non-intense mouse users. The combination of symptoms probably represented "normal" symptoms or effects of a constrained sitting posture caused by the VDT work.

The combination of symptoms located to the shoulder-scapular region and wrist and hand-fingers had a good internal consistency of 0,60 for the intense mouse users and a poor internal consistency for the non-intense mouse users of 0,38.

A possible explanation for this reliable combination of symptoms is that intense mouse use cause a static load on the shoulder -scapular region giving symptoms and also an ergonomic exposure on the right wrist and on the right hand-fingers.

One explanation for the shoulder- scapular symptoms is that possible posture strain in terms of low level static loading on the upper part of the trapezius muscle is induced by having the hand distant from the body when holding on to the mouse.

The posture strain may cause a low static loading of the upper part of the trapezius muscle during work and may result in a an overuse of the type 1 muscle fibers (2). The overuse may cause an ischemia and metabolic damage with release of metabolites such as bradykinin. These metabolites may sensitize pain-receptors and induce persistent pain (3). An important preventive measure may be to see to that work tasks involve different contraction levels, so that different fiber types are used. It may sound awkward but one preventive measure would be to increase the load in work so that the operators type 2 muscle fibers also are used. In practice this is obtained by creating jobs to have a variation of work tasks.

The symptoms from the wrist may be due to extreme position for the wrist. In computer mouse use an ulnar wrist deviation is common (4). Extreme joint positions have been shown to cause musculoskeletal pain rapidly possible by stimulating pain receptors in the joint capsula's or ligaments (5).

It is possible that the symptoms from the hand-finger may represent the strain of the exposure of click and drag operations. Perhaps due to strain caused by repetitive tendon tension especially in the tendon to the index finger during click-and drag operations when using a computer mouse. This may cause inflammation of tendons (2).

The internal consistency for the combination of symptoms in wrist and in hand-fingers was 0,66 for the intense mouse users and only 0,19 for the non-intense mouse users. Wrist symptoms may occur due to extreme position of ulnar deviation when operating the computer mouse. One possible explanation for the hand-finger symptoms was that this reflect the stress on tendons .

The present findings supports the idea that computer mouse use may cause symptoms not only in one part of the body but in many parts in specific combinations. If the suggested pathomechanisms are valid then it is important to recognize that three different morbid process may cause the symptoms associated to intense mouse use: a) shoulder-scapular pain

- static loading of type 1 muscle fibers-metabolic process? b) Wrist pain - extreme position (articular capsular strain?) c) hand-finger symptoms - extensor tendon inflammation?

The term syndrome is defined as the aggregate of signs and symptoms associated with any morbid process and constituting together the picture of the disease (6).

Thus since symptoms associated to mouse use may be caused by three different morbid processes the term syndrome does not apply

3.2 Is the use of combination of symptoms a better outcome to estimate the exposure hazards?

When the present study group was used to study the risk of symptoms related to intense mouse use and the exposure group was defined as having at least 10 hours of mouse use per week and the non-intense mouse users used as referents then we got the following results. The risk ratio would be 1,3 for having the single symptom in the shoulder - scapular region among the intense mouse users, 1,4 for having the single symptom in the wrist and 2,8 for the single symptom in the hand -fingers. If we instead study the outcome of grouped symptoms the risk ratio was 5,6 for having symptoms in all three regions the shoulder-scapular region, the wrist and in the hand-fingers for the intense mouse users. Similar the risk ratio for having symptoms in combination wrist and hand-finger region was 7,4 for the intense mouse users.

Traditional analysis of occurrence and association of work-related musculoskeletal symptoms usually focus on one body part at a time. Ergonomic exposure e.g. computer mouse use may cause symptoms not only in one part of the body but in many parts in specific combinations. The combination of symptoms may be an efficient way to assess the occurrence and associations of exposure - effect relationships and to evaluate preventive measures.

4 CONCLUSIONS

1. There are specific concurrences of some symptoms among intense mouse users. This concurrence could be used when evaluating exposure among computer operators using a mouse in health surveillance by questionnaires and also when evaluating preventive measures.

2. At present it seems likely that concurrent symptoms in computer mouse users may be the result of different morbid processes. Thus in the future it is recommended that the term "computer mouse syndrome " should be avoided or used with great caution

REFERENCES

1. SAS Institute Inc. SAS/Stat user's guide, version 6, fourth edition volume 1.Cary, NC, USA: SAS Institute Inc, 1989:773-821.
2. Hagberg M, Silverstein B, Welsh R, et al. Work related musculoskeletal disorders (WMSDs): a reference book for prevention. London: Taylor & Francis Ltd, 1995:421. (Kuorinka I, Forcier L, ed.

3. Hagberg M. Pathomechanisms of work-related musculoskeletal disorders. In: Rantanen J, Lehtinen S, Kalimo R, Nordman H, Vaino H, Viikari-Juntura E, ed. New Epidemics in Occupational Health. Helsiniki, Finland: Finnish Institute of Occupational Health, 1994: 42-53. People and Work;
4. Karlqvist L, Hagberg M, Selin K. Variation in upper limb posture and movement during word processing with and without mouse use. Ergonomics 1994;37:1261-7.
5. Harms-Ringdahl K, Brodin H, Eklund L, Borg G. Discomfort and pain from loaded passive joint structures. Scand J Rehab Med 1983;15:205-211.
6. Steadman TL. Steadmans medical dictionary. (23rd ed.) Baltimore: Williams & Wilkins Company, 1976.

APPLICATION OF A FUZZY MODEL TO A CONTROL-ROOM ERGONOMIC DESIGN

Lucio Compagno

Istituto di Macchine, Facoltà d' Ingegneria, Università di Catania
viale Andrea Doria 6, 95125 Catania, Italy

ABSTRACT

The importance of control rooms in actual industrial plants is due not only to the basic role that they perform in the manufacturing environment but mainly to the enormous and critical influence that human factors can have on processes, materials, equipments, and persons.

Thank to a classification of the ergonomic factors and of the characteristics of the operator, a fuzzy model is defined which, under simplified conditions, can manage at the same time both technical factors as well as human ones. The result of that model is a set of ergonomicity indicators which evaluate not only the global ergonomicity of the workplace but also the influence of the individual ergonomic factors and of the single characteristics of the operator.

Finally, some critical considerations are carried out, mainly concerning the calibration phase of the model.

1. INTRODUCTION

At the stage presently reached by the automation process in industrial plants the manufacturing computers network is controlled by a single supervisor computer. The human interface with such a system has typically the aspect of a control-room. The few operators working in that environment withstand the absence from the process and the great risk increase depending on the enlargement of the manufacturing factors that they control. Due to these reasons, control rooms are a critical aspect of the industrial processes, both from a technical point of view as well as from an ergonomic one.

It is to be remarked that where the automation is at the highest level and a deterministic behaviour is expected from the man-machine system, human factors largely influence the functional performance. Major effects are due to biomechanics, physiology, individual expertises, and temporary factors such as fatigue and health.

In addition, concerning that each operator builds an individual model of the process, it is very difficult to impose a particular functional model; that is due both to the individual mentality of the control room designer as well as to the fact that different operators will work in the same workplace.

This paper was partially granted by CNR (fund n. 93.00546.CT07).

2. CONTROL ROOMS ERGONOMICS

As carried out before [1], Ergonomic Factors in a control room can be classified in Ergonomic Groups as showed in table I.

Table 1
Classification of Ergonomic Groups

REF.	ERGONOMIC GROUP	ERGONOMIC FACTORS (example)
EG_1	control-room lay-out	shape, size, windows, ...
EG_2	air quality	pollutant concentration
EG_3	thermal environment	WBGT index
EG_4	noise	equivalent noise level
EG_5	lighting	average lighting level
EG_6	furniture (chairs, shelves)	sitting height
EG_7	general equipment lay-out	frequency of use
EG_8	equipment features	pushing force
EG_9	presentation and control software	number of menu levels
EG_{10}	mental workload	attention level

According with the type of an Ergonomic Factor, its analysis can be carried out in three different ways:

• measure of a quantitative parameter (e.g.: temperature),
• assessment of a qualitative parameter (e.g.: walls colour),
• complying with a design principle (e.g.: equipment positioning).

As agreed by many authors [3, 4], fuzzy theory suits quite well the ergonomic evaluation problems.

3. THE FUZZY MODEL

In a previous work [1] a complete model was proposed. In order to make easier the understanding of that model, some complexity reductions are primarily made:

• design and analysis are performed just in a single workplace;
• that workplace is independent from the other ones;
• just one job is carried out, ergonomically homogeneous (e.g.: watching and supervising).

Under that conditions, a simplified model is obtained whose basic elements are synthetically reported in table 2.

Table 2
Elements of the evaluation simplified model

SYMBOL	ELEMENT	QUANTITY
F_j	Ergonomic Factor	J
E_j	Ergonomicity Level related with F_j	J
b_j	Parameter related with E_j	J
C_k	Psycho-physiological Characteristic of the Operator	K
a_j	Parameter related with C_k	K
M_k	Partial Performance Degree related with C_k	K

The Partial Performance Degree, M_k, has the meaning of the way how a particular Psycho-physiological Characteristic of the Operator, C_k, influences the job execution.

In that model each F_j is related with the definition of a corresponding fuzzy set as follows:

$$\mathbf{B_j} \equiv \{ \text{universe of the possible values of } b_j, \text{parameter of } F_j \} \quad (1)$$

$$g_{Ej} : \mathbf{B_j} \to [0,1], \text{membership function of } b_j \text{ in } \mathbf{B_j} \quad (2)$$

$$\mathbf{E_j} \equiv \{ (b_j, g_{Ej}(b_j)), b_j \in \mathbf{B_j}\}, \text{fuzzy subset of the universe } \mathbf{B_j} \quad (3)$$

In the same way each C_k is related with the definition of a corresponding fuzzy set as follows:

$$\mathbf{A_k} \equiv \{ \text{universe of the possible values of } a_k, \text{parameter of } C_k \} \quad (4)$$

$$f_{Mk} : \mathbf{A_k} \to [0,1], \text{membership function of } a_k \text{ in } \mathbf{A_k} \quad (5)$$

$$\mathbf{M_k} \equiv \{ (a_k, f_{Mk}(a_k)), a_k \in \mathbf{A_k}\}, \text{fuzzy subset of the universe } \mathbf{A_k} \quad (6)$$

The ergonomicity of the workplace, related to an individual operator, is expressed by a fuzzy matrix, $[\mathbf{R_{jk}}]$, where:

$$[\mathbf{R_{jk}}] \equiv \{\mathbf{E_j}\} \times \{\mathbf{M_k}\} \quad (7)$$

$$\mathbf{R_{jk}} \equiv \{ (b_k, a_j, h_{Rjk}(b_k, a_j), b_j \in \mathbf{B_j}, a_k \in \mathbf{A_k} \} \text{fuzzy subset of the universe } \mathbf{B_j} \times \mathbf{A_k} \quad (8)$$

$$h_{Rjk}(a_k, b_j) \to [0,1], \text{membership function of } (a_k, b_j) \text{ in } \mathbf{R_{jk}}, \text{defined by:} \quad (9)$$

$$h_{Rjk} = h_{Ej} * M_k = \min \{g_{Ej}, f_{Mk}\} \quad (10)$$

Then the values of [R_{jk}] can be aggregated in (J+K+1) synthetical parameters through the fuzzy average operators (p_k and q_j are weight factors; α controls the type of the average operator):

$$S[F_j] = \Sigma_k \, (p_k \, hR_{jk}{}^\alpha)^{1/\alpha}, \text{ where: } p_k \in [0,1] \text{ and } \Sigma_k \, p_k = 1 \qquad (11)$$

$$S[C_k] = \Sigma_j \, (q_j \, hR_{jk}{}^\alpha)^{1/\alpha}, \text{ where: } q_j \in [0,1] \text{ and } \Sigma_j \, q_j = 1 \qquad (12)$$

$$S[R_{jk}] = \Sigma_j \Sigma_k \, (p_k \, q_j \, hR_{jk}{}^\alpha)^{1/\alpha}, \text{ where: } \Sigma_j \Sigma_k \, p_k \, q_j = 1, \text{ and } \alpha \in [-1,0[\, \cup \,]0,1] \qquad (13)$$

$$S[F_j] \in [0,1], \quad S[C_k] \in [0,1], \quad S[R_{jk}] \in [0,1] \qquad (14)$$

The meanings of that ergonomicity parameters are reported in table 3.

Table 3
Meanings of the ergomicity indicators

SYMBOL	QUANTITY	MEANING OF THE INDICATOR
$S[F_j]$	J	how the Ergonomic Factor F_j influences the ergonomicity of the workplace
$S[C_k]$	K	how the Characteristic of the Operator C_k influences the ergonomicity of the workplace
$S[R_{jk}]$	1	global ergonomicity of the workplace

The outlined model was tested by experimentally applying it in the control-room of a thermal electric power plant in two different ways:

• by comparing an old workplace with a new one (same operator);
• by comparing the fitness of two different operators (same workplace).

The old workplace was a traditional one ("needle" instruments and manual knobs). The new one was a last generation workplace (VDU's and keyboard).
Because of the intrinsic differences, a reduced analysis was carried out by examinating only a few Ergonomic Factors F_j, mainly belonging to EG5, EG6, EG7 Ergonomic Groups (see table 1). The value $\alpha = 1$ was chosen (that makes the fuzzy average an arithmetic one). The calculus was executed by a simple electronic spreadsheet.

4. CONCLUSIONS

The most difficulties arose firstly in the identification of the Ergonomic Factors F_j and in the definition of the related parameters b_j. After that, the construction of the fuzzy sets $\mathbf{B}_j$ and $\mathbf{A}_k$ resulted easier but very modeler-dependent.

Also the setting of p_k and q_j coefficients showed a large influence on the ergomicity indicators, $S[\mathbf{F}_j]$, $S[\mathbf{C}_k]$, $S[\mathbf{R}_{jk}]$. For these reasons, and thank to its capability to manage technical and human factors at the same time, the proposed model is, at the present stage, more a design tool than an evaluation one. A "standardization" effort should be done in order to extend it to other Ergonomic Factors and make it as objective as possible.

Since the dealt problem is quite complex it was necessary to treat it in a simplified way. For instance, the variation of the Characteristics of the Operator, during the work shift, was not considered.

The calibration of the fuzzy membership functions showed to be very delicate and influential on the model configuration. This phase could be aided by an expert system in order to code the human experience.

The optimal assignment of a set of different operators to the individual workplace shows to be a very interesting field of investigation, as well as the influence of long range factors, such as the specific experience and the age.

REFERENCES

[1] Compagno L., "Valutazione ergonomica fuzzy dei posti di lavoro nelle sale di controllo", V Congresso Nazionale SIE, Palermo, 4-7/10/1993.
[2] Ivergård T., "Handbook of Control Rooms Design and Ergonomics", Taylor & Francis, London, 1989.
[3] Karwosky W., Mital A., "Fuzzy Concepts in Human Factors/Ergonomics Research", Application of Fuzzy Set Theory in Human Factors, pp. 41-53, Elsevier, Amsterdam, 1986.
[4] Pacholsky L.M., "An Application of Fuzzy Methods in the Complex Ergonomics Diagnostics of Industrial Production Systems", pp. 211-226, Elsevier, Amsterdam, 1986.
[5] Wang M.J., Teh H.P., "A Knowledge Based System for Controls-Displays Selection", Advances in Industrial Ergonomics and Safety, Taylor & Francis, pp. 945-951, London, 1989.
[6] Klir G.J., Folger T.A., "Fuzzy Sets, Uncertainity, and Information", Prentice Hall, Englewood Cliffs NJ, 1988.
[7] Moray N., "The Application of Fuzzy Set Measurement to the Study of Mental Workload", Proceedings of the IAE XI Congress, p. 423-424, Parigi, 1991.

VDU workplace: Ergonomic evaluation between a VDU workplace and a CAE-CAD-CAM workstation.

L. Masseroni[a], M. Fregoso[a], G. Galletta[a].

[a] Environment, Health and Safety Service - ITALTEL SIT S.p.A. (IRI-STET).

1. INTRODUCTION

At the end of the '80s, Italtel* and the O.S.L.s (Workers Trade-Union Organizations) arrived at an integrative company agreement for addressing VDU work themes by means of an organic intervention, in line with the indications of the EEC draft Directive 90/270.
Given the number of installed machines and personnel involved (about 5,000 and 8,000 respectively), there were no reasonably certain elements upon which to base the daily management and future planning of the logistics, organisational and health-care aspects.
We recall that in those days there was abundant scientific production indicating that there were no "pathologies" that could definitely be attributed to working with VDU. Yet, there were contradictory voices, some even coming from authoritative sources, and these created videoterminal anxiety in the public at large. There was the risk of the problem becoming a clinical one, thus heightening the existing tensions.
We therefore felt we had to apply an overall approach which was technically correct and scientifically reliable. This approach, which was largely socialised and shared within our company, would permit us to skim off the false problems and boil everything down to the rational plane required for governing an industrial process.
Basically, the work program called for the following:
- training of and providing information to all VDU users;
- evaluation of the ergonomic requisites of the existing workplaces and establishment of company standards for corrective interventions or the realisation of future VDU workplaces;
- the possibility of permitting users to voluntarily access health checks regarding their visual and osteomuscular systems.

---

* **Italtel** (part of IRI-STET Group) is Italy's largest telecommunications manufacturer. It designs, manufactures and markets systems and equipment for public and private telecommunications, and realizes telecommunications networks and installations both in Italy and abroad.
Italtel main italian facilities are located in Milan, Settimo Milanese (Milan), Terni, Rome, L'Aquila, Santa Maria Capua Vetere (near Naples), Carini (near Palermo) and employs a total of about 15,000 people, half of which regularly use VDU in their work.

This report shows how the action taken resulted in the design, development and realisation of standards for jobs where the CAE-CAD-CAM workstations are used, particularly as concerns equipment characteristics (hardware and furniture).
There are other company standards which concern the environment (microclimate, illumination, noise) and the machine-man interface (software), but these are not considered in this report.

2. DESCRIPTION OF THE EXPERIENCE

During the definition of the applicable standards for realising new PC (personal computer) workstations or videoterminals, or for updating those already existing, it was pointed out the importance of the use of VDUs in Italtel (of approx. 5,000 installed video terminals, about 700 are CAE-CAD-CAM workstations).
It was therefore decided to also systematically approach this particular aspect and try to put to best use the experience obtained during the definition of the aforementioned standards.
CAE-CAD-CAM workstations call for the use of VDUs that are larger than those normally used by video terminals or PCs, and require more than one CPU, file holders and designs - some of which can be quite large and have to be consulted frequently - and various accessories, such as a mouse or graphics panel. In brief, the following activities are carried out in Italtel's workstations:
Software development: The operator's eyes are prevalently on the screen. Loading takes an average amount of time, with frequent interruptions for path selection. Data input is primarily by means of the keyboard. The workstation is used steadily throughout the year.
Design: The operator's spends about as much time looking at the screen as he does looking at the support document, and the keyboard and mouse are used to about the same degree for inputting data. The workstation is used sporadically but intensely.
Engineering: Most of the time the operator is watching the screen. It takes an average amount of time for loading, depending on the path selection. Either the mouse or graphics panel is used for inputting data. The workstation is used uninterruptedly throughout the year.
Documentation: Most of the time the operator is watching the screen. It takes an average amount of time for loading, and there are various opportunities for making decisions. The keyboard and mouse are used to about the same degree for inputting data.
In order to indentify the actual needs of the operators, we evaluated on the one hand, the difference between the sizes of the PCs or video terminals, and CAE-CAD-CAMs, and on the other, the operators' basic contributions, and the instrument and space requirements (1).

In brief, we found the following:
- hardware dimensions: monitor depths: 35 cm for PCs, 60 cm for workstations:
- space for computer accessories (one or more CPUs, mouse and graphics panel for the workstations) and required working space (including tables and filing cabinets) for PCs and workstations: about 7 and 9 square meters, respectively.

On the basis of this, the elements taken into consideration were the chair; the work surface height, length and width; and the layout of the workplace.

2.1. Chair

The chair characteristics had already been evaluated, tested and defined during the finalising of the company standards for activities involving the use of PCs or videoterminals.

Therefore, in this study, we just limited ourselves to submitting the proposed model to the operators for their approval. We felt the proposed model was also suitable for workstations because it fulfilled the minimum requirements specified in EEC Directive 90/270, as well as the indications that have matured at the scientific level. Moreover, it was already available on the market.

The main characteristics of the chair therefore met the following requisites:
- safety: must not be responsible for or cause accidents;
- practicality: must be easy to handle and have a hygienic covering;
- adaptability: must be dimensioned in relation to human measurements;
- comfort: must conform to human physical contours;
- solidity: must be wear resistant and have a long service life;
- suitability: must be suitable for the particular type of work and environment in which it is to be used.

2.2. Worksurface height

Establishing the best work-surface height was difficult because of the wide range of human morphologies. Nonetheless, the proposed fixed work-surface height was 72 cm. Workplace flexibility is assured by a chair, which can be easily adjusted in the vertical direction, and by a foot rest, used as required.

2.3. Worksurface width

We considered the "work area"; that is, the area in front of the operator between the elbows (the "elbow span" anthropometric parameter) and the comfortable-prehension area, which includes the area between the extended arms (the "large span" anthropometric parameter).

Since the work surface supports hardware, file holders, drawings and a considerable amount of other items, including special instrumentation, we selected a "large span" parameter value of 150 cm, which corresponds to 5% of the women.

2.4. Worksurface depth

Considering the different forearm length possibilities, we found we needed 15 cm of depth - which corresponds to half of the forearm length of 95% of all men - to provide proper support. In addition, we added 60 cm for the monitor, 20 cm for permitting the best screen-viewing distance), and 20 cm for the keyboard and/or mouse. These parameters established 115 cm as the minimum allowable work-surface depth for the workstation.

2.5. Layout of workplace with workstation

The various units - TV monitors, work surfaces, chairs, CPUs, file holders, designs, etc. - were laid out according to the job duties assigned to workplace.

3. CONCLUSIONS

Considering the 4 previously-indicated types of workstation jobs, we and the operators concerned realised two following workplace prototypes, and simulated the work to be carried out at them:
- a workplace for developing software and documentors, with a workstation table and a table for office work;
- a workplace for designers and engineers, with a workstation table and a table for consulting documents.

The results of the performed verifications showed that the proposed work-surface depth, screen-viewing distance, workplace flexibility, etc. all satisfactorily met the requirements, including being able to comfortably accommodate two operators and still provide sufficient space for consulting maps, drawings, and other documents.

REFERENCES

1. EPM, Ergodigit : For an ergonomic restructuring of the typist's workplace (1990).

Computers for social integration of the disabled people

A. Pedotti

Centro di Bioingegneria, Fondazione Pro Juventute Don Carlo Gnocchi I.R.C.C.S. - Politecnico di Milano, Via Capecelatro 66, I-20148 Milano, Italy

1. INTRODUCTION

Many factors are suggesting that in next years the attention of modern societies in terms of resources and structures of the health systems will progressively move from the problem of medical intervention in the acute phase towards the care of chronic diseases.
This change is mainly due to the increase of the number of people which are affected by more or less serious disabilities. Such an increase is the result of two main reasons:
- the improvement of the quality of the medical intervention in acute phase which allows to survive patients with very serious lesions;
- the increase of the mean duration of life which make our society composed more and more by elderly people who often are affected by some functional limitations.

This new scenario requires a new attitude and strategies for the National Health Systems. In the acute diseases, the goal of the medical intervention, despite the difficulty to be reached, is very clear and well defined: the defeat of the disease and the restoration of the original healthy condition.
In the chronic diseases the recovery of the patient cannot be the goal. In this case the efforts of the medical and social services are directed to keep or to restore a reasonable quality of life of the patient, that is a good level of autonomy, independence, capability of interaction with people social integration. The achievement of this goal is necessary not only for human reasons, but also to reduce the social costs related to the care of a completely "dependent individual".

There is also a second important difference. While in the treatment of acute diseases the patient can be considered a "passive" subject, the recovery of the autonomy of disabled people is a complex process in which the disabled is the actor himself who must play the main role.

In this context, the recent technological developments become an important tool to facilitate the social integration of disabled people [1, 2, 3, 4]. For instance, computers can be considered the present main technical aid for most disabled people: to communicate, to control the environment, to work, to facilitate the access to various routinely devices: telephone, television, remote data banks, etc.

On the other hand the technologies of microelectronics and telematics open new perspective for <u>teleworking</u> so that disabled people can be actively integrated in the production process in an easier way.

Another important role of informatics is the possibility to provide <u>computerised information</u> for the choice of the most appropriate technical aids to improve the level of autonomy of each disabled.

This structured information is absolutely necessary if we consider that there is a great variety of needs, depending on the disability, single or multiple, the age, the social environment, etc., and a great variety of possible technological solutions (fig. 1). To solve this problem a special data bank for information service has been created in Italy in connection with a European project [5].

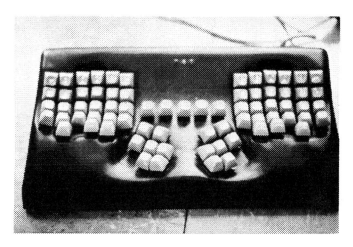

Fig. 1 Example of keyboard, originally developed for disabled persons, and also recommended for healthy ones, for a more ergonomic access to computer.

2. TECHNOLOGIES FOR TELEWORKING

Teleworking is an emerging opportunity in the Labour market which can expand dramatically the possibility of profitable employment of persons with disability. All those persons with impaired mobility resulting from a wide range of physical or sensory impairment can be considered as potential candidates to telework, in that the possibility to work at a distance can remove or overcome barriers and problems related to health conditions, safety, fatigue and stress, need for personal assistance, inaccessible transportation or architectural barriers. That means in general all the problems associated with moving from home to the workplace or from one town to another for work reasons.

Job integration is considered one of the main objectives of rehabilitation for the persons in working age. Various policies and initiatives try to address such objective in the various Countries, but consensus exists everywhere on the idea that the ultimate aim should be equal access to the largest spectrum of work opportunities rather than assisted employment in a limited range of jobs.

For the disabled, telework has to be seen as an integrated opportunity to profitable employment for a very extensive range of jobs, and as such it is likely to provide a great contribution to rehabilitation of a high number of persons:
- Integrated, because wherever a telework organisation exists the disabled teleworker can perform the same jobs as a non disabled one, the difference possibly being in the technology adopted for the telework workstation.

- Profitable, in that the investments for telework arrangements make sense in terms of effective (satisfactory for the user), productive (for the employer) and profitable (for both) job placement.
- Extensive range of job, due to the ever increasing number of computer-based or computer-related jobs offered by the current trends in the Labour market.

A large part of the disabled population, but especially those with the most severe physical disabilities, is expected to get substantial benefits from teleworking, and productive resources (which today are non-productive and have to rely mainly on assistance arrangements) can be unlocked in this way for employers and in general for the benefit of society.

An appropriate intervention in this area must be concentrated on teleworking based on multimedia platforms with on-line capability (home-based or from remote office). Therefore, the technological core of such initiative should be represented by the local telework computer station and by the associated telecommunication-teleinformatic facilities. These must accommodate in the whole the needs originating from either the job tasks (suitable multimedia environment and proper applications) or the user's disability (special or enhanced Input/Output devices, logistics, operational management, associated environmental controls for independence in the workplace). These should also provide effective solutions to the human interaction needs among teleworker, employer and co-worker which play a substantial role in creating the work environment.

3. DATA BANK FOR INFORMATION TO DISABLED PERSONS

S.I.V.A., which stands for *Technical Aids Evaluation and Information Centre*, was established in 1981 by the Don Gnocchi Pro Juventute Foundation, in cooperation with the "Polytechnic of Milano" University, with the aim of creating a nation-wide computerised information system and an advice service concerning the technical aids which contribute to rehabilitation and independent living of the disabled persons.

SIVA's current activities include:
- management of a computerised information system on technical aids (SIVA base);
- coordination of a national network of technical aids information centres, based on SIVA data bank and HANDYNET;
- educational programmes addressed to rehabilitation professionals;
- information and advice service;
- technical aids testing laboratory;
- a variety of special projects.

The team consists of 12 persons (1 engineer, 2 computer technicians, 2 documentalists, 2 occupational therapists, 3 physiotherapists, 2 secretaries). By concentrating in the same team all these activities SIVA aims at a comprehensive approach to the problems of information on technical aids and accessibility. In fact not only the pure aspect of gathering and disseminating products information is considered, but also:
- dissemination of other helpful information, like reference addresses, legislation, etc.;
- testing information (i.e. quality and functionality of technical aids);
- training of rehabilitation professionals to making the best use of the information system;
- development of models for information service delivery;
- provision of a highly specialised advice service addressed at the user, with a reference function for all the network.

3.1. The Information/Advice Service

Since its opening, SIVA has been providing over 8000 consultations to disabled persons, rehabilitation & health care professionals, teachers, architects, health authorities and even to manufacturers. The service is open every morning upon appointment, with an average of 15 clients.

Basic tools for the information/advice service are:
- SIVA computerised information system;
- the HANDYNET computerised information system;
- other databases (ABLEDATA from USA, REHADATA from Germany, the Educational Software BBS from the Italian National Research Council, etc.);
- a specialised library;
- the permanent exhibition of technical aids.

3.2. SIVA Information System and Network

The current version of SIVA base requires a DOS Personal Computer equipped with a standard VGA colour screen, 40 Mbytes hard disk and a 550 Mbytes CD-ROM player. The software interface has been developed on-purpose by the SIVA team: it is highly user friendly, its use does not require any informatics skill, its concept is especially addressed towards rehabilitation professionals.

At the present time the data bank contains extensive information on:
- some 6000 technical aids, each one described by a detailed technical record and by a computerised picture;
- some 3500 manufacturers, national suppliers or local dealers;
- some 3000 non-commercial organisations (including voluntary associations) involved in disability matters;
- some 800 national or regional legislation documents concerning technical aids and in general disability matters, including the official national register of prostheses or technical aids that benefit of financial support by the State;
- 2000 bibliographic documents concerning technical aids and environmental accessibility.

The data bank also includes:
- a guide to selection of technical aids, based upon the ISO 9999 International Classification of Technical Aids and SIVA's own thesaurus (controlled terminology);
- a special utility for keeping record of the counselling services given to the clients, whose processing provides statistics of the users profile, their impairments and pathologies, raised questions and proposed solutions.The update of the information system is carried out on a regular basis by a team of 5 full-time equivalent staff, mainly through contacts with manufacturers and suppliers.

While weekly updates are provided to SIVA information/advice service, the system is designed for external distribution through compact disks CD-ROM, issued every fourth month (every new release supersedes the older) subject to an annual subscription.

Subscribers are mainly rehabilitation services and resource Centres, where experts are expected to be prepared to act as counsellors to disabled clients. Up to now about 70 centres are accessing the system and thus take part in this network. Most of them have been set up inside Rehabilitation Units of Local Health Authorities: the remainder are information and Resource Centres set up by Municipalities, Associations and Universities (see Fig. 2).

Through a purpose-made software interface the Italian data are transferred to the HANDYNET information system whenever requested by the European Commission. The Handynet CD-ROMs are also distributed to all SIVA network in order to provide a additional information tool with European dimension.

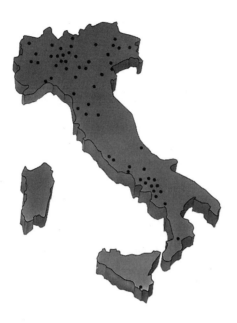

Fig. 2 Network of the Centers connected to SIVA Data Bank.

4. THE EUROPEAN PERSPECTIVE: HANDYNET

The Handynet Project, a section of the HELIOS programme of the European Commission, aims at establishing a European computerised information system concerning technical and social resources for the integration of the disabled persons into Society. Priority has been given to the Technical Aids information module and the first CD-ROM prototypes were produced in December 1991 and in May 1992.

Now the HANDYNET CD-ROM has reached its 6th release containing information on about 32000 products (technical aids) manufactured in the 12 European Countries and 15000 organisations (manufacturers, suppliers and non-commercial organisations).

The products covered by the system apply to any impairment (motor, visual, cognitive etc.) and fall into the categories defined by the International Standard ISO 9999 (now also accepted as European Standard EN 29999).

Over the years a number of feasibility studies, experimental pilots and technical developments have been carried out in order to set up the technical and organisational structure of the Handynet system. Complex problems were solved in order to comply with multilingualism so as to make information understandable to each other country through automatic translation; such a co-operative approach among Countries also encountered difficulties due to substantial differences among Health and Social systems.

As a result of these efforts an efficient network of data collection centres has been set up through official agreements between the European Commission and the member Countries; 12 National Data Collection Centres have been officially established which are also responsible for the national distribution of information: CEPIATH (Bruxelles, *Belgium*) for

French part, VLICHT (Leuven, *Belgium*) for Finnish part, Danish Centre for Rehabilitation and Education (Tastrup, *Denmark*), Handynet France c/o CNFLRH (Paris, *France*), Institut der Deutschen Wirtschaft (Köln, *Germany*), Disabled Living Foundation (London, *Great Britain*), ICS/FORTH, (Heraklion, *Greece*), National Rehabilitation Board (Dublin, *Ireland*), SIVA Fondazione Pro Juventute don Carlo Gnocchi (Milano, *Italy*), Centre de Coordination Handynet (Itzig, *Luxemburg*), Stichting Handynet Netherlands (Hoensbroek, *Netherlands*), Centro Nacional de Coordenaçao Handynet (Lisboa, *Portugal*), INSERSO/CEAPAT (Madrid, *Spain*).

Substantial step for the future of the HANDYNET is the recent approval of the European Commission Report by the European Parliament, which has assured the long-term maintenance and development of the system.

REFERENCES

1. A. Pedotti, R. Andrich (Eds.), Evaluation of assistive devices for paralyzed persons, Commission of the European Communities COMAC-BME, Edizioni Pro Juventute, Milano, 1984.
2. A. Pedotti, State and perspectives of mobility restoration for paralysed persons, R.B.M. Revue Européenne de Tecnologie Biomedicale, Ed. SEPFI, vol. 13, n. 1, 58-62, 1991.
3. A. Pedotti, Motor performance and aging, in: Gerontechnology, Studies in Health Technology and Informatics, vol. 3 H. Bouma and J.A.M. Graafmans (Eds.), IOS Press - Amsterdam (Publ.), 177-188, 1992.
4. A. Pedotti, Mobility restoration for paralysed persons, in: Advances in Biomedical Engineering, Biomedical and Health Research, vol. 2, J.E.W. Beneken and V. Thévenin (Eds.), IOS Press - Amsterdam (Publ.), 318-328, 1993.
5. A. Pedotti, R. Andrich (Eds.), European coordination of information concerning disabled persons, Commission of the European Communities COMAC-BME, Edizione Fondazione Pro Juventute - Milano, 1985.

Displays for visually impaired: Studies of cognitive and perceptual characteristics of speech synthesis

E. Hjelmquist and B. Jansson

Göteborg University
Department of Psychology
Haraldsg. 1, S-413 14 Göteborg, Sweden

Results are reported from an extensive experiment where speech syntehsis was compared to natural speech among a group of visually disabled persons in a recall study of connected prose. The results indicated effects of text type as well as of modality of text presentation. Speech synthesis gave equal, or lower, performance compared to natural speech. It was suggested that text type and training effects are important topics for future studies.

1. INTRODUCTION

The access to work possibilities for visually impaired and blind persons are critically dependent on the availability of displays which can present information in a way which does not rely on the visual system. Speech synthesis has been introduced as a possible means for overcoming the obstacles which a sensory handicap such as visual deficits present. The type of system discussed here is the text-to-speech conversion variant of speech synthesis. Over the last ten years there has developed a body of knowledge concerning cognitive and perceptual characteristics of such speech synthesis [1, 2, 3, 4]. It has been shown that present technical solutions work efficiently for certain purposes, though the quality of the speech synthesis signal is yet far from perfect. The comparison is made in relation to natural speech and empirical data show a rather clear picture to the effect that natural speech gives a better memory and understanding for certain types of verbal material than synthetic speech [1, 2, 3, 4, 5]. We were particularly interested in connected prose passages since differences between speech synthesis and natural speech concerning this type of material have sometimes transpired, sometimes not, in previous research. In work situations it could be of critical importance to correctly and quickly pick up verbal information presented with an electronic display. From the point of view of visually disabled persons' work possibilities, quality of synthetic speech used at work places is an urgent matter as far as its cognitive and perceptual characterstics are concerned. In this chapter findings from our own studies will be reviewed and discussed. Our studies have been conducted as laboratory experiments and interviews about subjective experiences and preferences. In this chapter we will report on results from the experimental studies.

The studies on speech synthesis as compared to natural speech also offer possibilities to investigate more basic questions of text processing. Therefore we used different types of text, viz. a number of texts from daily newspapers and another set of texts based on previous studies of text processing [6, 7]. It was hypothesized that the newspaper texts would be easier to process due to familiarity with that type of text and also due to the structural simplicity of those texts, compared to the other texts. We do not have any formal measures of the complexity of the texts and strictly speaking differences between text types should be interpreted with caution until further studies have been done.

2. METHOD

The intelligibility of texts was experimentally investigated. Fifty-three blind or severely visually impaired persons (60% males and 40% females) took part in the study. Two types of speech were used. Speech synthesis (VoxBox™ SA 201) was compared to a male human voice in a study of recall of different types of newspaper texts: editorials, news articles, and causeries/chat columns. The participant listened to a certain text, and immediately recalled as much as possible of the text. The recall study was performed at three occations with about six weeks between the recall trials. Between the recall sessions, the participants had access to computer based newspaper reading systems. Each participant listened to, and recalled seven texts at each trial. Thus, in total, each participant was to recall 21 texts. At each trial, the texts consisted of two editorials, two news articles, two causeries, as well as a standard text. The length of the target texts ranged between 267 to 665 words. The average length of the newspaper articles was 453 words.

The standard texts had the same story, or plot structure, but different content. The standard texts were modelled on a text, Circle Island, used in [7]. All three texts had a similar story grammar, including a setting, a theme, a plot, and a resolution. The length of the standard texts ranged between 167 and 186 words.

For each participant, half the newspaper texts were read by a human voice, and the other half by speech synthesis. The standard texts were all presented in the same modality for each participant. The speed of text presentation was fixed at the first and last trial, while the participants themselves could adjust the speed of the presentations in the middle trial. The fixed speech speed was about 140 wpm in both modalities. All 53 participants but seven took full part in the recall study. Altogether, about a thousand recalls were collected. In the present analysis, number of words in each recall was counted. Filled pauses or comments about the contents in the target text was excluded from word counting.

Analysis of variance with repeated measures was carried out on the number of recalled words. Further, the number of recalled words were divided by number of words in the target text. Thus, the absolute and relative number of recalled words were used as dependent variables. Three effects were considered, viz. modality, trial, and text type. Modality was a between groups factor when analyzing the standard texts, and a within group factor for the newspaper texts.

3. RESULTS

Analysis of variance with repeated measures of the two recall indices gave the following results. With the recall of the newspaper texts, there was no main effect of modality, but there was a strong main effect of text type, both for the absolute, F(2,90)=73.43, p<.001, and the relative measures F(2,90)=31.98, p<.001, see Figures 1a, b below. It should be noted that the

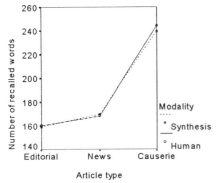

Figure 1a. Mean number of recalled words across article type and modality (N=46).

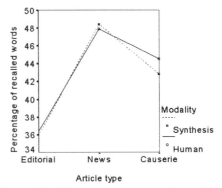

Figure 1b. Mean percentage of recalled words in relation to length of article across article type and modality (N=46).

news article type had largest effect when using the absolute measure. However, when using the relative measure recall of news was much lower. This reflects the fact that the news articles were somewhat longer compared to the other two types of articles. Considering the relative measures, causeries articles were more easy to recall than were the other two types of articles.

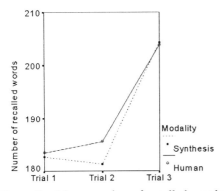

Figure 2a. Mean number of recalled words in relation to length of article across trial and modality (N=46).

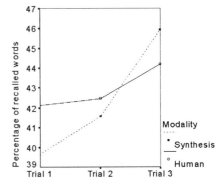

Figure 2b. Mean percentage of recalled words in relation to length of article across trial and modality (N=46).

Analyses of trial effects showed a positive trend for both the absolute ($F(2,90)=6.14$, $p<.01$), and the relative measure ($F(2,90)=3.90$, $p<.05$). Especially, the last trial differed from the first one for both indices. The last trial also differed from the second for the absolute recall measure, see Figures 2a, b above.

For both indices, it was notable that there were no interaction effects between modality and text type, or between modality and trials.

Thus, the results of the memory tests show a consistent pattern regarding the newspaper texts. There were no differences between the speech synthesis and the natural speech condition in any of the variables. The same pattern appeared independent of whether the absolute or relative number of words in recall were used as the dependent variable. There were no interaction effects. As to newspaper reading, it could be concluded that the intelligibility of the speech synthesis was good, or at least as good as the human voice, which also conformed to the subjective reports.

However, the results of the analyses of the "standard" texts showed a different pattern compared to the newspaper texts, viz. a consistent between group difference in recall performance to the effect that natural speech resulted in better recall, both with respect to the absolute, $F(1,44)=4.91$, $p<.05$, and relative recall measure, $F(1,44)=4.95$, $p<.05$, see Figures 3a, b below. Similar to the newspaper text condition, there were no interaction effects for the "standard" text condition.

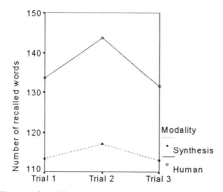 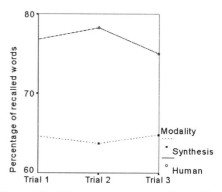

Figure 3a. Mean number of recalled words for "standard" texts across trial and modality (N=46).

Figure 3b. Mean percentage of recalled words for "standard" texts across trial and modality (N=46).

4. DISCUSSION

The studies presented here show clear results indicating that for presentation of prose passages of varying complexity, speech synthesis give rise to a somewhat lower recall performance than natural speech. However, the difference is not very large, and for one type of text there was nor difference at all. There are consequently strong indications that text type is of critcal importance for the applicability of speech synthesis.

From an applied point of view this is of course highly relevant. In situations, e.g. at work, where correct understanding and memory are critical for efficient performance, one should be aware that the use of speech synthesis might result in a somewhat lower perceptual and cognitive performance. On the other hand, in many other situations where text processing is not at a level where very high functioning is necessary, speech synthesis offers a reliable and efficient alternative to human voice presentation. It should be pointed out once more, that the subjects used in this study were fairly well acquainted with the technique and particularly at the end of the investigation had considerable experience of listening to speech synthesis.

Whereas the conclusions from a practical point of view of this study are rather clearcut, the theoretical conclusions are less obvious and rather point to the necessity of further research. In previous research lack of differences between speech synthesis and human voice have been reported [2, 5]. As pointed out in [4], these results have mainly been based on a test material where connected, extended prose passages have been included only to a minor extent. In our studies [4] the results showed a small but consistent recall advantage of presentation of text with natural speech. In that study prose passages from different genres of text were used to study recall as well as recognition performance.

The varying pattern of results found by different researchers demand further analyses and empirical studies. Altogether there are strong indications that text type is very important. On the other hand, subject variables, such as age, seem less important for the results. In the experiments in [4] it was shown that old persons did not perform relatively worse when listening to speech synthesis compared to younger subjects, though the old subjects performed on a generelly lower level, also when listening to natural speech.

Another finding is of interest viz. the pattern of results in Figures 2a and 2b indicating a clear training effect when listening to newspaper text irrespective of speech condition. There was no such trend for the standardized texts. Again, this pattern is compatible with effects of text type. It seems as if the more ordinary type of prose and prose content of the newspaper text leave room for further learning, whereas this is not the case for the other text type.

Finally, it should be noted that there was no interaction effect involving trial. In trial 2 the subjects were allowed to adjust speed of presentation themselves. This did not give rise to higher performance. Text type and training effects should be the focus of future studies of perceptual and cognitive aspects of speech synthesis.

REFERENCES

1. Greenspan, S.L., Nusbaum, H.C., & Pisoni, D.B. (1988). Perceptual learning of synthetic speech produced by rule. *Journal of Experimental Psychology: Learning, Memory, and Cognition, 14*, 421-433.
2. Schwab, E.C., Nusbaum, H.C., & Pisoni, D.B. (1985). Some effects of training on the perception of synthetic speech. *Human Factors, 27*, 395-408.
3. Hjelmquist, E., Jansson, B., & Torell, G. (1990). Blind persons' reading of daily newspapers with computer mediated technique. *Journal of Visual Impairment & Blindness, 84*, 210-215.
4. Hjelmquist, E., Dahlstrand, U., & Hedelin, L. (1992). Visually impaired persons' comprehension of text presented with speech synthesis. *Journal of Visual Impairment & Blindness, 86*, 426-428.

5. Pisoni, D.B., Nusbaum, H.C., & Greene, B.G. (1985). Perception of synthetic speech generated by rule. *Proceedingss of the IEEE, 73,* 1665-1676.
6. Thorndyke, P.W. (1979). Knowledge acquisition from newspaper stories, *Discourse Processes, 2,* 95-112.
7. Thorndyke, P.W. (1977). Cognitive structures in comprehension and and memory of narrative discourse, *Cognitive Psychology, 9,* 77-110.

Haptic devices in human-computer interaction

H. Luczak, M. Göbel and J. Springer

Institute of Industrial Engineering and Ergonomics,
Aachen University of Technoloy, Bergdriesch 27, 52062 Aachen, Germany

Survey of session 'Haptic devics in HCI' with contributions of

M. Akamatsu (AIST, MITI, Japan),

M. Dahm, H. Jansen-Dittmer,
D. Meyer- Ebrecht and K. Münker
(Aachen University of Technology,
Germany),

M. Göbel (Aachen University of
Technology, Germany),

V. Hedicke, J. Beimel, K. Kornblum
and K.P. Timpe (Berlin Technical
University, Germany),

G. Hommel, F.G. Hoffmann and J. Henz
(Berlin Technical University,
Germany),

H. Luczak (Aachen University of
Technology, Germany),

J. Springer (Aachen University of
Technology, Germany),

M. Tschelegi (University of Vienna,
Austria)

1. Introduction

In his introductory remarks to the session, *Luczak* pointed out, that interactions of humans with their environment are based on the perception of environmental information. This is required both for the recognition of the exterior situation and for the control of own actions. Visual perception allows the transmission of the most complex kinds of information. But due to the amount of information processing required for visual object recognition, the reaction delay is the longest of all senses. For spatial orientation visual perception is absolutely necessary and can not be replaced by other senses without accepting breakdowns in performance. Acoustic information usually originates by the touching of objects, and is therefore mostly used to indicate warnings and other critical incidents. Haptic perception consists of kinaesthetic (force) and tactile (vibration) perception. In real environment, these senses are used for object handling in addition to visual or auditive information. Only information of low complexity can be handled by haptic perception, but reaction time is very short and sensory signals are fed directly into human motor control. The different sensory modalites work in parallel, and are merged to a unique impression, if the transmitted information enables a consistent situation recognition.

Consequently, haptic perception might not be used to replace auditive or visual perception as it is with devices for non-handicapped persons, but is an important source of supplementary information, especially in the case of object handling. Input-devices with fixed functions (e.g. steering wheels and keyboards) make often use of it by a direct mechanical coupling. Computer input devices interacting with virtual objects - represented by software - would require a more sophisticated artificial generation of haptic information to complete human-computer-interaction according to the context of usage. The present paper is focussed on the actual researches and developments on computer controlled haptic devices, trying to enhance usability of interaction.

Haptic perception is of a bipolar character like many other modalities of somatosensoric perception. Additionally to the conscious perception of object-attributes it is used to regulate movements and other vegetative functions in an unconscious way. Orientation of perception is mostly object-related, but might also be body-related. Sensory stimulation may be caused actively by touching an object or passively by beeing touched by an object.

A measurement of the sensory qualities is only feasible in a direct way for tactile signals and for conscious detection. For this, basic characteristics of sensitivity and discriminability have been researched during the last decades, but the influence of haptic information on unconscious motoric regulation is only partially known yet. Further information about information transmission rates and pattern recognition is required to outline future application fields for human-computer-interfaces. As a first index, studies of vibrotactile speech transmission for deaf persons found a maximum information-transmission-rate of 20 to 60 bits/s using a single actuator and of 600 to 950 bits/s with multiple acutators [3].

Different typical prototypes in form of enhanced conventional input devices and new state-of-the-art data gloves will be presented down here to outline the latest developments in research of haptic devices, including possible benefits and bottlenecks.

2. Applications of haptic feedback for computer-mice and trackballs

The worldwide application of computer-mice and trackballs started with the introduction of graphical-user-interfaces. In contrast to text oriented displays, the whole screen surface is used for a set of virtual objects to interact with by a mouse or a trackball. However, no "touching" perception is conveyed to the hand or fingers on the input device while coming closer to or crossing over objects. This deficiency in information leads to an increasing workload due to the concentration on visual perception, which resources already have to be shared with the visual object recognition. Consequently an integration of visual and tactile information, beeing processed in parallel on the human side, should facilitate object manipulation and reduce visual loads.

Tschelegi presented a "Feelmouse" [9], which produces an active force on the left mouse-button depending on the display content. While moving the mouse across an object on the screen, the button moves actively and so stimulates a 'feeling' on the users' side. This supports the navigation within a window by lifting the mouse button slightly when touching the title or the scroll bar. For the scroll arrows, the button height changes in correspondance to the position within the whole document. In a second mode the force required to press the button may be varied, enabling to distinguish different situations and to protect the user against possible misuse. Furthermore, vibration behaviour is possible by an intermitting force change. This was tested for a delete button to emphasize the consequences if pressed. Object selection may further be supported by an adaptive feedback reaction for different types of objects. Several examples of using such a 'Feelmouse' demonstrated a better performance compared to the usage of traditional mice. This is true in particular for tasks with a high graphical complexity.

Akamatsu developed a 'multi-modal mouse' with a tactile display in form of a small pin projecting from a hole in the left mouse button [1]. When the cursor reaches an object on the screen, the pin presses against the finger positioned on the button. Thus the operator can confirm that the cursor is within a target, using both visual and tactile information at the same time. The effects on the behaviour of interaction were tested by a target selection task: The mouse cursor had to be moved as quickly and accurately as possible from a start point to the target area, followed by pressing the mouse button. The total operation time was recorded, completed by different detail measures of time sequence duration and position deflections. The results - obtained from ten subjects and twenty trials each- showed with tactile information a non significant reduction of 20 to 80 ms in total operation time. Although the duration of the ballistic part did not change significantly, there was a significant reduction of the cursor stop time ($p<0.01$), as well as of the clicking time ($p<0.01$). The distribution of the clicking positions within the target area was significantly enlarged with feedback. This suggests an increased performance during the corrective movements and facilitated response reactions if tactile information is availiable. A correlation between the cursor stop time, the clicking time and the distance of the clicking position could not be found, revealing that the effects of tactile sensory information correspond independantly to the different task sequences.

A different design was presented by *Göbel*. Instead of force or position feedback on one mouse button, a vibrotactile feedback was generated at both side-planes of the mouse-body [4]. If the cursor comes closer to an object on the screen, vibrotactile signals with increasing intensity associate a virtual energy-field being radiated by the object. A slightly different feedback intensity characteristic enables to distinguish the direction of the mouse cursor in relation to the object. The size of the vibrotactile detection area would decide if either the approximation or the exact positioning were predominantly indicated. To evaluate the influence of the additional vibrotactile feedback on task execution for different kinds of elementary movements, three types of experiments were performed: A continous tracking task to study controlled movements, a positioning task to study ballistic movements, and a selection task to study menu selection execution. During the tracking task, a vertical line moving in a horizontal direction on the screen had to be followed by the mouse-cursor as exactly as possible. The analysis of 22 subjects - each performing 6 trials - showed that the mean deviation increased by 5 % (not significant) if tactile feedback was present. The reaction delay after an abrupt change in movement direction was reduced, but the overswing amplitude increased at the same time. Explanations to such a reaction may be, that the adaptation of tactile feedback characteristic to the tracking task is not yet optimized. For the positioning task, the mouse-cursor had to be driven as fast as possible towards a vertical line after appearing on the screen. The time requirement for the whole task is then significantly ($p<0.01$) reduced with tactile feedback by 11 to 14% . The major factor for this effect is the 45% reduction of the reaction delay. For the selecting task, the mouse-cursor had to be driven into a field at the place of the line, and afterwards the left mouse-button had to be switched. Thereby considerable faster actions during nearly all movement sequences can be measured with feedback, resulting in a total reduction of action duration of 25% (p<0.01). In this case, the movements were less controlled and had a lower stability, but finally lead to a better total performance. Consequently the changes in reaction strategies suggested a more direct and intuitive reaction if tactile feedback is available.

Hedicke presented a trackball, enhanced by two kinaesthetic feedback modes [5]: The first one lifts the ball depending on the objects beeing touched, and the second one provides a controllable friction force while turning the ball. A series of experiments of the same types as they were used by Göbel was exectued by 11 male subjects, having only few experience to work with a trackball. When the lifting mode was applied, for all kinds of movements significantly worse performances were measured with kinaesthetic feedback. Obviously, the lifting of the ball on the target position led to a compensative finger force, which provocates a deviation movement from the target point. The application of the friction force feedback showed a different movement strategy for the tracking task, but finally no significant improvement in performance. For ballistic movements significantly faster task executions can be measured, especially due to the decrease in positioning time of 24 % for the selecting task and 30 % for the menu selection task.

3. New - multiple-dimension - input devices for free hand movements

Conventional input devices usually only have one or two degrees of freedom for movements. More complex forms of interaction, e.g. the manipulation of three-dimensional objects, require more sophisticated input devices for appropriate usage. Data gloves, capturing the human hand and arm motions in a direct way, might be one of the standard input devices for applications in virtual reality, telerobotics, space technology and medicine. Due to the higher number of dimensions for interaction, the meaning of non-visual feedback to support movement control even increases.

Although great in number, only few devices meet the joint requirements of accuracy, robustness and simple usage [2]. To achieve this goal, the 'TU Berlin Sensorglove' was developed by *Hommel et.al.* It consists of a glove with 24 integrated sensors and an ultrasonic range finder. Ten position sensors are fastened to the glove's back and measure finger flexion, and two additional sensors are applied to obtain the thumb rotation. These sensors rely on the inductivity change of a coil in an oscillator, ensuring a high resolution. Twelve additional capacitive pressure sensors - two sensors per finger and two on the palm - are placed on the glove's inside and detect the pressure distribution if an object is grasped. An ultrasonic range finder has been developed to detect the position and orientation of the Sensorglove in space. It is expected to achieve an accuracy of approximately 1 mm in position and 1 degree in orientation. Connection to a host computer is realized by an external controller and a serial data-communication enabling 30 measures per second for each sensor and 10 measure per second for the range finder.

In the field of telerobotics, the 'TU-Sensorglove' is used to control a dextrous robot hand [6]. An operator controls handling tasks by wearing the Sensorglove that are performed by the dextrous hand. Possible applications for this are the machine-control in industrial environments or the control of medical instruments for minimal invasive operations. Therefore, the synthesis of special grasping algorithms is developed through the analysis of human grasping behaviour. In another interdisciplinary project the glove is used for the input and subsequent recognition of hand gestures. For this purpose, the command language will be formalised and the vocabulary has to be defined in a gesture dictionary. The adapted signal processing and classification algorithms including stochastic models, neural networks, genetic algorithms and fuzzy logic models are actually developed, including the enhancement of the Sensorglove with additional acceleration sensors.

Another example of application is the manipulation of sculptured surfaces in a CAD system as reported by *Springer*. This normally requires a high mental effort of the designer, including the mathematical understanding of surface definition and manipulation. Because of the broad application of sculptured surface systems within domains where the manual abilities of the worker plays an important role for task fulfilment, sculptured surface modellers should enable to use these qualification. Direct Manipulation of objects in a CAD system, which is used instead of or beside other dialog techniques corresponds very closely to the "tool idea" of design tasks. One idea of using Direct Manipulation as a realistic dialog technique for geometric design problems is based on tools, which - on the basis of a flexible rough geometrical topology - generate a new volume by distortion of the part or cutting or adding material to a new volume [7]. Processes of by-hand geometric modelling are transformed directly to software. Application areas for a free and by-hand modelling process are industrial design or the design of casts. But still an essential barrier in the handling of such a system consists in the missing feedback of the object's characteristics when manipulating the object. To improve the tasks of qualitative topology description by a CAD-system and software-control, a concept was developed which combines the by-hand abilities and the tactile-kinaesthetic experience of the designer with the Direct Manipulation characteristics of the CAD-system. The existing system consists of an easy-self-developed sculptured surface system with an EXOS-data-glove (Exoskeleton HandMaster^{TM}), used to control the modelling as well as systems functions (e.g. zooming and rotation of the visual CAD model). Switching between both modes is realized by gestures. The properties of the modelling material are characterised by a set of parameters, defining the simultaneous movements of neighbouring points on the manipulated surface and, with that, the extent of the area manipulated. The feedback, which is controlled by the surface model, was realized by tactile feedback in the glove when modifing the surface. Actually the application of a kinaesthetic feedback on a pneumatic basis is tested. The main problem of this device is to transmit fairly high forces into the fingers with lightweight actuators. Such a device will give the possibility to simulate material characteristics for getting a more realistic impression while using Direct Manipulation techniques in the design and manipulation of sculptured surfaces.

To handle digital X-Ray images in medical applications, a new approach to the user interface was presented by *Dahm* [8]. The nature of high-definition digital images, in particular their excessive range of grey shades and their sheer size, prohibits to make use of established workstation concepts from the office automation or CAD domain. The developed concept yields into the interpendence between work, organisation and communication and also justices the different structures of subjective experience of specific users. It was found, that it is efficient to stick the functional seperation between interaction and task - which is typical for established computer workstations - enabling an intuitive link between the interaction and the task performed for the sake of the hand-to-eye-coordination. This requires a dedicated high power image computer for short system response delays.

4. Conclusion and future perspectives

The recent developments of input devices and research on haptic feedback - in addition to visual control - underline the importance of more sophisticated means to support the control of input movements in accordance with the human resources. In several studies, combining conventional computer mice or trackballs with additional forms of haptic feedback, it is shown that significant changes in movement behaviour occur, leading partially to increased task performances. The application of multi-dimensional input devices for Direct Manipulation applications in a three-dimensional work-space emphasizes even more the meaning of an additional haptic feedback to support movement control and object handling. For this, the development of light-weight actuators and sensors with acceptable performance in terms of signal intensity and resolution will be a demanding technical approach to enhance the usability of manual input devices.

All these attempts have to be considered as first experiences for the design of haptic feedback characteristics, but there is still a large lack of knowledge about the detailed mechanisms of human multi-modal information processing and integration, which will be required to design optimized haptic devices. The very different approaches to apply haptic feedback demonstrate, that the design of the feedback characterstics further has to rely very close to the individual task and the individual operations Future devices might provide an adaptive haptic feedback, whose character depends on the actual task as well as on the users' behaviour.

References

1. M. Akamatsu, The influence of combined visual and tactile information on fingerand eye movements during shape tracing, Ergonomics, 35 (1992).
2. S. Aukstakalnis, D. Blatner, Silicon mirage: the art and science of virtual reality, In: Stephen F. Roth (Ed.), Peachpit Press, Berkely, 1992.
3. H.-J. Blume, R. Boelcke, Mechanokutane Sprachvermittlung, Fortschrittsberichte VDI, Reihe 10, Nr. 137, VDI-Verlag Düsseldorf, 1990.
4. M. Göbel, H. Luczak, J. Springer, V. Hedicke and M. Rötting, Tactile Feedback applied to Computer-Mice, Int. J. of Human-Computer-Interaction, 1995 (in press).
5. V. Hedicke, J. Beimel, K. Kornblum and K.-P. Timpe, Kinesthetic feedback for trackballs, In: Grieco, A. , Molteni, G., Occipinti and E, Piccoli, B., 4th Int. Scientific Conference on Work With Display Units, Book of short papers, University of Milan, Vol. 2 (1994).
6. J. Henz, R. Zijal, G. Hommel, Intelligent Manipulation Control for an Imprecise Dextrous Robot Hand solving a High Precision Task, Singapore, ICARCV, 1992.
7. S. Houde, Iterative Design of an Interface for Easy 3-D Direct Manipulation, In: P. Bauersfeld, J. Bennet and G.Lynch, Striking a Balance, Proceedings of the conference on Human Factors in Computing Systems CHI '92 Reading, Mass., Addison Wesley, 1992
8. D. Meyer-Ebrecht, PACS-Picture Archieving and Communication System for Medical Application, Int. J. Biomedical Computing, 1994, in press.
9. M. Tschelegi, The Feelmouse: Applications of force feedback in modern user interfaces, In: Grieco, A. , Molteni, G., Occipinti and E, Piccoli, B., 4th Int. Scientific Conference on Work With Display Units, Book of short papers, University of Milan, Vol. 2 (1994).

The Popularisation of Ergonomics

T.F.M. Stewart,

System Concepts, 2 Savoy Court, Strand, London WC2R 0EZ, UK

There has been a major increase in the public recognition of Ergonomics. Ergonomics has become the buzzword of the nineties. Advertisements for everything from office chairs and computer keyboards to tennis rackets and garden tools now claim to have been 'ergonomically designed'. Ergonomics comes from two Greek words, Ergon - work, and Nomos - law, and involves applying scientific knowledge about the strengths and limitations of people to the design of equipment, workplaces and environments.

'Ergonomically designed' should mean that a product has been designed and tested to be suitable for people to use effectively, efficiently and comfortably. Ergonomics requirements are now incorporated in Standards and in Legislation (both International and National) as well as in every day speech and advertisements. People now take ergonomics seriously and even hard-nosed management is prepared to invest in it as never before. The introduction of ergonomics into regulations and standards has also helped provide a disciplined framework for communicating and formalising ergonomics knowledge.

1.   **ERGONOMICS VS HUMAN FACTORS**

Ergonomics used to have a poor public image and often seemed to mean that someone had replaced the simple styling of a product with ugly but hand sized controls - usually missing the point of the product in the process. The problem with ergonomics as a term is that it is typecast as small scale, focusing on details. In the UK, some ergonomists have started to favour the American term Human Factors as suggesting a broader based discipline which addresses all the aspects - physiological, psychological, sociological and more. Curiously, in the USA, Human Factors Engineers are moving towards the term ergonomics for exactly the same reason. The professional body in the US is now confusingly called the Human Factors and Ergonomics Society.

The term 'human factors' may be attractive in Europe but, in English at least, runs the risk that it is too similar to conventional usage. Television programmes about 'the human factor' inevitably deal with the unpredictability of people, the apparent irrationality of human behaviour and the importance of 'being nice to people'. The professional term 'human factors' is rather different and is more about methods of increasing the predictability of human behaviour and of designing products and systems to capitalise on such prediction. 'Being nice to people' is no bad thing and I believe we could do with rather more of it, but in practice it is not the reason why management should take account of ergonomics. The reason why ergonomics is of vital concern for industry is that without adequate attention to human factors, technology simply does not work properly, nor deliver real benefit, or worse, can be unsafe.

2. WHY WAS ERGONOMICS IGNORED BEFORE?

First, I believe that it important to dispel a myth common amongst ergonomics enthusiasts. Industry does not just ignore or undervalue ergonomics. There are many other good practices which industry in general fails to exploit properly. These include project management, time management, energy efficiency, operational research, management information systems, industrial and graphics design and so on.

Secondly, the costs of poor ergonomics are seldom attributed accurately. How many times is 'pilot error' blamed for technology design failures? How many systems fail because the users never learned to use them properly? How many new products are withdrawn because people found them unacceptable?

The problem is epitomised by a comment made to me by an engineer who built radar consoles when he discovered that I was an ergonomics consultant. He said 'why does the ergonomic solution always conflict with the technical solution?' He was complaining about conflicting requirements of squeezing technology into a small space (the technical solution) with laying the displays and controls out so that the user could work effectively (the ergonomic solution). His frustration was understandable but misplaced. The real problem is that his training, experience and job pressures prevent him from seeing his job as creating a radar console which could be used. Packing in the technology should not have been the objective, only a means to an end.

Finally, many human factors specialists do not practise what they preach. As a human factors practitioner, I am well aware of the importance of understanding the user's needs in the design of products and services. As a business consultant, I am well aware of the importance of understanding my customer's needs if I wish to be paid and gain repeat business. However, I am constantly struck by the failure of some of my colleagues in human factors to recognise that these are both the same point. Our 'users' have important needs which we must appreciate if we are to help them achieve successful change. We are happy to tell designers to pay attention to their users, to use systematic methods of collecting data, to perform pilot studies and trials and to be responsive to feedback. But we are often not very good at selling ergonomics ideas ourselves.

3. WHY ARE ERGONOMISTS BAD AT SELLING ERGONOMICS?

I suspect one reason might be that ergonomists do not have the personality to be salespeople. There has been considerable research by occupational psychologists on the personality traits found in salespeople. Two main traits have been identified - empathy and ego strength.

3.1 Empathy

Empathy means understanding the customers and seeing it from their point of view. Ergonomists seem to be good at empathy. Indeed, one of the major roles of the ergonomist is to 'put him or herself into the user's shoes' and represent the user's position early in the design process.

However, when it comes to selling ergonomics, the ergonomist's empathy may be misplaced. Our empathy needs to be with our customers, for example managers or designers, not just with the end-users of the equipment. Our record for empathy with designers is poor. We are always telling them how they must behave.

Taking this a little further, we tend to view the people that use our services at users. Instead, I would argue that we should see them as customers. As CUSTOMERS, the USERS are still there, but they have some additional characteristics.

C stands for choice. The term user implies that the most important aspect is the use. Customers have other attributes and choosing to buy ergonomics is only one of their options. We have got to help them to make the choice to use us.

T is for trust. Customers buy something with the firm expectation that it is going to work. They trust the supplier. You buy a washing machine, and it washes clothes. If it does not then you often have rights to get your money back. But in information technology, you buy a computer and in order to get it to do anything useful, you also have to buy software and then find out how to use it and so on. Ergonomists can be just as bad at delivering what the customers expect. How often do we avoid giving clear recommendations?

O is for objectives. Unlike a user, the customer's objectives lie outside mere use. They are not interested in the 'ergonomics answer' if it ignores other vital considerations such as economics. Recognising the objectives of our customers gives us a much better chance of delivering something that is genuinely useful to them.

M is for Money. The final point is that customers have money. It is interesting how having to pay for something focuses attention on the essentials. When people do pay for ergonomics, they expect it to be useful, correct and delivered on time. Our professions record in this respect is not always as good as it should be.

3.2 Ego strength

On the question of ego strength, there would seem to be no problem there - plenty of 'egos' in ergonomics. However, again our ego strength may be misdirected. The ego strength in the salespeople is important, because they are committed to achieving successful sales. Failing to sell is a personal affront. I do not think all ergonomists feel that way. How often do we hear 'but they did not use our results' or 'we could not persuade them to adopt an ergonomic approach' reported as though that was normal and acceptable. Good salespeople do not view failure that way.

Our approach often follows a medical model in which we are the specialist doctors and our customers are patients. I have called it **'white coat' ergonomics**. There are a number of characteristics of this approach. We keep the specialist knowledge to ourselves. We encourage mysticism, we use obscure language, and we keep ourselves separate. Furthermore, we misunderstand the purpose of ergonomics for our 'patients'. "The operation was successful, but the patient died", a surgeon might say, so too will ergonomists. "The product failed but we did a good ergonomics study", and we do not seem to care.

What we need to do is to learn the lessons we preach to other people, and consider the need of our users and customers. We must adopt a different model, I call it **shareware ergonomics**. Shareware is a term from the computer industry for a type of software which people are encouraged to copy. Rather than protect their products, the designers encourage you to copy it and send to your friends. You can try it and use it without penalties. If you like it, you are then expected to send some money for the latest version and the documentation. The software designers survive on their merits. We should do that more often with ergonomics. We should spread the word. We should also encourage amateurs to use ergonomics properly. They will try to use ergonomics anyway.

We should not be defensive and worry about protecting our own interests. I believe the outcome will be the 'survival of the useful'. If we have something useful to offer, we will survive. The marginal, the doubtful and the obscure will suffer and may die, because neither amateurs nor professionals want it. If we are professional, we will continue to work and be busy, but only by delivering added value.

As I have said already, we are better at telling other people how to behave, rather than following our own advice. We must understand our own customers to succeed. I would like to suggest four key points to remember when talking to our customers.

- **LISTEN!** I suspect many ergonomists treat consultancy as an opportunity to show how much they know about a topic. It is a little like students who do not read exam questions properly. They treat it as though it said 'write as much as you can about one of the words you recognise in the question'. In dealing with our customers, we must listen to learn what their requirements are and pay close attention.

- **CARE!** We should be offended if they do not use our product. We presumably believe in ergonomics - I do. We must communicate this enthusiasm. We should be 'grabbing their attention' to persuade them and use all the techniques we can find to get them adopt what we believe is right.

- **SELL!** Selling is not just the listening and the caring, it is also closing the deal - a financial transaction. In that transaction, we have to specify our part of the contract in terms which are meaningful to the customers and at a price they are willing to pay.

- **DELIVER!** There is no point in selling ergonomics as 'hype'. If we sell but fail to deliver, then we set back the cause of good ergonomics and discredit our profession.

4. POPULARITY HAS ITS 'DOWN SIDE'

There is also a negative side to increased public demand for ergonomics. Manufacturers are more likely to use the words 'ergonomically designed' in their advertising than apply an ergonomics approach to their activities. Some of the public attention is little more than lip-service and in many organisations, ergonomics is being entrusted to marginalised individuals who have little real authority or power to influence the business. Even worse, unworkable laws may bring ergonomics into disrepute and the discipline is being hijacked by opportunists.

To address this challenge, ergonomists are organising themselves and improving the professionalisation of their discipline. But we must not forget to support this popularisation and professionalisation by more active and equal collaboration with other professionals.

5. COLLABORATION IS VITAL

Our record for collaboration with other professionals is not good. We are happy to complain about the way designers do not appreciate what we are offering, cannot apply themselves to learning even the simplest of experimental techniques and keep asking ridiculous questions with unrealistic expectations about the speed with which we can answer them. We complain about territoriality in other disciplines yet fail to notice our own 'ergocentricity'.

One answer, it seems to me, at the risk of being provocative, is that there must be less 'us and them' and a great deal more of the 'how can we help you solve these problems?' This involves a degree of mutual respect and mutual confidence. It also requires a degree of self confidence. That self confidence is not well served by endless agonising about whether what we are doing is 'proper' science, psychology or engineering?

Problems tend to be multidisciplinary, yet cutbacks in academic funding seem to have encouraged a retrenchment to core disciplines in funding both research and teaching. This was probably not intended but as funds become more limited, who is going to risk research proposals which 'fall between the cracks'? In the UK, the Joint Councils Initiative on Cognitive Science was a welcome move to buck the trend but may not have helped to support genuinely 'fringe' activities. The scientific parameters on which research quality was judged may still have tended towards the traditional physical sciences. To me, a key ingredient in genuine inter- or multidisciplinary activity is that it involves teamwork and mutual respect for participants.

In addition, there is an urgent requirement to develop education and training for users of ergonomics, to develop sensible ergonomics tools and to make ergonomics knowledge more usable. As ergonomics consultants, we often see investment in expensive furniture wasted because the staff do not know how to use the adjustability provided. Even when the furniture is old, there is much that staff can do to get the best out of it, if they have some ergonomics skills themselves. In 1987, recognising our clients' need for ergonomics training for their in-house staff, we established The

Ergonomics Training Centre, which is now based in the Business Design Centre in North London. We run regular office and industrial ergonomics training courses both in-house and for public consumption. Two of our most popular courses were originally developed by the Joyce Institute in the US. The Datahealth™ course is aimed at VDT users themselves and is very practical. It recognises that individual solutions may vary widely. Thus the morning classroom session (conducted on-site) is followed up by workarea consultations where the trainer helps the staff apply the general principles to their own workplace. Practical Office Ergonomics™ is a two day course which covers the key ergonomics principles associated with the European Directive on display screen work and trains individuals to carry out workplace assessments using practical checklists.

Our experience with these courses suggests that many individuals are interested in ergonomics and are willing to learn to apply it properly to their own workplaces. Some might argue that by providing such training and encouraging ergonomics self reliance, we are doing ourselves out of business. That is neither our belief, nor our experience. We really do believe that ergonomics is too useful and too important to be kept to ourselves.

6. BEWARE THE 'COWBOYS'

We have already seen signs of 'ergonomics consultants' who barely know how to spell ergonomics let alone practise it professionally. These cowboys tend to be cheap (in every sense of the word) and may win contracts against reputable ergonomic consultants. The poor service these people offer sometimes results in increased work for other ergonomics consultants picking up the pieces. But more often, the clients become disillusioned with ergonomics itself. In the longer term, we all run the risk that 'ergonomics consultant' will become a term of abuse and ergonomics itself discredited. We cannot afford to keep ergonomics to ourselves. We must popularise. We must respond to the demand. If ergonomists do not seize this opportunity, others will.

Ergonomics on video display units - lessons at the federal high school for officials of non technical administration in Germany

Hildegard Schmidt

Ausbildungsabteilung, Bundesverwaltungsamt, 50728 Köln, Germany

1. STARTING POINT

After a study of the German Institute of Occupation (Bundesanstalt für Arbeit) it is forecasted that in the year 2000 more than two third of German employees will work more or less with a computer to get their work done. The institute of occupational education in Berlin has presented the results of an examination in Germany in the year 1992 concerning the influence of technical devices at the workplaces, which showed that working at a video display unit has dominated the work of more than 5.3 Million people[1].

Especially in the administration we can recognize a rising tendency of using a computer. The federal high school for officials of non technical administration in Cologne is teaching every year about 11.000 students. This university should become a platform to perform the teaching of ergonomics on video display units to fulfill article 6 of the directive 90/270/EEC.

As soon as the students will have finished their education, they will work in classic bureaus. Most of this work will be done in a sitting posture in front of a VDU. It is proved that non-ergonomical devices, wrong behavior at the VDUs, bad working-conditions and software which doesn't suit for the task, can cause a lot of diseases, like work related musculoskeletal disorders (WMSD). For 1991 the WHO - Collaborating Center in Essen found out, that 850 days of temporary disablement have been caused by WMSDs for only 100 assured persons. More than 30% of all work related disorders are in Germany caused by WMSDs with rising tendency. Therefore the prevention is most important and should be performed as early as possible.

So the federal high school was supposed to be the best place to start with teaching ergonomics on video display units in November 1993.

2. ORGANIZATION

The students had the option to choose either an ergonomic-course with 20 units (one unit was 45 minutes) in three days, a course about hard- and software and ergonomics for seven days or single lessons about ergonomics on VDUs.

During a short period of three month more than 250 participants joint the classes.

3. GOALS OF THE EDUCATION

Teaching ergonomics on VDUs as a part of the occupational education is the most effective and therefor economical way to help young officials to prevent workplace-related complaints.

Sensibilization for the responsibility to take care of one`s own body and to prevent oneself before diseases, to give knowledge how a VDU should be designed, how to organize one`s work in a healthier way and gaining experience under different working conditions are the main objects of these lessons.

The participants filled out a form to control the teachers work. They had to answer questions concerning the methods of teaching and a question concerning the subject itself: "Do you think the lessons about ergonomics on VDUs will help you to improve your later workplace conditions?" 80% answered with yes; 10% with no; 10% had no opinion.

4. THE CONTENTS

The course is composed out of modular components. This was helpful because of the different wishes of the classes to work out a theme more than an other. For example, I trained a class of former officials of the german postal services who had already classes in this organization about ergonomical VDU, so we skipped that module and talked about the influence of new technologies (haptic devices etc.) on VDU-workers.

4.1. Human factor

What is the meaning of health (WHO); the different components are presented, which are necessary to get satisfied employees.

The effects of non-ergonomic workplaces like unadjustable equipment, wrong positions of monitors or monotone sequences of operations, the influence of the light are discussed.

We talk about the costs for medical treatment, social-health insurances and overall relations between health, productivity, economy and technology.

The aim is to show that taking care for the work environment and handling devices in an ergonomical way is the most economical one for each organization and most satisfying for the employer.

The students design their own catalogue of requirements during this chapter[2].

4.2. Monitor

What are the characteristics of a good ergonomic video display?

The definition and content of MPR II, TCO, the technology, different types of monitors, radiation and the positioning are themes of the chapter.

The aim is to explain the differences between the security protocols TCO and MPR II and the DIN/ISO/CEN - standards. The students are taught to recognize the absence of quality and they learn how to examine the quality of the monitor and how to position it.

In this chapter all participants have used with big success the TCO-Monitor-Checker, a tool to examine the video display combined with a checklist[3].

4.3. Workplace-design

What are the essential requirements to an ergonomicly designed workplace with or without a VDU?

The environment like lightning, noise, climate, smell and the workplace-design in relationship to the work organization are subjects of this module. The students design workplaces, we visit organizations to examine the workplaces "on the job" and lightning and noise are measured.

In a practical way the students should "learn by doing" what are the main influences on a VDU and what can be done to avoid problems like current air, noise and bad light conditions.

After the students work out these themes, they are offered to evaluate workplaces and architecture-plans, to use magnetic boards for the arrangement of VDUs or to visit a company for bureau-furniture.

4.4. Software-ergonomics

What characterize a well designed software?

Communication with the computer is only effective and satisfying, if the software is easy to use independent of the usergroup. The main features of the human-machine-interface, the spreadsheet, the organization of a program, the use of the colors, aid-functions, the presentation of letters and numbers and so fare are worked out with the help of examples. We discuss ISO 9241 part 10 and its practicability for employees working on video display units.

The students learn how to deal with uncomfortable programs and they are supposed to recognize the advantages of a well designed ergonomical software product.

4.5. Prevention and health

Is it unhealthy to work at a video display unit? What can I do to keep me healthy while working with a computer?

Psychological and physiological complaints caused by long-term working on VDUs are shown. Possible sources and the prevention of discomforts are discussed and put into practice. We exercise sitting in the right position and the use of the chair. Next to the right handling of devices it is necessary to keep one`s body in shape by exercise.

In this chapter we point out that while working with a computer, it is healthy to periodically interrupt the work and do exercises to prevent diseases.

The most attractive method is the use of the interactive software product PC-FIT USER SAVER (Humanware, Vienna), an award winning educational tool from Austria. It animates the employee to stretch and strain the muscles but also to take a break for relaxation. And it also informs about the main subjects concerning the work with display units[4].

4.6. Analyses of workplaces

Final examination to prove the knowledge of the students. This chapter gives the opportunity to examine and evaluate a workplace of one`s choice. This is practiced with different tools like the TCO-Monitor-Checker, checklists or interviews. After the analyze of the VDU, we evaluate the results and develop solutions.

The aim was to check if the students have understood the main contents of the subject ergonomics on video display units. And if they therefor will be able to evaluate their later workplaces in the administration.

The young officials work together in groups and are free in the choice of the examination method.

4.7. Excursion

The students visit the Deutsche Arbeitsschutzausstellung, Dortmund, which has been created in the name of the ministry of occupation and social affairs to inform about all kinds of workplaces. One big part of the exhibition is devoted to video display units with all kinds of monitors, software application, bureau furniture and workplace design, test fields for stress enviroment and unhealthy forced posture, a noise channel and much more to discover.

5. CONCLUSION

The courses ergonomics on video display units at the federal high school for non officials of the federal government have shown that there is a big interest in handling the devices of a VDU in an ergonomical way. It was amazing to recognize that a lot of students were interested because they had the feeling that someone cares for their health or their coming situation at work.

REFERENCES

1. R.Jansen and F. Stooß, Qualifikation.BIBB, Berlin, Germany, 1993.
2. W.Duell and C.Katz, Ratgeber., Fa 24 BAU, Dortmund, Germany, 1992.
3. TCO Zentralorganisation der Angestellten und Beamten, Monitor, Stockholm, Sweden, 1993.
4. Humanware, PC-FIT Begleitbuch, Vienna, Austria, 1993.

Country-specific aspects of computer/VDU safety information

A. Donagi and M. Chereisky

Israel Institute for Occupational Safety and Hygiene,
22 Maze St., Tel-Aviv 61010, Israel

All working tools and workplaces have their problems relating to safety, physical health and psychological comfort of the users. Computers and their user-facing components - VDU - are no exception. Moreover, it seems that never in human history has a machine or technology spawned such a multitude of safety concerns that later turned out to be exaggerated, or even non-existent.

This may be partly explained by the fact that the extensive introduction of computers and VDU into various fields of human activity came almost unexpected by the mass psyche. Interestingly, such a psychological unpreparedness had found its expression in a nearly complete absense of computers or similar machines in the world's science fiction literature before the 40s, and the subsequent flood of "cyber-apocalyptic" works.

As a technologically developed country with a culturally heterogeneous population, Israel has its share of problems related to VDU safety and human factors, some typical for all developed nations, and some more country-specific. Being a public institution providing information, consultation, training, publishing and coordination services to the country's industries, education and R&D systems and general public, the Israel Institute for Occupational Safety and Hygiene (IIOSH) is in a good position to assess and comprehend these problems.

This paper represents an attempt of such multi-faceted analysis. Understandingly, it only touches several aspects of the issue, and more in a qualitative rather than quantitative fashion. We also consider some specific problems of safety-related communication in Israel from the viewpoint of an information provider.

1. COMPUTER SAFETY IN THE MIRROR OF INFORMATION REQUESTS

The primary job of the IIOSH information center, which is a major national provider of OSH-related information, is responding to requests coming in virtually non-stop by mail, fax and telephone from all over the country and from abroad. The center makes use of an extensive information base including specialized library, numerous CD-ROM databases, and a computer-abstracted archive of more than 7,000 answers and resumes. On-line connections are maintained with major international information networks.

Analysis of the information request flow has shown the potential hazards of the work with computers and VDU to be a matter of certain concern for Israeli industry and general public. The table shows the number of VDU safety-related requests received and answered during the 1989 - 1993 period.

Table 1
Number of VDU safety-related requests

Year	1989	1990	1991	1992	1993	Total
No. of requests	13	15	25	41	45	139

A steady rise (obviously reflecting growing public interest and concern) is apparent; however, the number of such requests accounts for just over 2 per cent of the total of 7,010 OSH requests handled by the the information center during this period. One should note that Israel is a heavily computerized, "VDUized" and media-permeated country with a higher-than-average health awareness and alarmist tendencies.

More detailed analysis by subtopics (such as "General Safety Information", "Radiation", "Workstation Ergonomics and Human-Computer Interface", "Eyesight Problems", etc.) reveals that the interest in computer/VDU safety tends to be more specialized: the share of "General Safety" requests has dropped from 46% in 1990 to 23% in 1994, while both absolute numbers and percentage shares of "Radiation Hazards from VDU", "Ergonomics" and "Pregnancy" questions have risen significantly. This fact may be explained by:

- Familiarization with computers/VDU as an indispensable part of working environment;
- Fast-growing computer literacy of the population;
- More mature appreciation of involved (or supposedly involved) safety problems.

However, continuing flow of requests on such topics as "Pregnancy Effects" and "Radiation Hazards" - long considered somewhat obsolete by VDU safety specialists - show that the fear of alleged health hazards, especially VLF/ELF radiation, is more ingrained in computer users than might be expected. Below, we attempt to present some explanations for such persistence.

2. SAFETY COMMUNICATION IN A MULTI-CULTURAL ENVIRONMENT

A continuing significant demand for more deep and substantiated information on VDU safety poses a new challenge to an information provider, owing to a number of reasons:
- Huge number of reference sources (over 1,000 since 1989 in the NIOSHTIC and CISDOC databases alone);

- Undecisive and sometimes controversial nature of many articles and surveys;
- Relatively high attention paid to this problem by the mass media;
- Questioners' expectations of "plain and clear" answers;
- Traditionally active attitude taken by the country's powerful trade unions in the workers' safety and health issues.

There are also some country-specific aspects of safety information providing, important for its efficient delivery to people who are affected (actually, potentially, or allegedly) by occupational hazards, including those associated with computers and VDU.

Work safety information describes potential hazards at a work-place, means of accident and health risk prevention, and minimization of their consequences. The wellbeing, and often the life, of working people greatly depend on timely delivery of safety information (SI) by a SI provider (SIP) and its adequate comprehension.

Assurance of the SI availability and efficiency requires significant efforts and planning on the part of a SIP. The problem seems demanding enough even when a target population is more or less homogenous with regard to its professional status, educational level, cultural and linguistic background.

But in many cases additional complications arise due to the cultural diversity of the audience whose members belong to different (sometimes very distant) cultural traditions and are native speakers of totally unrelated languages (e.g., Polish and Amharic). Normally, they share common socially institutionalized language(s) - in the case of Israel, Hebrew (which is also the native or preferred language of the majority of population) and sometimes English. However, the level of command and communicating skills of "language minorities" members vary greatly.

In such a multi-cultural environment, a SIP is confronted with an uneasy choice, as witnessed by long-time experience of the IIOSH Information Center:

- To present information in the majority (official) language, with possible concessions to an anticipated inability of a part of the target population (i.e., "occupationally-wise") to adequately comprehend it; or
- To dissect the targeted population into culturally homogenous subgroups ("linguistically-wise") and to address each sub-group separately.

The choosing of the first ("occupationally-wise") option calls for a number of factors and demands to be taken into account by the SIP:

(1) Optimal degree of language simplification, sufficient for understanding by non-fluent recipients, but not over-simplified to impair the contents and to annoy fluent recipients.

(2) Probable incongruity between professional and intellectual level of a recipient and his/her language skills (typical for many new immigrants).

(3) Careful selection of technical terms, possibly in favor of those sounding more "international", instead of indigenous equivalents.

The second ("linguistically-wise") option also involves serious problems:

(1) Problems of translation, including selection of appropriate technical terms and expressions:

- Different terms with the same meaning used by a local "language minority" and their "metropolia brethren" (e.g., the Russian-speaking populations in Israel and in Russia);
- Varying meanings and usage of the same terms ("Translator's false friends");
- Differences in the perception of expression style and symbolics, crucially important due to a vital and time-pressing nature of SI;
- "Language generation gap" between specialist translators (typically veteran citizens, whose terminology, style and usage concepts are outdated) and their newcomer-comprised audience.

(2) Methodological and logistic problems of addressing a population the characteristics and distribution of which across the national economy are difficult to evaluate.

(3) Economic considerations and probable unwelcoming attitude from the society at large.

In our opinion, efficient solutions for the problem of safety communication in a multi-cultural environment should be as pluralistic and diversified as the environment itself. A scientifically and practically based combination of these two major approaches, based on additional research, would help SIPs to effectively provide working people of different origins with health- and life-saving information.

3. DELIVERING THE MESSAGE

Efficient provision of the computer/VDU safety information to its targeted recipients, taking into accounts the above-discussed country-specific factors, involves a number of activities:

- Continuous close monitoring of the worldwide trends in research and improvement of computer/VDU safety. With all due respect and atention to the efforts in this direction undertaken by European countries (including those aimed towards implementation of the EEC Directive into national legislations), a non-European country such as Israel, whose own research resources and facilities are limited, should rely on universally accepted evaluations and judgements of internationally recognized bodies, like ILO. This organization regularly addresses the issue of VDU safety. Its 1989 publication *Working with Visual Display Units* [1] was followed in 1994 by the more specific and conclusive *Guidance* on VDU radiation safety [2], which contains highly useful list of typical questions and answers. Among numerous national publications on VDU safety, we would like to cite the New Zealand *Code of Practice* [3], which can serve as an example of objective, careful and unambiguous presentation, well suited for the needs of a small non-European (at least geographically speaking) country. Proceedings of international scientific forums are also an important source of solid information, particularly those of WWDU conferences - see, e.g., proceedings of WWDU '92 in Berlin [4].

- Preliminary processing of information: selection of suitable publications, their careful evaluation, referencing, abstracting, and incorporation into the information base. The selected items are being made available to the IIOSH staff and to a number of organizations and individual specialists collaborating with the Institute. Due to a small size of the country, a college-like atmosphere may be maintained of largely informal professional communication, which greatly facilitates and expedites the exchange of data and opinions;
- Digesting and translation of selected information into Hebrew and, sometimes, into other languages widely spoken and read in Israel (especially Arabic and Russian). Experience shows that translation into "minority languages" should be made directly from the source language (mostly English), rather than from a "mediator language", i.e. Hebrew;
- Publication of translated, as well as original, material in various forms: reviews and analytical papers in professional journals; "Data Sheets" distributed among industry plants and other major employers (universities, government-owned corporations, defence forces); articles in the general press, etc. For example, a paper reviewing the up-to-date results in the field of computer and VDU radiation safety has been published recently in the broadly circulating Hebrew-language *Occupational Safety* journal [5]. A similar publication is also to appear in a locally published English-language medical science journal. Sometimes the issue is presented for coverage by radio and television, which is especially efficient for delivering the up-to-date information to the owners and users of a very large number of computers in homes, schools and small businesses. It is clear, that these groups of users are less approachable through regular publication channels. Efficient appreciation and distribution of safety information is facilitated by the fact that the IIOSH staff comprises native speakers of at least eight languages;
- Actions aimed at appropriate updating of curricula of educational and professional training institutions, primarily of the Safety Instruction Center operated by IIOSH and conducting courses and seminars at different levels.

The recent developments in the field of computer/VDU safety and human factors justify more extensive and deep research of the involved country-specific factors. In addition to those already mentioned, subjects calling for investigation include:

- Effect of local/regional environmental conditions upon work with computers and VDU;
- Special aspects of bilingual user interface, including subjective preferences;
- Efficiency and safety of computer/VDU use by "white-collar" migrant workers (typically well-educated but language-deficient and computer-illiterate);
- Introduction of computer-based technologies into "low-tech" industries, psychological effects upon conservative workforce and methods of professional retraining (with computer/VDU as either a new working tool or a training tool); and others.

These problems may prove actual for other countries as well, in view of massive post-Cold War economy restructuring and workforce migration. In our opinion, their solution should be pursued within the framework of international multi-disciplinary research collaboration, of which the WWDU Conferences have become an important forum.

REFERENCES

1. Working with Visual Display Units (Occupational Safety and Health Series, No. 61). International Labour Office, Geneva, 1989.
2. Visual Display Units: Radiation Protection Guidance (Occupational Safety and Health Series, No. 70). International Labour Office, Geneva, 1994.
3. Approved Code of Practice for the Safe Use of Visual Display Units. Occupational Health and Safety Service, Department of Labour, Wellington, New Zealand, 1993.
4. Work with Display Units 92. Selected Proceedings of the 3rd International Scientific Conference on Work with Display Units (Berlin, 1992), North-Holland, Amsterdam, 1993.
5. A. Donagi, S. Weissman and M. Chereisky, On the Problem of Electromagnetic Radiation Emitted by Computers: An Information Update, Btichut (Occupational Safety), No. 235 (1995) [In Hebrew].

A Systems Analysis for Integrating Macroergonomic Research into Office and Organizational Planning

M.M. Robertson[a] and M.J. O'Neill[b]

[a]University of Southern California
Institute of Safety & Systems Management
Los Angeles, California 90089-0021

[b]Herman Miller, Inc.
Research and Design
P.O. Box 205, #0440, Zeeland, Michigan

1. INTRODUCTION

Researchers have noted that the traditional ergonomic approach to VDU research emphasizes the microscale or microergonomic aspects of the work environment (e.g., keyboard, screen image, manuscript placement, etc.). This approach needs to be broadened to include an understanding of other physical variables, (e.g., layout, storage, and adjustability) organizational design, and psychosocial variables and their relationship to stress, health and effective work (Brill, Margulis, Konar, & BOSTI, 1984; Bradley, 1989; Hedge, Sterling, Sterling, 1986; Carayon, 1992; Sauter, Dainoff, & Smith, 1990; Robertson, & Rahimi, 1990). Relatively few studies have taken such a macroergonomic approach (Brill, et.al., 1984; Bradley, 1993; Sauter, Dainoff, & Smith, 1900; O'Neill, 1994). This research suggests that there is potential for translating the findings from a macroergonomic approach into relevant office design, and organizational planning interventions.

Since stress and performance problems are complex and multivariate in nature, many of the underlying causal factors in an analysis of the work place may be under-identified or completely omitted. As a result, only the more obvious symptoms of computer intensive office workers have been studied, which can lead to superficial solutions. To address this issue, this paper describes the application of a systems analysis model, coupled with research findings derived from a broader, macroergonomic framework, to provide a process for more comprehensive, systematic solutions (Robertson & Rahimi, 1990). The application of this systems model is targeted at solving office workers' performance and effectiveness problems within intensive office technologies environments and providing realistic solutions for improving performance.

2. SYSTEMS ANALYSIS MODEL

This paper describes and demonstrates the first three steps of a seven step system analysis model. This model is a modification of one proposed by Mosard (1982) which is based on earlier work in systems engineering by A.D. Hall (1969). The proposed system analysis model consists of seven steps. These are: 1) defining the problem; 2) setting the objectives and developing an evaluation criteria table; 3) developing alternatives;
4) modeling alternatives; 5) evaluating alternatives; 6) selecting an alternative; 7) planning for implementation, evaluation, & modification.

2.1 Defining the problem

A high level of complexity is generally inherent to large scale problems and issues. This in turn necessitates a formal, systematic analytical approach to problem definition (Mosard, 1982). Thus, step 1 in the systems analysis approach involves defining the problem. Warfield (1974) proposed an analytical tool that has proven useful in defining large complex problems, called a "problem factor tree," which develops the problem, sub-problems, and causal factors, including their interrelationships. In this process, the major problem is broken into smaller sub-parts (Mosard, 1982).

To develop a problem factors tree, the problem factors are precisely stated and carefully linked together through an iterative process (Mosard, 1982). The lower level problem factors in the model contribute to the major problem. Feedback loops may also be incorporated. Thus, the problem factor tree depicts a hierarchical, logical structure for understanding the elements of a problem. Figure 1 depicts the defined problem of "an increase in absenteeism and turnover, and a decrease in performance and effectiveness of office workers." It is hypothesized that the problem is caused by occupational stress from office technologies, and workplace design. Three major sub-problems thought to contribute to the main problem, and supported by several research studies are defined: health problems, psychosomatic stress and physiological stress. For psychosomatic stress two sub-problems are defined: pyschosocial disturbances, and perceived lack of environmental control. Figure 1 shows numerous causal problem factors which contribute to the major problem. Lack of job content, poor job design, and lack of flexible workstation design are the last three causal problem factors depicted at the base of the hierarchical structure.

There are many sub-problems identified in regard to physiological stress. Some of these include visual discomforts and musculoskeletal discomforts. Numerous causal problem factors are shown, contributing to both sub-problems, with the last problem factors being lack of flexible workstation design, improper VDU screen design and improper layout and design of workstation.

This problem factor tree depicts the causal factors and sub-problems that represent the integration of microergonomic and macroergonomic office and job design issues.

2.2 Setting the Objectives and Developing Evaluation Criteria

In step 2 of the systems analysis method, the objectives and evaluation criteria are developed for use in selecting the best alternative for achieving the objectives. An "objective tree" is created as part of this process (se Figure 2). An objective tree is a hierarchal, graphical structure of objectives that addresses the problems that have been identified (Mosard, 1983). The objective tree is created by first identifying the major needs, goals, objectives and sub-objectives. The objective tree for the proposed problem

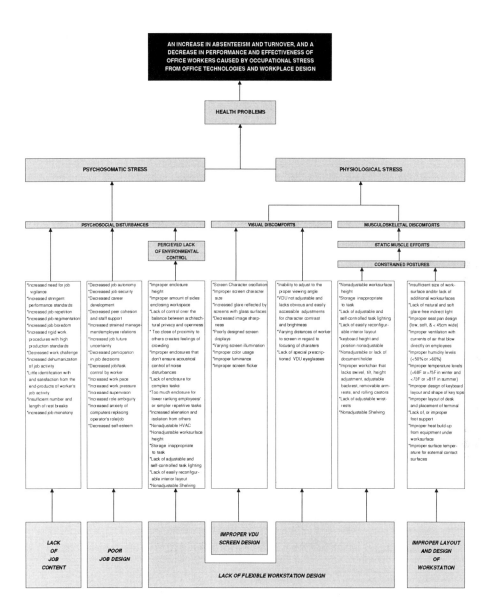

Figure 1: A depiction of the problem factor tree. The major problem is defined at the top with the sub-problems and causal factors shown below indicating the hierarchical, logical structure of the encompassing problem elements.

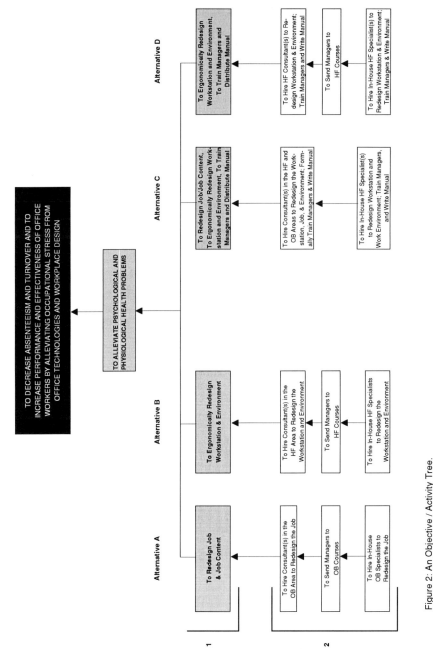

Figure 2: An Objective / Activity Tree.

Note: 1 = Objective Tree
2 = Alternative / Activities Tree

is depicted in the upper half of Figure 2. The major goals identified are to "decrease absenteeism and turnover, and to increase performance and effectiveness of office workers by alleviating occupational stress from office technologies and workplace design."

In the objective tree, the lower level objectives contribute to the attainment of the middle level objectives, which in turn contribute to the upper level needs or goals (Warfield, 1972). The objective shown in Figure 2 is to alleviate psychological and physiological health problems. Four sub-objectives are defined (e.g., to redesign the job and job content, to ergonomically redesign the workstation and environment, to redesign the job, to ergonomically redesign the workstation and environment and to train managers in job and workstation redesign and awareness and to distribute a manual).

To facilitate the development of the objectives tree, the degree of interaction between objectives, constraints, and the persons/groups involved in the process should be analyzed (Mosard, 1982).

2.3 Developing alternatives

Step 3 of the systems analysis approach involves developing alternative approaches to attaining the objectives and sub-objectives. Alternatives are defined as a specified set of activities or tasks designed to accomplish an objective (Mosard, 1982). The objective/activity tree in Figure 2 illustrates four alternatives (A through D), along with their appropriate set of activities. Hybrid alternatives may be created which incorporate the best features of several of the initially identified alternatives. Alternative C is a hybrid alternative representing only one of the many possible combinations of common activities that could be specified. The four alternatives depicted here were derived from case studies and field research representing typical approaches implemented by organizations to achieve the objective listed at the top of Figure 2.

After the objectives and alternatives are selected, a preliminary decision criteria table is developed. This criteria table is used to evaluate the usefulness of each of the alternatives as methods for accomplishing the objectives. Decision criteria typically include risks, costs, benefits, and measure of effectiveness, which may be based on short-term and long-term perspectives (Mosard, 1982; 1983).

While not described in this paper, the complete systems analysis model can also be used to analyze the relative effectiveness of alternative design interventions, provide a cost/benefits analysis, establish the relative importance of each evaluation criteria and a plan for implementing and evaluating the selected alternative.

3. CONCLUSION

This paper described and demonstrated the use of a systems model incorporating the findings of empirical and field research, as well as case studies collected from a worldwide sample. This approach identifies the salient variables which influence health and performance. Typically, companies focus on narrow solutions to reducing occupational stressors associated with intensive VDT work. This results in ineffective solutions. The important benefit of the systems model described in this paper, is the integration of micro-ergonomic and macro-ergonomic approaches for solving organizational problems. Companies are now at a point where they are willing, due to rising health costs and legislation, to allocate resources in order to adequately address office technologies problems. Applying this systems analysis approach can enhance an organization's competitive edge by improving the fit between the office worker, the job, and the physical environment, resulting in a more healthful and effective work environment.

REFERENCES

Bradley, G. (1989). *Computers and the Psychosocial Work Environment*. Taylor and Francis, London.

Brill, Margulis, Konar, & BOSTI, (1984). Using office design to increase productivity. Vols. 1 and 2. Buffalo, NY.: *Workplace Design and Productivity*.

Carayon, P. (1992). A longitudinal study of job design and worker strain: Preliminary results. In J. Quick. L. Murphy, J. Hurrell Jr. (Eds.) *Stress & Well Being at Work: Assessments and Interventions for Occupational Mental Health*. APA, Washington, D.C., Brown-Brumfield, Inc. MD.

Hall, A.D., (1969). A three dimensional morphology of systems engineering. *IEEE Transaction System Science Cybernetics*, Vol. SSC-5, pp. 156-160.

Hedge, Sterling, Sterling, (1986). Evaluating office environments: The case for a macroergonomic systems approach. In O. Brown, Jr. and H. W. Hendrick (Eds.) *Human Factors in Organizational Design and Management - II*, Elsevier Science Publishers B.V. (North-Holland), 419-424.

Mosard. G. (1982). A generalized framework and methodology for systems analysis. *IEEE Transaction Engineering Management*, Vol. EM-29, pp. 81-87.

O'Neill, M.J., (1994) Workspace adjustability, storage and enclosure as predictors of worker reactions and performance. *Environment and Behavior*, 26 (4), 504-526.

Robertson, M. & Rahimi, M. (1990). A systems analysis for implementing video display terminals. *IEEE Transactions Engineering Management*, 37(1), 55-61.

Sauter, S.L., Dainoff, M.J., & Smith, M.J., (1990) *Promoting Health and Productivity in the Computerized Office*, London: Taylor & Francis.

ACKNOWLEDGEMENTS

The authors would like to express their appreciation to Alex Ritzema for his efforts in data collection, and development of the graphics presented in this paper.

FINDINGS OF THE OFFICE ERGONOMICS RESEARCH COMMITTEE

R. F. Bettendorf, Executive Secretary
One Bonnet Street, P.O. Box 1267
Manchester Center, VT 05255

1. Introduction

The Office Ergonomics Research Committee was formed in April 1991 by a group of U.S. companies that were concerned by reports of an increasing number of upper extremity musculoskeletal disorders (UEMD) among office workers. The committee's objective is develop an understanding of office related upper extremity musculoskeletal disorders (UEMD) with an emphasis on determining the effect that office work has on causing or exacerbating them, what interventions are successful in preventing or resolving them and what treatments are recommended in dealing with them. Current members include: Apple Computer, AT&T Global Information Solutions Corporation, The Center for Office Technology, Compaq Computer Corporation, Details, Inc., Herman Miller, Kensington Microware, Key Tronic, Keyboard Productivity Inc., The Knoll Group, Lexmark International, McClatchy Newspapers, Microsoft, Steelcase, UNISYS and USAA.

Initially, the committee developed twelve questions that needed to be answered to develop an understanding of the causes of and strategies necessary to deal with these disorders. These questions dealt with the type and frequency of the disorders in the office environment; their causes and the interventions required to address them; the role that input devices, workstation ergonomics, exercise and psychosocial factors play; the medical aspects; and, how to communicate the intervention strategies that will successfully address them.

The approach taken was to establish and add to a UEMD knowledge base concerning these questions by literature searches, the opinions of experts brought in to address specific questions or topics and by investigations conducted by committee members. A major contributor to this knowledge base was the collective experiences of member companies in dealing with musculoskeletal disorders in their employee populations.

To fill in the gaps, the committee has funded significant research studies, research symposia and literature analyses on the association between keyboards, mice, office furniture, psychosocial factors and these disorders.

Progress has been made in developing the answers to many of the answers to these questions. The following sections outline the committee's major findings as of January, 1995.

2. Extent of the problem

The U.S. Bureau of Labor Statistics (BLS) reports yearly on the number of newly reported occupational injuries and illness in private industry workplaces.[1] Table 1 contains the latest BLS data.

Table 1
U.S. Bureau of Labor Workplace Injuries and Illnesses

Category	1991	1992	1993	Delta
Total Injuries & Illness (thousands)	6,345	6,799	6,737	-1.0%
Total Illness	368,000	457,000	482,000	+5.5%
Repeated Trauma Cases	224,000	281,800	302,400	+7.3%
Repeated Trauma Incidence Rate - All Industries (per 10k full time worker)	29.7	36.8	38.3	+4.1%
Repeated Trauma Incidence Rate F/I/RE Industries * (per 10k work years)	8.6	19.2	23.7	+23.4%

* The Finance, Insurance & Real Estate Industries are white collar industries and may be indicative of rates for all office workers

The above shows that repeated trauma illnesses are only a small (4.5) percent of all occupational illnesses and injuries but they increased while total injuries and illnesses declined. However, the 7.3% rate of increase is a decline from the rates of 25% and 18% in 1992 and 1991.

The repeated trauma incidence rate per 10,000 full time workers in all industries increased slightly. Of concern to the committee is that the rate in the white collar finance, insurance and real estate industries increased at a far greater rate of 23.4% in 1993. The Bureau also reported that 12% of the repetitive motion problems were in typing or key entry tasks and that 21% of all these disorders were in the white-collar occupations of technical, sales and administrative support.

3. Input Device Research

In 1991, the committee was disappointed when it found that the body of existing keyboard research dealt primarily with the human factors criteria of speed, error rate and whether operators liked the feel of the keyboard. They did not address the UEMD question.

Though keying force was being identified as a potential risk factor, there was no standard approach to measure static keyboard force. Confirmed methodologies to measure dynamic keying force did not exist. The actual forces being applied by users and how these forces compared to the force required to activate the key switch had not been determined. However, approaches to measure keyboard force being applied by typists were evolving in the laboratories of the Universities of Michigan and California-San Francisco.

Since then significant progress has been made in this area, partially due to committee funding of several keyboard projects.

The committee developed keyforce/displacement curves for the major types of key switches: buckling spring; rubber domes; mechanical switches; and linear springs. The characteristics of each varied significantly. Since no common terminology or methods of measuring static key forces existed, the committee has proposed a methodology and terminology standard to the International Standards Organization. The purpose of this standard is to help ensure that the static keyboard force measurements by manufacturers and universities are consistent and comparable.[2]

The committee findings to date indicate that users hit the keys much harder than is necessary to activate them.

A study by M. Feuerstein of the University of Rochester, funded by the committee, found that users strike the keys four to five times harder than is necessary to activate the key switch.[3] This replicates the earlier work of Armstrong and Remple that found that their subjects' average force ranged from 2.2 to 4.7 times the force required.[4]

Contrary to expectations, the Feuerstein study found no correlation between typing speed and force applied. It also found that subjects with UEMD symptoms hit the keys significantly harder than those without symptoms.

From discussions at research symposia, the committee has confirmed that dose response relationships between keying force or repetition rate and the onset of UEMDs have still not been established.

However, assuming that less force is better than more force, the committee has funded a pilot study with the University of Wisconsin. The objective of this study is to determine the extent that key switch activation force and key displacement influence force applied by users in a tapping experiment. Approaches to study user keying behavior and how to modify keying habits are also being considered.

Due to funding limitations, the committee has relied on the work of others to form its conclusions on the value of alternative keyboards in helping prevent these disorders.

A study by the Lawrence Livermore National Laboratory and the University of California-San Francisco evaluated an Apple Adjustable Keyboard on subjective preference and observed joint angles during typing.[5] It concluded that the subjects in the study rated the Apple Adjustable keyboard as being more comfortable and easier to use than a standard keyboard. However, the ulnar deviation measured on the split keyboard was not significantly reduced vs the standard keyboard which casts doubts on the claim that split keyboards will reduce ulnar deviation.

An IBM Technical Report reviewed and critically examined the split keyboard literature.[6] It was based upon 44 works published from 1926 to 1993. This study found no scientific evidence to support the contention that the use of split keyboards either corrects the symptoms of or prevents the onset of cumulative trauma disorders. It also found no scientific evidence that the use of standard keyboards contributed to their onset. Further there was no compelling evidence that split keyboards improved performance but that they might improve typing comfort.

4. Workstation Ergonomics

The committee agrees that effective use of workstations, ergonomic accessories and personal computer equipment can reduce on-the-job discomforts. However, the relationships between discomforts, UEMDs and disabilities are not known. The committee observes that ergonomic chairs, workstations and devices are proliferating with many conflicting claims concerning their value in reducing musculoskeletal risks.

The committee funded a literature review by the University of Vermont. This review concludes that there is a paucity of scientific studies relating ergonomic factors to upper extremity musculoskeletal disorders in the office environment. Future publication of this study is planned.

One of the committee's member companies, The Knoll Group, conducted a study to determine the segments of the U.S. population that may be properly accommodated by various workstation keyboard surface heights.[7] Previous studies have demonstrated that within the constraints of ANSI/HFS 100-1988, substantially the entire adult US population can be accommodated at a 73.5cm (29") high worksurface by a combination of adjustable seating, footrests, and changes in forearm angle.

This study examined the consequences of the currently accepted ergonomic advice that the forearm should be parallel to the floor while typing to reduce wrist deviation. An elbow angle of ninety degrees plus or minus 5 degrees was assumed. This study demonstrates the need to provide either adjustable worksurfaces or adjustable keyboard supports to achieve a forearm parallel posture. The study also found that adjustable workstations set at 29" are too high. A height of 69 cm (27") will accommodate 92% of the males and height of 64 cm (25") accommodates 54% of the females.

5. Psychosocial Influences

To better understand the role that psychosocial factors play in the experiencing or reporting of upper extremity musculoskeletal disorders, the committee funded a symposium of seventeen international experts that was hosted by Dr. Samuel Moon of the Duke University Medical Center. These experts were from many disciplines including: social and organizational psychology, occupational medicine and safety, office ergonomics, industrial engineering, job stress, neuromuscular research, occupational rehabilitation, orthopedics, and health care economics. The symposium focused on the importance of psychosocial influences on broadly-defined aspects of this problem, mechanisms by which such influences may act, and implications for research and prevention. The presentations and discussions underscored both the importance and complexity of the psychosocial factors on the experiencing or reporting of cumulative trauma disorders. A publication of the proceedings is planned by mid-1995.

The committee recognizes the importance of these factors but has concluded that the relative importance of each factor and the mechanisms involved are not well understood.

6. Medical Considerations

The committee agrees with the contention of medical experts that many UEMD cases never receive a firm diagnosis but are put in catch-all categories such as overuse syndrome, cumulative trauma disorder, etc.[8] For diagnosed disorders such as tendinitis, tenosynovitis, epicondylitis, etc., treatment protocols exist and conservative rather than surgical treatments can be effective in most cases.

The committee also finds that the incidence of carpal tunnel syndrome among office workers is greatly overstated by the popular media.[8] In the NIOSH Newsday Health Hazard Evaluation only twenty-one reports were made of symptoms consistent with carpal tunnel syndrome. This represents 6% of all participants who reported symptoms and only 2.5% of the study's population.[9] A study of three newspapers found that the prevalence of probable carpal tunnel syndrome was only 1.6%.[10]

The committee also recognizes the importance of personal factors such as obesity, age, general physical condition, degree of coordination, stress, hobbies, etc., and predisposing medical factors such as diabetes, thyroid conditions, arthritis, use of birth control pills, pregnancy, hysterectomy, etc.

The committee is also concerned that many primary care practitioners lack the training to properly treat upper extremity musculoskeletal disorders. It urges employers to align themselves with practitioners or clinics that can provide prompt, effective and conservative treatment for employees reporting these disorders.

7. Summary

The committee has found that many misconceptions exist as to the severity and the types of disorders that U.S. office workers are experiencing. There is little scientific evidence on the causes of these disorders and the values of commonly prescribed interventions. Research is starting but it is still very limited. A long term, international research strategy is required to fill the voids in our understanding.

This is a multi-factorial problem for which there is no single solution. All elements of the equation must be included when dealing with an outbreak including equipment and workstation ergonomics, individual personal factors plus individual and organizational psychosocial factors.

References

1. United States Department of Labor, Bureau of Labor Statistics, USDL-94-600, Workplace Injuries and Illnesses in 1993, December 21, 1994.
2. Edwin T. Coleman, Lexmark International, Inc., Keyboard Key Force/Displacements Measurements: Proposed methodology and terminology, Marconi Keyboard Research Conference, 1994.
3. Michael Feuerstein, Tom Armstrong, and Paul Hickey, Keyboard Force, Fatigue and Pain in Symptomatic and Asymptomatic Wordprocessors. 12th Congress of the International Ergonomics Association, Toronto, Canada, 1994.
4. David Rempel, Jack Gerson, Thomas Armstrong, Jim Foulke, and Bernard Martin, Fingertip Forces While Using Three Different Keyboards. Proceedings of the 1991 Human Factors Society 35th Annual Meeting, San Francisco.

5. P. Tittiranonda, S. Burastero, D. Rempel, Ergonomic Evaluation of the Apple Adjustable Keyboard, IEA 1994, Vol. 4: Ergonomie et Design.
6. James R. Lewis, A Critical Literature Review of Human Factors Studies of Split Keyboards from 1926 to 1993, IBM Technical Report-TR54.853, August 3, 1994, IBM Boca Raton, Florida.
7. Karl Konrad, Population Segment Accommodation for Keyboard Entry at Various Workstations, The Knoll Group, 1992.
8. Nortin M. Hadler, Arm Pain in the Workplace: A Small Area Analysis, Journal of Occupational Medicine, February, 1992.
9. NIOSH, Health Hazard Evaluation Report, Newsday, Inc. HETA 89-250-2046, May 1990.
10. Newspaper Association of America and the University of Iowa, Multi-Site Newspaper Study, Results - Phase 1.

Round Table: An unholy alliance - experience of the development and implementation of standards and legislation on display screen equipment in Europe- The CEN/ISO experience

T.F.M. Stewart

System Concepts, 2 Savoy Court, Strand, London WC2R 0EZ, UK

The purpose of this round table was to assess the impact of the display screen directive EEC/90/270 and its relationship with ergonomics standards, particularly ISO 9241/EN 29241. This Directive is the latest and most far reaching of a number of approaches to VDU regulation and some of the current difficulties in interpretation and implementation stem from its interaction with earlier approaches. At the Round Table, two participants reviewed the current situation in their own countries and relate it back to earlier attempts to regulate display screen work through national standards, (Ahmet Cakir - the DIN experience) and through specific national legislation, (Tomas Berns - the Swedish Ordinance experience). Two further participants reviewed the history and implementation of European wide measures including guidance based on extensive research programmes (John Ridd - the researchers experience) and the Directive itself (R Hoftijzer - the EC experience). There was also a Discussant, Per Gunnar Widebeck, who has long experience of ergonomics standardisation. This paper deals with experience in developing European and International standards.

Ergonomics standards play an important role in improving the usability of systems, through improved consistency of the user interface and improved ergonomic quality of interface components. They give managers confidence that the systems they buy will be capable of being used productively, efficiently, safely and comfortably.

The work of the International Organisation for Standardisation is important for two reasons. Firstly, the major manufacturers are international and therefore the best and most effective solutions need to be international. Secondly, the regional European Standardisation Organisation (CEN) has opted for a strategy of adopting ISO standards wherever appropriate as part of the creation of the single market. CEN standards replace national standards in the EC and EFTA member states. This has greatly increased the significance of standards in Europe and as a result has placed significant pressure on ISO.

ISO and CEN have signed a formal agreement (The Vienna Agreement) to ensure effective collaboration and this has given Europe a unique position in international standardisation activities. This should not disadvantage non-Europeans in terms of ergonomics standardisation, since ergonomics aims to address the needs of a range of users and the workforce itself is becoming increasingly international and mobile. With the exception of products that are only used by a very restricted population, good ergonomics standards should cater for as great a range of human variability as possible.

The ergonomics committee in ISO (TC 159) has a sub-committee which deals with human-system interaction (SC 4). It is this committee which has developed ISO 9241. Its members are representatives of the national standards bodies of member countries and meetings involve national delegations in discussing and voting on resolutions and technical documents. The primary technical work takes place in eight Working Groups (WGs) and each of these has responsibility for different work items.

WG1 is responsible for ISO 7249 and ISO 9355 which deal with fundamentals of displays and controls. WG 7 deals with terminology and is currently dormant. WG8 is concerned with ISO 11064, the ergonomics design of control centres.

ISO 9241, which deals with ergonomics requirements for office work with visual display terminals, has been developed by five working groups, WGs 2 to 6. See Table 1.

Table 1.   ISO 9241 Ergonomics requirements for office work with visual display terminals (VDTs)

	Status	Estimate for DIS
Part 1: General Introduction	IS/EN	6/94(Rev)
Part 2: Guidance on task requirements	IS/EN	
Part 3: Visual display requirements	IS/EN	
Part 4: Keyboard requirements	2nd DIS/prEN	5/95
Part 5: Workstation layout and postural requirements	2nd DIS	2/95
Part 6: Environmental requirements	DIS/prEN	5/95
Part 7: Display requirements with reflections	3rd CD	2/95
Part 8: Requirements for displayed colours	2nd DIS	2/95
Part 9: Requirements for non-keyboard input devices	CD 10/94	5/95
Part 10: Dialogue principles	DIS	3/95 IS
Part 11: Guidance on usability specification and measures	3rd CD	2/95
Part 12: Presentation of information	CD 10/94	6/95
Part 13: User guidance	CD	2/95
Part 14: Menu dialogues	3rd DIS	2/95
Part 15: Command dialogues	CD	2/95
Part 16: Direct manipulation dialogues	2nd CD 10/94	9/95
Part 17: Form filling dialogues	CD 12/94	12/95

ISO 9241 contains different types of information to be considered and used (where appropriate) when designing the ergonomic aspects of products, or assessing the ergonomic properties of a system. Some parts provide general guidance to be considered in the design of equipment, software, and tasks. Other parts include more specific design guidance and requirements relevant to current technology, since such guidance is useful to designers. However, ISO 9241 also emphasises the need to specify the factors affecting the performance of the user, and to assess user performance as a basis for judging whether or not a system is appropriate to the context in which it will be used.

As the different parts of ISO 9241 are approved and published as International Standards, they will be adopted as European Standards and become EN 29241 following the Vienna agreement between ISO and CEN.

WG 6 is concerned with how 9241 can be used and also with a new work item on Human-Centred Design of Interactive Systems. (ISO/NP/13407). The purpose of this standard will be to provide support for those responsible for managing design processes to ensure that proper attention is paid to the human and user issues.

Although the main users of the standard will be managers responsible for design and development of interactive systems, the standard will also be useful for specifiers and procurers of systems as well as for developers themselves. The standard will enable users of the standard to assess the benefits of taking account of ergonomic principles and will specify essential activities necessary to ensure human-centred design. It will also provide a framework for reporting that all necessary activities have taken place. For example, although the standard is still at an early stage, it is envisaged that it may contain checklists covering such issues as:

- Has the context of use (users, tasks and environment) been clearly understood or are there explicit plans to gather relevant information as part of the project?
- Is there an appropriate allocation of function between system and user? For example, is the system perceived as a helpful tool to support task performance or is the user relegated to being an input device to the system?
- Is there an explicit and adequate usability requirements specification?
- Is an iterative design process proposed (design-implement-evaluate)?
- Are there plans to prototype the human-system interface and has sufficient time been allowed to incorporate any results?
- Are there adequate procedures proposed for the systematic collection of user input? For example, this may involve a variety of different methods from seconding user representatives onto the design team, through structured trials or prototype systems to user questionnaires and surveys.
- Are established sources of human factors knowledge clearly identified or are there explicit plans to gather such information as part of the project? For example, published national and international standards, in-house style guides, codes of practice etc.
- Is there a usability evaluation plan?

It will therefore be a valuable management tool and will provide guidance on relevant sources of information and standards and on applying the user performance approach to system development. There are already many regulatory and other constraints on system design, therefore this standard complements existing approaches and methods rather than attempting to provide a competing methodology. The underlying motivation for the standard is a recognition that existing design methods take insufficient account of ergonomic requirements. User-centred design offers benefits of increased productivity, enhanced quality of work, reductions in support and training costs and improved user health and safety.

A new Japanese Industrial Standard (JIS) corresponding to Part 3 of ISO 9241 (visual display requirements) — JIS Z 8513-1994

N. Koizumi*

Research and Development Center, Futaba Corporation
1080 Yabuzuka, Chousei (village/county), Chiba 299-43, Japan

1. INTRODUCTION

The last year (1994) became a memorable year for the Japanese Industrial Standard with the completion of a framework regarding ergonomics-related standards, i.e. **JIS Z 8500** through **8599**. Formerly, **JIS Z 8907**-1987 in relation to ISO 1503 (and IEC 447) was the only "JIS", however ISO 1503: 1977 was not an outcome of ISO TC 159 (Ergonomics), but of ISO/STACO originally. On March 1st 1994, **JIS Z 8500**, the first ergonomics-related standard was established[1] in relation to ISO/DIS 7250.2, and published on May 31st, 1994. As the second and the third ones of **85XX** series, **JIS Z 8502** corresponding to ISO 10075: 1991 and **JIS Z 8513** corresponding to ISO 9241-3: 1992 were drafted[2] by separate drafting committees by the end of March 1994, and were established on December 1st 1994. The first edition of **JIS Z 8513** was published on December 31st, 1994.

2. MY UNDERSTANDINGS ON LEGISLATION AND STANDARDS

More than five years have past since my participation in the activity of ISO TC 159 in Japan, as an engineer in the field of emissive flat panel display technology.

Also, since 1990, as a member of sub-committee on the liquid crystal displays under the technical committee on electronic display devices in Electronic Industries Association of Japan (EIAJ), I have been involved in the domestic activity for IEC SC 47C/WG 2, semiconductor optoelectronic and liquid crystal devices. Through such activities and social trends, I got knowledges of the relation among the legislation, standards and guidelines, not only from technological and scientific viewpoints, but also from political ones[3].

As for ISO 9241 series, the special issue on the EC directive on display screen equipment in a British magazine[4] was the most instructive to me.

Table 1 shows relations between various categories of ISO / CEN activities and corresponding legislations originally prepared for my oral presentation in WWDU '94. It was also shown by the transparency in the morning "round table" session on October 4th, 1994, before my presentation in that afternoon.

---

*706 - 10, Shimo-Nagayoshi, Mobara, Chiba 297, Japan (home address in case of after retirement)

Table 1
Various ISO / CEN TC vs BS / UK regulations (S.I.) / ISO / EN & EC OJ,

TC No.	ISO TC 159 Ergonomics (CEN TC 122)	ISO TC 176 Quality management & QA (CEN CS F20)	ISO TC 181 Safety of toys (CEN TC 52)	ISO TC 199 Safety of machinery (CEN TC 114)	ISO TC 207 Environmental management (no TC in CEN)
	ISO CD 9355-1~3	transfered from CEN TC 114 to ISO TC 159		(prEN 894-1~3)	
STD / S.I. No.	(BS 7179-1~6 ··· obs.) ISO 9241-1(~17) EN 29241 series *Part 3 → JIS Z 8513* (ISO CD 13406-2 for FPD)	(BS 5750) ISO 9000~9004 EN 29000~29004 JIS Z 9900~9904	S.I. 1989 / 1275 ISO (not avail. yet) EN 71-1~6 JIS S (not avail. yet)	S.I. 1992 / 3073 ISO *TR* 12100-1,-2 EN 292-1,-2 JIS B/C (not avail. yet)	(BS 7750) ISO 14000 series no EN standard JIS Z? (not avail. yet)
EC OJ etc.	⑤ 89/391/EEC Health & safety directive ↓ *WWDU* *90/270/EEC* DSE* directive *: DSE (display screen equipment) ≈ VDT / VDU ② 89/336/EEC EMC directive ↔ S.I. 1992 / 2372 UK Regl. (EMC) BS EN 50081/2 (CLC TC 110) (IEC TC 77) ④ 73/23/EEC LVD directive	Conformity Assessment Procedures in Community Legislation ⑥ 93/465/EEC Annex	① 88/378/EEC Safety of toys directive ⑤ 89/391/EEC Health & safety directive (Joint task) ⑥ 93/465/EEC CE conformity marking decision 93/68/EEC CE marking amendments**	③ 89/392/EEC Machinery directive	Council regl.(EEC) No. 1836/93 "EMAS" (eco-management and audit scheme) ⇨ C€ **: 87/404/EEC, ① 88/378/EEC, 89/106/EEC, ② 89/336/EEC, ③ 89/392/EEC, 89/686/EEC, 90/384/EEC, 90/385/EEC, 90/396/EEC, 91/263/EEC, 92/42/EEC, ④ 73/23/EEC

The italicized parts in the table (i.e. *Part 3 → JIS Z 8513*, <u>WWDU</u>, and *90/270/EEC* in the column of ISO TC 159, and *TR* in the column of ISO TC 199) were originally printed in red colour with the same font as others to express the main title and points of my oral presentation.

I only listed five ISO TCs which my affiliation should have some concerns but I am confident that "Ergonomics", "Quality (of the product)", "Safety" and "Environment" are all deeply related to the "tenderness to the mankind and the earth" and all industries in the world must take care of such viewpoints from now on.

3. THE ACTIVITY OF THE JIS DRAFTING COMMITTEE

As reported intermediately in my previous short paper[2], the drafting committee of **JIS Z 8513** was composed by eighteen members chaired by Dr. S. Saitoh beside the Japanese Ergonomics National Committee on ISO TC 159/SC 4.

For the period of eight months from July 1993 through February 1994, eleven sub-committee meetings together with six plenary meetings were held to complete the final draft to be submitted to AIST / MITI.

My personal opinion which was somewhat of minority in the committee was revealed as some part of the technical report[3] of the second Asian symposium on information display, which was held in Hamamatsu, Japan about three weeks later than WWDU '94, titled "Reconsiderations of the VDT ergonomics standards from technological, scientific and Asian cultural viewpoints, but not political ones". However, as the report includes the problems not only for Part 3, but also for Part 6 and 8 of 9241 series, here in this article I would like to introduce some contents of the "explanatory notes" for **JIS Z 8513**, which will be attached to the text as a supplement, when the standard will be published later.

As this explanatory notes are *neither* a part of provision, *nor* a part of the standard itself, English texts of them are usually unavailable even when the English version of **JIS Z 8513** will be published in the future. Actually, the draft of this explanatory notes is prepared by Sub-Group 1 of the Japanese Ergonomics National Committee on TC 159/SC 4, apart from the JIS drafting committee (the most member coincide), around July through September 1994.

The contents in English (if translated, with some summary) are itemized as follows.

1. The purport of establishment
2. The circumstance of establishment
3. The items especially argued during the discussion of the draft
   3.1 Problems regarding the original international standard
       (1) Applicable types of display devices
       (2) Luminance and luminance contrast
   3.2 Relation to the existing national standard, **JIS X 6041**-1987, titled in English, "CRT display and keyboard units for business use"
   3.3 Problem regarding the vertical way (from top to bottom) in reading and writing directions of sentences in Japanese language
   3.4 Explanatory note for some technical terms and their definitions and descriptions
       (1) office work,   (2) angle of view,   (3) between-character spacing,
       (4) legibility / readability,   (5) character format,
       (6) workstation,   (7) others (reference tables of the terms attached)
4. Scope (including the list of the titles of seventeen parts of ISO 9241 series)
5. The contents of stipulated items
   5.1 The ground of stipulated values regarding "Kanji" and "Kana"
       (1) character height,   (2) character width-to-height ratio
   5.2 Comparison between **JIS Z 8513** and **JIS X 6041** (shown as a table)
6. Pending items
   6.1 Items to be studied successively
   6.2 Items to be proposed by Japan hereafter to ISO as our national opinion
       (1) Luminance and luminance contrast,
       (2) Chinese / Japanese / Korean (CJK) in relation to ISO/IEC 10646-1
7. Decay characteristics of phosphor materials and the prediction of flicker (Annex A)
8. Composition table of drafting committee members

4. EXAMPLES OF THE TEXT DIFFER FROM CORRESPONDING IS

In Figure 1, the first page of the final draft is shown in reduced size with the numbers ①, ②, ③ and ④ for their explanations. The translation or explanation for each item in English will be as follows;   (continued to the second next page)

日本工業規格　　　　　　　　　　　　　　JIS

人間工学 — 視覚表示装置を用いるオフィス作業 Z 8513-1994
　　— 視覚表示装置の要求事項　　①

Ergonomics — Office work with visual display terminals (VDTs)
— Visual display requirements　②

日本工業規格としてのまえがき

この規格は，1992年第1版として発行されたISO 9241-3 Ergonomic requirements for office work with visual display terminals (VDTs) — Part 3: Visual display requirementsを翻訳し，原国際規格の様式によって作成した日本工業規格であるが，規格内容の一部を我が国の実情（日本文の文書）に即して変更した。
なお，この規格で点線の側線又は下線を施してある箇所及び参考（附属書の前）は，原国際規定の規定内容を変更した事項，又は原国際規格にはない事項である。

---

0. **序文**　オフィス作業システムにおける作業性 (performance) は，人々の快適性と同様に，視覚表示装置（以下，VDTという。）の画面上の情報表示方法，及び作業場の視環境によって影響される。
個々の作業者の要求の満足度は，アプリケーションに高く依存する。ここに規定する推奨事項及び要求事項は，ISO 6385に規定する人間工学の原則に基づく。

1. **適用範囲**　この規格は，単色及び多色のVDTの設計及び評価のための画質の要求事項について規定する。この要求事項は，性能上の規定として記述され，評価については試験方法及び適合を規定する。

　この規格で推奨する事項は，欧字及びアラビア数字に基づいているが，特に断りがない限り，漢字及び仮名にも適用できる。
　参　考　原国際規格では，"欧字"を具体的に"ラテン文字，キリル文字及びギリシャ系のアルファベット"と記している。　③

　作業性及び快適さに影響を及ぼす他の要因としては，輝度，明滅 (blinking)，色などによるコーディング，書式及び情報の表示の様式がある。これらの視覚上の側面以外の項目は，この規格では扱わない。
　この規格は，オフィス作業用の電子式ディスプレイの人間工学上の設計に適用する。VDTを用いるオフィス作業とは，データ入力，文書処理及び対話形問合せのような活動を含むが，CAD（コンピュータ援用設計），プロセス制御のような，他の特定のアプリケーションに対する推奨事項は含まない。　④
　そのようなアプリケーションについての推奨事項は，別個に制定する計画である。

2. **用語の定義**　この規格で用いる主な用語の定義は，次のとおりとする。
2.1 **観視角 (angle of view)**　視線と表示面との交点において，表示面の法線と視線とのなす角。
2.2 **アンティエイリアスフォント (anti-aliased font)**　例えば，階調を付けるなどによって，文字の線を滑らかに見せる技法を用いた文字記号。

Note: The text of the published JIS Z 8513 is printed in a different format from the one shown above, submitted to AIST / MITI in February 1994.

Figure 1. Example of the final draft (the first page in reduced size with ①〜④)

①: There is no indication of the corresponding international standard with parentheses, i.e.(ISO 9241-3:1992), just below **JIS Z 8513**-1994, because **JIS Z 8513** is *not* exactly same as ISO 9241-3, as explained in ② and ③.

②: This part in the solid frame is "Foreword as a Japanese Industrial Standard", followed by the explanation below:

This standard is a Japanese Industrial Standard compiled in the form of original international standard, translating the first edition of ISO 9241-3 : 1992 (E) ··· *title is abbreviated* ··· , but the contents of the standard was changed partially to match the actual circumstances (documents in Japanese language) of our nation.

By the way, the part with dotted side lines or dotted underlines, and the reference (before the Annex) are the items where the specified contents of original international standard were changed, or there was no such item in original international standard.

③: This part is translated as follows;

The recommendations in this standard are based on European characters and Arabic numerals (originally), but as long as there is no remark, they are able to be applied to (the Japanese) "Kanji" and "Kana" characters, too.

  Note In the original international standard, "European characters" are described definitely as "Latin, Cyrillic, and Greek origin alphabetic characters".

④: This part is the explanation of "anti-aliased font", saying "by using the gradation, etc. for example,".

5. PROPOSALS FOR THE REVISION OF JIS Z 8513 IN THE FUTURE

As I reported previously[3], I have the opinion that the original ISO 9241-3: 1992 should not be IS (international standard) but TR (technical report) so long as it is applicable to flat panel displays along with cathode ray tubes.

At the same time, the existing national **JIS X 6041**, which was once affirmed on June 1st, 1992 must be reviewed according to the Article 15 of Industrial Standardization Law in Japan, whether it can be affirmed as it was, it is necessary to revise or it shall be withdrawn, within five years from the date of affirmation.

So, **JIS Z 8513** itself should also be reviewed sooner or later, especially when the status of the above mentioned related international and/or national standards have changed.

I am not saying Kenzaburo Oe's line, but the applicability of ISO 9241-3: 1992 to flat panel displays is somewhat "ambiguous" because the standard is deeply inclined to cathode ray tube technology in terms of display devices.

Regarding flat panel displays, apart from 9241 series, ISO TC 159 / SC 4 / WG 2 is now preparing ISO CD 13406-2.

Therefore, if technological and scientific "ambiguity" is unfavorable, in the future, 9241 series should be preferably confined to cathode ray tube technology, leaving flat panel displays to 13406 series. Of course, such international trend must be reflected to the revised edition of **JIS Z 8513** accordingly.

6. CONCLUSION

Finally, I would like to conclude this paper with my personal opinion on the international standardization as well as the internationalization of "JIS".

Traditionally, we, Japanese tend to consider that the overseas decisions can not be changed easily regardless of their conformity, not contributing sufficiently to such decisions beforehand, partly because of the problem of the language, which obstructs mutual understandings internationally.

As the result, such decisions become so called "Gai-atsu" (外圧), meaning outer (外) pressure (圧) to Japan from foreign countries.

I believe such attitude is far from the internationalization of "JIS" and our nation must contribute to the international standardization more actively.

To do so from now on, it is necessary to revolutize to remove the delusion of persecution from our consciousness, and also, to establish the system to encourage our experts participating in the international standardization activity both morally and financially.

I hope most industries in Japan as well as in the world are awakened to the principle of the charge of the beneficiary, so long as the industrial standards are concerned.

I will be very glad if this paper could increase the transparency of this **JIS Z 8513** for the people other than Japanese.

7. ACKNOWLEDGEMENT

The author wishes to thank related members of SG 1 of JENC on TC 159/SC 4, as well as of another JIS (believed to be **JIS Z 8512**-1995) drafting committee, which will be identical with ISO 9241-2: 1992.

REFERENCES

1. K. Tanii, The Japanese Journal of Ergonomics Vol. 30, No. 4 (1994) 255 (in Japanese)
2. N. Koizumi, Fourth International Scientific Conference (WWDU '94) Book of short papers Vol. 2 (1994) A 13
3. N. Koizumi, Technical report of IEICE, EID94-49 (1994) (in English)
   ⋯ also numbered IDY94 - 120 as ITEJ Technical Report
4. DISPLAY Technology and Applications Vol. 13 No. 3 (1992)

Implementation of the EC-directive 90/270 in the Netherlands

Ir. P. Voskamp R.e., Drs. R.H. Hagen, Drs. P. Biemans

Ministry of Social Affairs, Postbus 90801, 2509 LV Den Haag, The Netherlands

INTRODUCTION

Just like in any other memberstate of the European Community, the EC-directive 90/270/EEC on the *minimum safety and health requirements for work with display screen equipment*, needed to be implemented in the legislation of the Netherlands. On December 30, 1992, - one day before the final date for implementation - this has been achieved with enforcement of a special decree for VDU-work (Besluit Beeldschermwerk), based on the Working Environment Act (Arbeidsomstandighedenwet). The 'VDU-work Order' is founded on most of the articles of the EC-directive. Some smaller alterations have been made because of the general wording in the EC-text. To avoid opinion and interpretation differences, the Dutch Labour Inspectorate published an information sheet (P 184). In this guidebook all articles of the 'VDU-work Order' are clarified and, if possible, attached to a national or international standard (EN or NEN).

1. The VDU-Work Order

The definition of worker in the EC-directive is: 'any worker (...) who habitually uses display screen equipment as a significant part of his normal work'. In the 'VDU-work Order' of the Netherlands this definition is: 'a worker who in course of this work usually uses display screen equipment for at least *two hours per calender day*.' The word 'habitually' is applicable where VDU-work consists of an major component of the employee's function. This definition has been introduced to exclude negligible display screen work. Taken into account the evidence from ergonomic research that indications of injury may significantly arise at sustained VDU-work, a criteria of two hours per calendar day has been adapted. Accordingly, the VDU-Work Order becomes relevant for 1,8 million employees (43% of the total number).

Article 7 of the EC directive contains the requirements on work organisation. The article is relevant because of its impact on the number of hours that people work with Visual Display Units. It states that the employer needs to plan the employee's activities in such a way that daily work on a display screen is intermitted by breaks or changes of activity, reducing the workload. In the 'VDU-work Order' this article is transformed into: 'The employer should plan the employee's activities in such a way that any work at a display screen for *two successive hours* or more, will always be alternated by seperate tasks or a rest period, reducing the workload'.

The explanatory notes to this article stress the necessity to prevent people from working with VDU's during the entire working time. Interruptions in working with display screen equipment over the working day are essential, at least after every two successive hours. Seperate work patterns are preferable during these interruptions. Alternation with work of a different kind, requiring different physical and mental effort, is an appropriate way to relieve the stress due to display screen work. If no other kind of work is available, display screen work must alternate with regular breaks. The duration of the other tasks to be performed or the length of the breaks must be sufficient to reduce stress from VDU-work. The need to relieve the stress of display screen work by alternation with seperate working tasks is indicated by evidence from literature that five or six hours of VDU-work is ergonomically inappropriate for a working day of eight hours. This in no way detracts from the requirement that employees should not spend more than two successive hours working without interruption at a display screen. If display screen work alternates with breaks, the breaks should preferably last at least ten minutes.

2. Information-sheet 'Work with VDU's' (P 184)

The information-sheet 'Work with VDU's' of the Labour Inspectorate was published in 1993. In this year almost 11.500 copies of this guidebook were sold. Early 1994 an inquiry has been conducted to evaluate the effects of the VDU-Work Order and the publication of the guidebook. The guidebook P 184 provides useful information about requirements in the annex of the EC-directive. In the subsequent cases it was possible to attach the general wording of the annex-rules to a standard:

Requirements for the VDU: NEN ISO 9241/EN 29241 part 3
"   "   " chair: NEN (Dutch Standard) 1812
"   "   " table: NEN 2449
"   "   " lighting situation: NEN 3087
"   "   " soft-ware: ISO 9241 part 10-19

The guidebook also gives information on health problems related to work with VDU's. Furthermore, many requirements and recommendations are presented - based on legislation of the EC-directive - to avoid health problems due to VDU-work. The guidebook also contains a checklist, that may support the employee to examine one's own workstation according to the requirements and recommendations in P-184.

An inquiry has been conducted in order to evaluate policy outcome. Effects of the widespread publication P-184 on the actual working conditions are discussed. Important questions are:

- Who are the purchasers of *P-184*?
- Does the content of *P-184* meet the expectations of the purchasers?
- Does *P-184* have a positive effect on working conditions with Visual Display Units?
- Have VDU-workstations been adapted to the requirements of the Dutch government?
- How does working conditions policy compare with complaints of employees?
- Will these complaints give rise to an overall improvement of workstations?

A questionnaire has been sent to a random sample of 469 purchasers of the guidebook. The response rate turned out to be 43.5 percent. Fairly representative data have been obtained for the total group of buyers, although relatively few reactions were obtained from the category banking, insurance business and commercial services.

3. Conclusion

In the Netherlands the implementation of the EC-directive has been implemented with exact definitions of working time and breaks and also with references to standards for the ergonomic aspects of the VDU-work.

Generally speaking, the guidebook meets to a large extend the expectations of its purchasers. They appreciate the way the information is presented. Yellow borders in the left margin of the text, demonstrate the difference between requirements and recommendations. The difficulty level of the guidebook corresponds to the average education level of the readers, which is rather high. The checklist is also of significant value. About one third of the readers uses the checklist to examine the overall quality of VDU-work in the organization. According to the buyers the main deficiencies of the guidebook are the bad binding, the glaze of the paper, the lack of a summary and clear directions for improving the working conditions.

Many Dutch VDU-employees receive information on the VDU-work Order via the guidebook, published by the Labour Inspectorate. However, only a small number of guidebooks have been sold to small companies (1-9 employees), compared to medium sized companies (10-99 employees) and large industrial corporations (100 employees or more). The small organisations might be reached through the overall line organisations. A special manual could be made for this target section, which includes a summary of the requirements and recommendations next to a checklist and clear instructions about how to improve working conditions.

The buyers of *P-184* are very actively engaged in the quality of work with VDU's. The 'VDU-work Order' gives, as the complaints of the employees do, a big impulse towards improvement of the working conditions of VDU-employees. The guidebook has demonstrated its value for remedial purposes. To remedy the complaints of employees by improving the working conditions is seen as more important than solely adjusting the working conditions to the requirements of the Order. Next to the major concern for furniture, screen, possibilities for interruptions, lighting and guidance, the environmental factors climate, workspace and noises become more important. Improvements that are harder and more expensive to accomplish are easily postponed. About one-third of the users of *P-184* give low priority to the improvement of the working conditions. Extensive formal procedures and lack of financial support are the major hindrances for improving the quality of VDU-work.

Ninety percent of the buyers of the guidebook bear in some way responsibility for the working conditions of their colleagues. Generally speaking, they find it hard to estimate the effects of ameliorations. A extensive survey on VDU-work before and after improvements are realized, may demonstrate whether improvements serve the goal to reduce the number of health problems among VDU-employees. These evaluations need to focus on specific shortcomings of VDU-working conditions and complaints of employees. This way the success of pursuing the goal of optimum working conditions may become clear to the users of *P-184*.

So far the Dutch Labour Inspectorate has spent little attention to the subject of work with VDU's. This is probably a consequence of the fact that all VDU-workstations have to be adapted to the requirements of the Order only by January 1 ,1995. In view of the fact that there are 1.8 million VDU-workers in the Netherlands, and the direct relationship between VDU-work characteristics and health problems, the Labour Inspectorate could spend some more time on this subject. During the inspections the features of VDU-work that are hard to improve need to get special attention, because improvements on these features are often delayed.

The guidebook has demonstrated its value for remedial purposes. Nowadays people tend to adapt their work environment to legislation requirements. On the other hand, care for good work conditions in an early stage - the design of offices - may be more beneficial compared with this remedy-approach. Besides, improvement in an early stage is less expensive and easier to accomplish. For that reason prevention of physical and mental health problems need special emphasis in any work environment policy.

The improvement of the working conditions may also result in positive side-effects. The attention for the improvement of working conditions may have a positive effect upon the reduction of sick-leave. Furthermore, it may prevent the loss of skilled and experienced employees who become unfit for the VDU-work. This means that there is a positive effect on the costs of labour and the productivity, by which the (maintenance of) employment will be stimulated in a durable way.

REFERENCE

Ministerie van Sociale Zaken en Werkgelegenheid, Werken met Beeldschermen (Work with Visual Display Units) P 184, Sdu Uitgeverij, Den Haag 1993.

PC-FIT User-Saver® - VDU Ergonomics for Users

S. Bachinger[a], W. Hackl-Gruber[b],
M. Molnar[a], A. Pribil[b].

[a]human-ware, scientific consultant in ergonomic VDU workstation design,
Burggasse 88, A-1070 Vienna, Austria.

[b]Institut for Industrial Science, Technical University of Vienna,
Theresianumgasse 27, A-1040 Vienna, Austria.

1. INTRODUCTION

Various empirical studies have shown that there is a connection between specific conditions at the computer workstation and the incidence of certain health problems, especially those concerning the eyes, skeletal and motor systems and also mental stresses. A comprehensive international bibliography from Siegried Grune dated 1990 (!) included a collection from more than 12.000 titles dealing with video display terminals.

With the increase in the amount of work being carried out at the computer the need for preventative health measures has also increased. This is reflected directly in EC Directive 90/270/EEC which outlines minimum requirements for safety and health protection at VDU workstations. It is binding for EC Member States and companies working in them.

1.1. Preventative Strategies

Preventative Strategies have two main points of intervention. On the one hand it is possible to concentrate on hardware and environmental criteria. This means planning display units, screen and input media, user interface, chair and desk design, room lighting on ergonomic principles.

On the other hand the working process and the worker's activities can be organized so as to reduce workload, strain and stress and to avoid negative health effects. Especially to teach workers in safety and health is one of the main goals. Let us take out two articles of the Directive:

Article 6:
"... workers shall receive information on all aspects of safety and health relating to their workstation."

Article 7:
"The employer must plan the worker's activities in such a way that daily work on a display screen is periodically interrupted by breaks or changes of activity reducing the workload at the display screen."

The EC-Dircetive 90/270/EEC calls for companies to take a number of measures for prevention in the areas of health protection and work safety for computer workers.

1.2. Problems to be solved

This means a lot of material, organisational and financial resources. The need for practical and at the same time effective and economic health protection instruments is becoming more and more important. There are hardly any safety education and training tools available for putting the various measures into practice.

The devising of generally accepted strategies in this respect involves a number of problems, for example general usability and motivation of VDU workers-

2. OBJEKTIVES AND CONCEPTION

There are two particular problems which need to be solved in this respect: Firstly, users must be suitably informed and made aware of the problem: Secondly, measures must be developed which effectively achieve their desired aim. Based on the practical problems concerned with the avoidance of unhealthy workload at display units, we have devised a solution - **PC-FIT User-Saver**® - in which the computer itself looks out for the user´s health.

We realize that user awareness, motivation and competence are contingent on information and knowledge about preventative measures. With **PC-FIT**® this information ist available where it is required - at the workstation itself.

The software package **PC-FIT**® was developed in collaboration with experts from the fields of industrial medicine, ergonomics, orthopaedics, psychology and physiotherapy.

2.1. Description

The program offers three options which can be selected by the user as required:

1.It can be used like an alarm clock to remind the user to interrupt VDU work or to take breaks. One can be reminded to take breaks as a function of the amount of time spent without a pause at the screen , or at fixed times or time intervals.

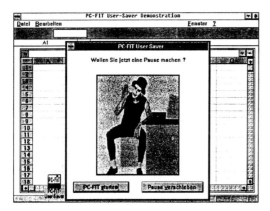

Figure 1. Break Reminder.

2. It offers 30 physiotherapeutic exercises for various parts of the body (including the eyes) designed to counter physical stress imbalances.

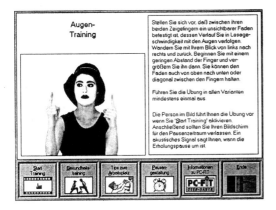

Figure 2. Exercise.

3. It provides information on the ergonomic design of workstations and work procedures, listed under headings (e.g. chair, lighting, software ergonomics, etc.) with practical tips for a better self management.

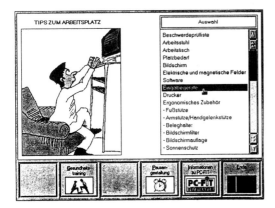

Figure 3. Information and tips.

The software is supplemented by an information booklet with articles written by experts about the various aspects of ergonomics and health. **PC-FIT**® provides specialist information and also, by using different didactic tools (for example moving pictures and cartoons.) encourages users to employ preventative strategies at their own workstations.

3. EVALUATION AND RESULTS

An systematic evaluation study of this teaching and health provision instrument (including test/control group and before/after comparisons) have been carried out in collaboration with the Institute for Industrial Science at the Technical University of Vienna.

The main question was, do and how do users use this instrument? The case study included psychological tests and questionnaires about stress and strain, health and wellbeeing, obkective ergonomic evaluation methods and the installation of a logfile. The testperiod lasted 12 weeks and took place at office workstations. The testgroup consists of 14 persons, the control group of 35 persons. All persons of the test and control group have been informed before starting by an extensive information session and took part in the study voluntarily.

We will give you a short overview about results, statistically generated from the questionnaire and the logfile (descriptive statistics, significance tests, univariate and multivariate statistics):

Table 1
Questions and main results (in percent)

	yes (%)	competly (%)	partly (%)	no (%)	no answer (%)
Programm was easy to handle	85	-	-	-	15
Use of "health exercises" (user's preference list: back, neck, shoulders etc.)	55	-	-	45	-
Use of "tips on the ergonomic design of workstations" (user's preference list: electromagnetical fields, software, chair, desk etc.)	-	46	46	8	-
Use of "break reminder"	42	-	-	58	-
Reading of "information booklet"	-	31	23	46	-
Did learn something new	67	-	-	25	8
Did optimize something at my workplace	17	-	-	83	-

The rate of general health problems and especially back pain was reduced significantly in the **PC-FIT®** user group.

Futher research is just going on at two German universities.

4. CONCLUSION

PC-FIT® and this paper is less interesting as a scientific approach than as a practical strategy for safety and health management at VDU. The transfer of research and theoretical preventative concepts into practical form is an important necessity. **PC-FIT®** is not just a software but a strategy. It does need an organizational frame as for example health and safety workgroups.

External and internal health managers are offered a ready-made tool for protecting the health of computer workers. The program can be used for information, enlightenment and motivation, thereby fulfilling the demand in the EC Directive for informing and training users.

Our approach to safety and health management seems to be a good one. **PC-FIT®** took part in an European competition looking for safety education and training products. This competition was organised by the International Social Security Association in partnership with the Commission of the European Communities as part of the European Year of Safety, Hygiene and Health Protection at Work. **PC-FIT®** was the winner of the first prize within the EFTA-countries.

REFERENCES

1. European Council Directive 90/270/EEC on the minimum safety and health requirements for work with display screen equipment.
2. Grune Siegfried: Video display terminals. A comprehensive international bibliography, 2nd, rev. and enlarged edition, Grulit, Bochum-Wattenscheid, 1990.

Testing Conformance to Software Standards: A Usability Evaluation of ISO 9241 DIS Part 14 - Menu Dialogues

R.E. Granda and S.L. Stanners[1]

IBM Corporation, Somers, NY, USA

1. INTRODUCTION

ISO 9241 is an ergonomics standard for office work using visual display terminals (VDTs). It consists of requirements and recommendations that address user tasks, environment, computer hardware and software. ISO 9241 consists of seventeen parts; Parts 3 through 9 are considered to be hardware oriented while Parts 10 through 17 are considered to be software oriented (Bevan, 1991).

A critical aspect of standards is the conformance/compliance section. The parties that are expected to comply should be able to do so in well defined steps and with procedures and methodologies that have been researched, tested: the methods must be reliable, valid as well as relatively easy to administer and implement. A demonstration of such capabilities is especially important in the human-computer interaction area which is still in the early stages of developing objective, quantitative protocols and methodologies.

In the case of Part 14, the immediate need to demonstrate inter-rater reliability and usability of the conformance methodology is necessary since no formal exercise appears to have been conducted. The importance of performing this exercise becomes even more critical as it appears that a similar conformance methodology is planned for Parts 15, 16, and 17 covering the areas of command language, direct manipulation and form filling dialogues.

This paper reports the results of an evaluation of the inter-rater reliability and usability of ISO 9241, Draft International Standard - Part 14: Menu Dialogues (June 7, 1991). The objective of the evaluation was to determine the feasibility of applying Part 14 (the content and supplied checklist) to the design and evaluation of software programs using menu dialogues.

2. PROCEDURE

2.1 Phase I

Two interface standards experts participated in the initial in-depth evaluation. Their goal was to become expert in the evaluation of software menu dialogue interfaces using Part 14. They spent approximately two months in this phase.

---

[1] This work was conducted when both authors were affiliated with IBM Corporation. Dr. Stanners is presently working for Sensormatic Corporation, Boca Raton, FL, USA.

During this time they studied the draft standard, and engaged in extended discussions with selected members of the working group (developing the standard) and other Human Factors experts knowledgeable in human-computer interface standards.

To investigate the practical applications of Part 14, the participants applied Part 14 to the menu dialogues of DOS (5.0). Before they could begin the DOS menu evaluation, they determined they had to take some steps that are not described in Part 14. First they learned that they would have to enlist the assistance of some DOS interface experts to conduct the evaluation accurately. The second step of the evaluation requires the evaluator to determine whether the software product complies to the applicable requirements and recommendations. Since compliance judgments are only made for applicable requirements and recommendations, it is critical that applicability judgments be accurate.

For this step, the participants determined it was necessary to develop a strategy to evaluate the menus in groups. Part 14 does not contain a strategy to evaluate menus in groups, therefore it appears that evaluators are supposed to evaluate each menu individually. However, this is not practical for many professionally written, commercial software applications, which may contain hundreds and even thousands of menus. Additionally there are sections of Part 14 that require the user to evaluate *groups* of menus. For example, evaluators are asked to make judgments on menu categorization, grouping (3.1) and consistency (3.3.1).

After developing a grouping strategy, the participants used the checklist supplied in Informative Annex A of Part 14, to document their applicability and compliance judgments.

2.2 Phase II
The objective of Phase II was to obtain expert reviews of Part 14 from IBM Human Factors experts regarding the usability of Part 14. To meet this objective the seven test participants (internal IBM Human Factors experts) reviewed the requirements and recommendations of Part 14 for clarity and usability. Each participant documented their opinion in a short, written report.

2.3 Phase III
The objective of Phase III was to evaluate whether IBM Product Interface Designers would agree on which of the requirements and recommendations in Part 14 were applicable to menus in the OS/2 2.0 Workplace Shell. The test administrators instructed five OS/2 2.0 Workplace Shell interface developers to use Part 14 to evaluate the OS/2 2.0 Workplace Shell. The test administrator instructed the participants to document their applicability judgments on the checklist included in Part 14. The developers gave the test administrator written or verbal comments on the content and usability of Part 14.

2.4 Phase IV
The objective of Phase IV was to compare the usability and reliability of two checklists (the checklist included with Part 14 and an internal, experimental

version) used to document applicability judgments for ISO 9241, Part 14. The second checklist was designed to address some of the problems test participants reported in Phases I, II, and III. Since the major problems discovered in Phases I, II and III were a general lack of usability and low inter-rater reliability, this phase covered step 1 (applicability judgments) only.

2.4.1 Subjects
Five people participated individually in the comparison test. All were full time employees of IBM and described as DOS interface experts by their managers. All had worked on DOS products for a minimum of two years.

2.4.2 Material
All participants used the same IBM PS/2 Model 70 computer, with a 386 processor and VGA graphics on an 8514 display to conduct the evaluation. All participants had written instructions telling them how to complete the evaluation, a copy of Part 14, and a copy of an internal, experimental checklist. The test administrators created the internal, experimental version of the checklist in an attempt to make the entire evaluation process for Part 14 easier, more accurate and reliable.

The internal, experimental checklist differed from the original checklist in several ways. One difference was that, while the original checklist allowed users to document both applicability and conformance judgments, the internal, experimental checklist was actually split into two checklists - one for "applicability", the second for "compliance" judgments.

Second the test administrators attempted to simplify the format of the applicability checklist by eliminating the "and/or" conjunctions and making the statements into simple questions. For example, 6.1 is the group of requirements titled "Option accessibility and discrimination". On the checklist, the first several requirements in the group read:

```
6.1.1 Critical Options continually displayed.  AND
6.1.2 Frequent usage options placed in a screen area which
will not obscure task data.  AND/OR
6.1.3 Occasional usage menus presented on demand   AND
6.1.4 Available options presented only unless information
concerning other options required   OR
```

The same group for the internal, experimental checklist read:

```
6.1.1  Are critical options continually displayed?
6.1.2  Are options that are used frequently placed in areas
that will not obscure task data?
6.1.3  Are options that are used occasionally presented on
demand either via pop-up/pull-down menus or in a dedicated
area of the screen?
```

2.4.3 Procedures
Each participant used both checklists to evaluate part of the DOS interface. The order of use was counterbalanced to eliminate effects of practice. Participants evaluated a different group of menus with each checklist and all used the same two groups of menus.

All participants read a set of instructions before beginning. The instructions suggested that participants read the introduction of Part 14 as well as sections 3 and 6. Participants were only asked to evaluate DOS menus against approximately half of the content of Part 14 (sections 3 & 6) to shorten the time necessary for the test. The instructions also informed participants that they could refer to Part 14 as they completed their applicability judgments and that they should feel free to ask questions throughout the test. The instructions said that participants should notify the test administrators when they finished reading Part 14 and were ready to begin making applicability judgments.

Participants used a checklist to document their applicability judgments. After each participant completed one checklist, the test administrator changed the interface to bring up a second set of menus and gave them the second checklist to complete. After each participant completed both checklists, they answered questions regarding the usability of the checklists.

3. RESULTS

3.1 Phase I
Participants concluded that it would be necessary to utilize product interface experts to conduct the evaluation. Without an expert knowledge of the interface being evaluated it was impossible to determine accurately the applicability of the requirements and recommendations in Part 14. They also determined it was necessary to develop a strategy to evaluate *groups* of menus, since Part 14 did not contain such a strategy. Evaluating each menu individually was not a practical way to apply the standard, nor was it possible since some of the requirements pertain to *groups* of menus.

3.2 Phase II
The Human Factors experts found the organization of the standard confusing. The need for a "fast path" set of instructions on how to use Part 14 was emphasized. The applicability (or lack of it) of specific recommendations to Graphical User Interface style software applications was cited as a potential confusion factor. Included below are samplings of typical comments:

- The organization of the standard is confusing.
- How do I understand quickly how to get through this? I need a fast path so I don't have to muddle through the whole document to understand how to begin.
- Software developers and designers will NOT use this to design. It is too hard to follow.
- It barely seems to apply to today's interfaces (GUI, Pen).

- It is hard to apply these to the shallow menus for OS/2 (and other GUI menus) except in a superficial way.
- There is not much guidance here - really it is very basic. What difference does it make if analysis is done by "observation" or by "documented" evidence. If it is right, who cares?
- This is not written for GUIs.
- It doesn't cover direct manipulation at all.
- The "and/or" logic in the checklist is confusing and not consistent with the document.
- What is "conventional" / "logical"? Something that is conventional / logical to me might not be to a UNIX user.

3.3 Phase III

The average inter-rater reliability of the participants' judgments (Fleiss, J.L., 1981, Lewis, J.R., 1992) for applicability of the requirements and recommendations (step 1) was poor (kappa = .252). This means the developers did not agree on the requirements and recommendations that were applicable for the software interface they evaluated.

Participants commented that Part 14 was very difficult to understand and apply. Some reported reading the entire document as many as three times and still were not sure how to conduct the evaluation. Participants agreed that most developers would not spend the time that they felt would be necessary to use Part 14 accurately. Participants also felt that Part 14 seemed to apply to character based applications instead of GUI style applications. Some typical product interface designer comments are given:

- It seems to apply to character-based applications rather than GUI style applications.
- I didn't understand the "and/or" system for the checklist. I understand how to use logical conditions, however this was very difficult to interpret.
- I didn't understand the "methods used" section of the checklist.
- The inter-rater reliability of our judgments was very poor. This must be quite bad for an international standard.
- Participants found the exercise to be tedious and not helpful.

3.4 Phase IV

The participants spent between 10 and 45 minutes reading Part 14. The shortest times were for two participants who quit reading Part 14 in favor of using it as a reference while they completed the checklist. Four of five participants said that the revised checklist was easier to use than the original. The reliability scores for both checklists were poor. The kappa score for the original checklist was .216 and the kappa score for the revised checklist was .230. Another score was calculated to compare the ratings of the participants to those of an expert on Part 14 and DOS 5.0. The average percent of correct responses (as compared to the expert) for the original checklist was 62%. The average percent of correct responses for the revised checklist was 67%.

The following findings for Phase IV are noted:

- Inter-rater reliability of applicability judgments was very low.
  There were many items that participants could not agree on, both in the pilot and the checklist tests. We believe that the reliability problem is due primarily to the ambiguous wording of many of the recommendations.
- Many of the participants' judgments of whether a recommendation or requirement was applicable didn't agree with experts judgments.
  The test participants did not have the time that the experts had to educate themselves about Part 14. Consequently we would not expect their judgments to be identical, however they should not be as different as they were. Sixty-two percent of the participants responses were identical to the responses of the experts, for the original checklist and, 68% for the revision. The differences in opinion between expert and novice users of the standard are certainly not desirable and probably not acceptable.
- All participants ignored the "and/or" structure of the checklist.
  When queried about their interpretation of the "and/or" structure, 4/5 participants said that they paid no attention to it. As a consequence they completed each line of the checklist. Even when the recommendations were connected by "or" (meaning they did not need to judge applicability for all the recommendations, but pick the one that was applicable) they judged the applicability of all of the recommendations.
  The effect of eliminating the "and/or" structure was tested by asking participants to use a revision (without the "and/or" structure) of the original checklist and compare the usability of the two. Participants rated the usability of the revision higher than that of the original; however, there was only a slight improvement in reliability. it appears that the "and/or" format was not the main inhibitor to inter-rater reliability.
- All participants said that the abbreviations, representing the methods used to determine applicability or compliance, were hard to associate with their meaning.
  The abbreviations of methods used to determine applicability or compliance are one or two letters located at the top of the checklist. The key to their meaning is located at the bottom of the page. The key defines the abbreviations, but this was not at all apparent to the test participants. Most participants paid very little attention to them and did not bother to indicate a method used.
  After using the checklist for two lengthy evaluations we recommend that this requirement to specify a method be removed.
- Participants did not read Part 14 thoroughly.
  Two participants spent less than 10 minutes reading Part 14 and skipped immediately to the checklist. One of the two complained that it was incredibly hard to read and that he didn't know of any developers who would bother reading it. These same participants complained that some of the terms were too vague to apply.
- Participants liked the concise matrix style of the checklist.
  When the current format was compared to a lengthier but more explanatory format all participants said they liked the conciseness of the current (matrix style) format.

4. DISCUSSION

The present evaluation underscores the scientific necessity for rigorous testing of proposed protocols and testing methodologies used in the ergonomics evaluation of human-computer interfaces. Part 14 cannot be used in its present form by software designers or evaluators with a high degree of accuracy, efficiency and consistency. If this protocol is adopted for Parts 15, 16 and 17, we predict similar results. Extensive testing is recommended prior to adoption of any required protocols in this area.

As a first step, a review of existing and potentially applicable methodologies is needed. Until such a review is completed, the long-term impact of imposing mandatory requirements using inadequate methodologies through ergonomics standards should be fully understood by standards making bodies. The question of whether or not a standards development body is an appropriate setting for specification of evaluation protocols without the proper independent scientific/technical research support appears to be answered in the negative - at least for this type of application within the human-computer interface area.

There is a real danger that this lack of attention to scientific principles could result in negative repercussions to the acceptance of 'standards' in the human-computer interaction (HCI) area. We recommend that other courses of action be explored as ways of encouraging designers/developers to apply and implement human-computer interaction principles to the development of software applications. These should emphasize iterative designer/user interactions rather than edicted, compulsory requirements.

5. CONCLUSIONS

Part 14 could not be used in the form presented in the 21 June, 1991 version by software designers or evaluators with a high degree of accuracy, efficiency and consistency.

The insistence on protocols involving untested and unproven schema to evaluate human-computer interfaces as a means of indicating standards compliances is premature and potentially counter-productive to acceptance and use of HCI principles.

REFERENCES

Bevan, Nigel, 1991. Human Aspects in computing: Design and Use of Interactive Systems and Work with Terminals. H.J Bullinger (Ed.) Standards relevant to European Directives for display terminals (pp.533-537) Elsevier Science Publishers B.V.

Fleiss, Joseph L., 1981. Statistical Methods for Rates and Proportions - 2nd Edition. New York: John Wiley & Sons.

ISO Draft International Standard 9241 - Ergonomic Requirements for Office Work with Visual Display Terminals, Part 14: Menu Dialogues (7 June 1991)

Lewis, J.R., 1992. The Kappa Measure of Interrater Agreement: Two BASIC Programs. Boca Raton, FL: IBM Corp. Technical Report TR-54.695.

A general modeling framework for the human-computer interaction based on the principles of ergonomic compatibility requirements and human entropy

W. Karwowski

Center for Industrial Ergonomics, University of Louisville, Louisville, KY 40292, USA

1. INTRODUCTION

The present state of knowledge suggests several cause-effect relationships between the visual display units (VDU) design characteristics, body posture and perceived postural comfort of the operators [1, 2]. Working with video display terminals (VDTs) may lead to several adverse health effects such as visual problems or work-related musculoskeletal injury [3]. Many studies of postural problems experienced when working with VDTs emphasize physical design of hardware including adjustability of computer workstations, task workload, task variability and duration, work practices and work organization, and environmental and psychosocial factors [4]. It was also shown that cognitive task requirements of the computer tasks may also affect postural loading of the human operator [5, 6]. As pointed out by Grieco [7], the human interaction with VDTs should allow for dynamic muscle work in order to prevent constrained postures that increase static muscular loading and the risk of related incidence of musculoskeletal disorders among the VDT operators.

2. OBJECTIVES

Although a large amount of scientific data have been gathered about many different aspects of people working with visual display terminals, a unifying framework for integrating such data into a comprehensive model of the human-computer interactions, that would allow to examine critical risk factors of the related musculoskeletal problems experienced by the VDT operators, has not yet been developed. The objective of this paper was to propose the foundations for such a framework in view of the fundamental concepts of the science of ergonomics [8, 9], including the notions of the system interactions, complexity, human and system entropies, ergonomic compatibility requirements, and human adaptation.

3. VDT SYSTEM INTERACTIONS AND COMPATIBILITY REQUIREMENTS

As discussed by Karwowski [9], ergonomics/human factors focuses on investigating the (ergonomic) interactions between the people and other (relevant) system elements. Ergonomics investigates such relationships at the human-machine-environment sub-systems with different levels of complexity. Therefore, any theoretical framework of the science of ergonomics should be based on the notion of ergonomic interactions that affect the system compatibility, or those that define the ergonomic compatibility requirements {CR} of the system.

It should be noted here that according to the *Complexity-Incompatibility Principle* [10], as the (ergonomic) system complexity increases, the ergonomic incompatibilities between the system elements, expressed through their interactions at all system levels, also increases, leading to the greater ergonomic (non-reducible) entropy of the system, and decreasing the potential for effective ergonomic regulation (intervention efforts).

As discussed by Dainoff [11], the VDT operator engages in a controlled interaction with the surfaces of support (chair seatpan, backrest, floor, work surface) with the goal of maintaining dynamic equilibrium. The structure of this interaction is determined by four classes of constraints: 1) system goals 2) workstation characteristics, 3) operator characteristics, 4) chair characteristics. The nature of the task may require very different postural orientations depending on the viewing distance to the copy/screen, physical dimensions of the VDT operator, and the nature/range of VDT workstation adjustments. Within these constraints, it is assumed that an operator will minimize muscular efforts in order to maintain an equilibrium.

In view of the complexity-incompatibility principle [10], the VDT operators are trying to locally minimize the incompatibilities at different levels of the system, i.e. at those interactions that are possible for them to use and modify. This process of human adaptation to the VDT task can be considered the last resort solution when the system incompatibility cannot be further reduced. In this case the human operators attempt to change the structure of their physical interactions with the computer workstation, i.e. the VDT and chair components (machine subsystem). From the operator point of view (human subsystem), the easiest interaction to modify in order to minimize the perceived muscular discomfort and stress, is the postural interaction, aimed at control of their own body.

4. A FRAMEWORK OF THE ERGONOMIC SYSTEM

As discussed by Karwowski et al. [8] and Karwowski [9], the ergonomic system (S) is a construct developed for the purpose of scientific investigation of human work systems. The ergonomic system contains the human subsystem (H), machine/task subsystem (M), the environmental subsystem (E), and a set of the (ergonomic) interactions (I) occurring between different elements of these subsystems in time. Further discussion on this subject can be found in [9]. The set $I = \{i_1, i_2, ..., i_n\}$ } is viewed here as the set of all possible interactions between people, machines and working environments that are present in a given state of the HME subsystem. These interactions (i_n) reflect the existence (or non-existence) of the relationships between the subset of all relevant human characteristics $H = \{h_1, h_2, ..., h_i\}$, such as anatomical, physiological, biomechanical, or psychological, the subset of (ergonomic) characteristics of a machine/task $M = \{m_1, m_2, ..., m_j\}$, and elements of the set $E = \{e_1, e_2, ..., e_k\}$, representing the subset of environmental conditions (E), such as physical environment characteristics, social support, organizational structures, etc.

5. SYSTEM ENTROPY AND INCOMPATIBILITY

5.1. System and human entropies

Following the concept of the ergonomic system [9], the entropy (E_S) of the ergonomic system (S) can be modeled using the entropies (E) due to the human-related interactions (H-subsystem), machine/task-related interactions (M-subsystem), environment-related interactions (E-subsystem), and time (T). In view of the above, the system entropy (E_S) can be defined as a function of entropy of the set of ergonomic interactions (E_I) and time (T) as follows:

$$E_S = \mathbf{f}[E_I, T] \tag{1}$$

Since the set of ergonomic interactions (I-subsystem) consists of the possible relations between the subsystem elements of {H}, {M}, and {E}, the entropy of {I}, (E_I), can be expressed as follows:

$$E_I = \{E_H, E_M, E_E\} \quad (2)$$

where:

$E_H = \{h_1, h_2, ... h_i\}$ = contributing entropy due to the human subsystem,
$E_M = \{m_1, m_2, ... m_j\}$ = contributing entropy due to the machine/task subsystem,
$E_E = \{e_1, e_2, ... e_k\}$ = contributing entropy due to the environmental subsystem,

and $E_I = \{i_1, i_2, ... i_n\}$, with $n = \{i, j, k\}$.

It should be noted that E_H, or *the human entropy*, is interpreted here as the entropy due to those system interactions which affect the compatibility of the ergonomic system (structure) with the given human characteristics from the subset (H). Such entropy is a measure of the system incompatibility. For ease of description, the E_S and E_I can be rewritten and referred to as follows:

$$E(S) = f[E(I), T], \text{ and } E(I) = \{E(H), E(M), E(E)\}. \quad (3)$$

The entropy of an ergonomic system depends on the variety and complexity of all relevant interactions for the subsystems H, M and E [10, 8]. Any manipulation of elements of the human-machine-environment system may result in subsequent changes in the number or structure (or both) of other interactions, and, therefore increase (or decrease) the system's entropy.

5.2. Complexity, compatibility requirements, and system regulation

The structure of system interactions (I) at the given system level, induces complexity of that system. It is the complexity of the {M} and {E} subsystem interactions that defines the ergonomic compatibility requirements {CR} of the system.

In general, the greater the system compatibility requirements {CR}, the greater the need for the ergonomic intervention efforts, called here the *system regulation*. Therefore, it follows that an entropy of the machine-environment {M, E} system, or the system regulator, E(R), is also defined by the system's structure complexity. It should be noted that the optimal (ergonomic) system is the one with minimal ergonomic compatibility requirements, i.e. minimal system incompatibility. The optimal ergonomic system satisfies most (if not all) of the compatibility requirements of the system.

6. A general modeling framework for the human-computer interaction

As discussed above, the machine/task (M) and environmental (E) subsystems can be regulated (controlled), and are jointly called the system regulator (R). Consequently, the sum of their respective entropies defines the entropy of the system regulator E(R):

$$E(R): E(R) = E(M) + E(E) \text{ or equivalently:} \quad (4)$$

$$E(R) = E\{(M) + (E)\}, \text{ denoted as } E(R) = E(M,E). \quad (5)$$

The sum of E(M) and E(E) also defines the system's compatibility requirements {CR}, and the entropy of the ergonomic system regulator E(R). At a given the level of human entropy E(H), the entropy of the ergonomic system regulator E(R) leads to the specific outcome of the (ergonomic) system regulation process, i.e. determines the ergonomic system entropy

E(S).

The above can be illustrated as the process of ergonomic system regulation, with E(H) as the system input, E(R) as the system regulator, and system entropy E(S) as the output, or the regulation outcome (new state of the ergonomic system structure) as follows:

```
              |   E(R)
       _____|_____
              |
       E(H)   |   E(S)
```

7. THE PRINCIPLE OF HUMAN ENTROPY DETERMINATION

7.1. System regulation and entropy

For the system regulation structure shown above, the system entropy E(S) can be defined as follows [12]:

$$E(S) >= E(H) + E(R) - E_H(R), \quad (6)$$

where $E_H(R)$ is the joint entropy of the machine/task and environment {M,E} subsystem, represented by the regulator (R) when the state of the human subsystem (H) is known.

When $E_H(R) = 0$, i.e. when the regulator subsystem R={M, E} is a determinate function of the human subsystem (H), the above equation transforms as follows:

$E(S) = E(H) + E(R)$, and consequently it follows that:

$$E(H) = E(S) - E(R), \quad (7)$$

The above equation shows that the human entropy E(H) is defined by the difference between the system entropy and the entropy of the system regulator. The above also indicates that the entropy of the system E(S), if minimal at a given stage of the system design, can only be further reduced by a corresponding increase in the entropy of the ergonomic system regulator (R).

7.2. Limitations of ergonomic system regulation and human adaptation

According to the above presented framework, the human entropy E(H), i.e. the entropy due to those system interactions which affect the compatibility of the ergonomic system (structure) with the given human characteristics of the subset (H), can be reduced only by increasing the entropy of the system regulator E(R), as defined by its complexity, which implies the need for increasing the system's compatibility requirements {CR}.

Following the Ashby's [12] law of requisite variety, this can be called the law of requisite complexity, which states that only complexity can reduce complexity. The above means that only added incompatibility (entropy) of the regulator (R), expressed by the system compatibility requirements {CR}, can be used to reduce the ergonomics system entropy (S), i.e. reduce the overall system incompatibility, expressed by the human entropy E(H).

It should be noted that the minimum value of the system entropy $E(S)_{MIN}$, equal to the human (interaction system) entropy E(H), occurs when the value of E(R) = 0, indicating that no further system regulation is possible. This is called the *ergonomic entropy* of the system.

$$E(H) = E(S)_{MIN} \text{ when } E(R) = 0. \quad (8)$$

As discussed by Karwowski et al [9], the ergonomic entropy $E(S)_{MIN}$ is the 'non-reducible' level of system entropy with respect to ergonomic intervention (regulation) efforts. It should be noted, however, that this entropy can be modified by the non-ergonomic means, that is through the human, rather than system, adaptation efforts. This can be done by reducing the value of human entropy E(H), through improvements in human performance and reliability by training, motivation, or skill conditioning.

8. THE HUMAN-COMPUTER INTERACTION SYSTEM (HCIS)

Based on the concepts outlined above, one can formally define the human-computer interaction system HCI-S as follows:

[HCI-S] = {(H), (R={K, M, E}), (I), (T)}, where: (9)

H - a set of human operator characteristics (perceptual, physical and cognitive, etc.),
K - a set of task requirements (physical, sensory, perceptual, cognitive, psychosocial, environmental, etc.)
M - a set of computer characteristics (hardware and software including computer interfaces)
E - an environment,
I - a set of interactions between H and R, and
T - time.

The set of interactions {I} embodies all possible interactions between H, K and M of the regulator {R} in a given environment subsystem {E}, regardless of their nature or strength of association. Such interactions can be elemental, i.e. one to one association, or complex, such as an interaction between the human operator, a particular software that is used to achieve the desired task, and available physical computer interface(s).

8.1. VDT ergonomic system characterization: example

An example of the physical interactions of the chair-human operator subsystem in VDT work is presented in order to illustrate the theoretical framework presented above. Let the ergonomic entropy of the VDT system be defined on the subsystems of E_S as follows:

$E(S_{HCI})$={user (H), R = {task (K), M={workstation (W), (VDT), chair (C)}}, (T) }, (10)

where K and M subsets of the system regulator (R) are the ergonomic design variables.

Let us consider the postural strain at the VDT work due to physical interactions. If K and W are assumed to be constants, i.e. their values are set before the VDT operator starts working with the system, then the chair characteristics (C) can be considered as the system regulator (R), which design parameters directly affect the interactions between the system and the user. The complexity of interactions (between H and C) define the current compatibility requirements {CR} of the system. The above allows to simplify the considered entropy of the examined ergonomic system (HCIS) as follows:

E(S) = E{H, R=chair}. (11)

According to equation #7, i.e.: E(H) =E(S) -- E(R), the human entropy of the system (as defined by the physical interactions between the human operator and the chair) equals the user-chair system entropy E(S) minus the entropy due to specific chair design or regulator E(R). The value of E(R) is determined by the chair compatibility requirements {CR}, and the consequent (resultant) level of complexity of the regulator (R) (new system design concept). In order to satisfy the compatibility requirements of the chair, i.e. to make the chair more compatible with the user, or simply to make the chair better fit the user and assure more comfort, one has to increase the number of adjustable features (degrees of freedom) of the chair, thereby increasing its complexity and entropy E(R). In other words, in order to reduce E(H) one needs to increase E(R).

It should be noted that this increased system complexity may significantly reduce effectiveness of the ergonomic intervention, as the user may be unable to deal with the added system complexity, i.e. may not be able to properly adjust variety of chair features (adjustments) to assure his/hers comfort. It should also be remembered the ergonomic compatibility requirements are subject to changes over time.

9. CONCLUSIONS

The interactions between system elements constitute the basic entities that need to be considered when studying any ergonomic system. In this context, the theoretical basis of the science of ergonomics must be based on such interactions, and aim to explain their dynamic nature. It is hoped that the proposed general modeling framework for the human-computer interaction, based on the principles of ergonomic compatibility requirements and human entropy, will help to improve our understanding of the underlying structure of the VDT-human interactions and the nature of ergonomic system regulation. Such understanding should in turn allow to develop and apply appropriate intervention measures to optimize the computer environments for human use.

REFERENCES

1. A. Aaras, R.E. Westgaard and S. Larsen, Postural load and the incidence of musculoskeletal illness. In S. Sauter, M.J. Dainoff and M.J. Smith (Eds.) *Promoting Health and Productivity in the Computerized Office,* London, Taylor & Francis (1990) 68-93.
2. W. Hunting, T. Laubli and E. Grandjean, Postural and visual loads at VDT workplaces. Part I: Constrained postures, *Ergonomics,* 24 (1981) 917-931.
3. M.J. Dainoff, Occupational stress factors in visual display terminal (VDT) operation: a review of empirical research, *Behavior and Information Technology*, 1 (1982) 141.
4. M.J. Smith, Mental and physical strain at VDT workstations, *Behaviour and Information Technology*, 6(3) (1992), 243-255.
5. W. Karwowski, R. Eberts, G. Salvendy and S. Noland, The effect of computer interface design on human postural dynamics, *Ergonomics,* 7(4) (1994) 703-724.
6. M. Wærsted, R.A. Bjørklund and R.H. Westgaard, Shoulder muscle tensions induced by two VDU-based tasks of different complexity, *Ergonomics*, 34(2) (1991) 137-150.
7. A. Grieco, Sitting posture: An old problem and a new one, *Ergonomics*, 39 (1986) 345.
8. W. Karwowski, T. Marek and C. Noworol, Theoretical basis of the science of ergonomics. *Proceedings of the 10th Congress of the International Ergonomics Association,* Sydney, Australia, London, Taylor & Francis (1988) 756-758.
9. W. Karwowski, Complexity, fuzziness and ergonomic incompatibility issues in the control of dynamic work environments, *Ergonomics,* 34 (6) (1991) 671-686.
10. W. Karwowski, T. Marek and C. Noworol, The complexity-incompatibility principle and the science of ergonomics. In F. Aghazadeh (Ed.), *Advances in Industrial Ergonomics and Safety VI*. London, Taylor & Francis (1994).
11. M.J. Dainoff and J. Balliett, Seated posture and workstation configuration. In M. Kumashiro and E. D. Megaw (Eds.), *Towards Human Work: Solutions to Problems in Occupational Health and Safety*, London, Taylor & Francis (1991) 156-163.
12. W.R. Ashby, *An Introduction to Cybernetics*, London, Methuen & Co Ltd. (1964).

HUMANIZING WWDU'S: A MACROERGONOMIC TQM STRATEGY FOR WORK SYSTEM AND JOB DESIGN

H. W. Hendrick

Institute of Safety and Systems Management, University of Southern California, Los Angeles, CA 90089-0021, USA

Work system and job characteristics related to WMSDs in VDT work are gleaned from recent studies. Traditional design practices that lead to dehumanized and WMSD-related work systems and jobs are noted. Macroergonomics is proposed as a design strategy that avoids the pitfalls of traditional work system and job design approaches. Job characteristics related to improved QWL and low incidences of WMSDs, and ways of achieving them in VDT work systems, are described.

1. INTRODUCTION

During the past two decades, perhaps the primary ergonomic occupational health issue in industrialized countries has been work related musculoskeletal disorders (WMSDs). It is not that the WMSD problem is new. WMSDs related to manual materials handling have been recognized as a major ergonomics problem since the formal beginnings of ergonomics as a profession in the late 1940s. What appears to be the major contributor to the widespread *increases* in WMSD's in the 80's and 90's is the progressively increasing introduction and use of video display terminals (VDT's) in the workplace (e.g., see Bammer, 1987).

Historically, conventional ergonomic interventions frequently have proven effective in reducing WMSDs in manual materials handling situations. In contrast, VDT related WMSD's do *not* appear readily correctable solely by conventional workstation (micro) ergonomics. For example, Bammer (1990) conducted a meta-analysis of field studies of work-related neck and upper limb disorders reported internationally during the 1980s. Results of her analysis showed no consistent relationship of non-work factors to employee musculoskeletal disorders. The data on biomechanical factors led her to conclude that (ergonomic) efforts to effect biomechanical improvements are important and should be encouraged; but, by themselves, these improvements are insufficient to reduce work related musculoskeletal disorders. She concluded that "improvements in work organisation to reduce pressure, and to increase task variety, control, and the ability for employees to work together must be the main focus of prevention and intervention." She further notes that "ironically, such improvements in work organisation generally also lead to increased productivity ." (Bammer, 1993, p. 35).

In essence, what Bammer has identified as the key correlates of WMSDs are what industrial and organizational psychologists commonly identify as the dehumanizing characteristics of jobs and work systems - characteristics that reduce psychological meaningfulness, felt responsibility, and knowledge of results; and that often lead to high stress, demotivated employees, job dissatisfaction, absenteeism, and reduced productivity (Organ and Bateman, 1991). Bammer's conclusions are further supported by a more recent major U.S. study by NIOSH in collaboration with U.S. West Communications and the Communications Workers of America (Hales, et. al, 1992). This study involved 533 workers from five distinct VDT operator job classifications at three U.S. West metropolitan locations. In an attempt to reduce WMSDs, U.S. West previously had made a major investment in ergonomically improving VDT operator work stations and lighting. Over a year later, there was no significant reduction in the incidence rate of WMSD symptoms (which were prevalent in over 20% of the operators). As a result, NIOSH was asked to conduct this more extensive, *macroergonomic* type of investigation. In addition to several demographic, medical history, work practice, and VDT work time factors, the NIOSH study identified seven psycho-social variables significantly related to the incidence of WMSDs. The researchers concluded that "...This study adds to the evidence that the psychosocial work environment is related to the occurrence of work-related upper extremity musculoskeletal symptoms." (Hales, et. al, 1992, p. 4).

2. VDT WMSDs AND COMMON WORK SYSTEM DESIGN PRACTICES

From over thirty years of organizational and ergonomic design, consulting, and teaching experience, I have become convinced that a major part of the VDT-related dehumanized work and associated WMSDs problem lies in three interrelated work system design practices. These are *technology-centered ergonomics, the "left over" approach to function and task allocation,* and a *failure to integrate the sociotechnical characteristics of the system into its organizational and work system design.*

2.1 Technology-Centered Ergonomics

When a new technology is developed, designers typically focus on incorporating it within some form of hardware or software to achieve some desired transformation or outcome. If consideration is given to those who must operate or maintain the newly developed products, it typically takes the form of determining what skills, knowledge and training will be necessary to utilize them. Often, even this kind of consideration is not systematic or well thought through. If ergonomic factors *are* considered, it usually takes the form of designing human-system interfaces for the *already designed* hardware and software to minimize human error and improve physical comfort. Rarely are the intrinsic motivational aspects of the jobs, psycho-social characteristics of the work force, or other related organizational and work system design factors considered. Yet these are the very factors that are critical to humanizing WWDUs.

2.2 The "Left Over" Approach to Function and Task Allocation

In system design, when a purely technology-centered approach is taken, the focus is on assigning to the "machine" any functions or tasks which its technology can enable it to accomplish. Then, what ever is "left over" is allocated to the persons who must operate, maintain, or be serviced by the system. This, by far, has been the most common means of function and task allocation in exploiting new technology (Bailey, 1989). Because this approach fails to adequately consider the characteristics of the work force and related environmental factors in allocating functions and tasks, the result usually is a suboptimally designed work system. A fundamental empirically derived principle of sociotechnical system design is that optimal effectiveness of the system requires *joint optimization* of the personnel and technological subsystems; and that this is achievable only through *joint design* of the two. When we attempt to optimize just the technical subsystem we force the personnel subsystem to have to accommodate (DeGreene, 1973). In essence, this becomes a "fitting square pegs into round holes" situation (Hendrick, 1986a&b). Put in ergonomic terms, joint optimization requires a *human-centered* approach. Bailey (1989) refers to this method of function and task allocation as a *"humanized task* approach", and states that "this concept essentially means that the ultimate concern is to design a job that *justifies* using a person, rather than a job that merely can be done by a human. With this approach, functions are allocated and the resulting tasks are designed to make full use of human skills and to compensate for human limitations. The nature of the work itself should lend itself to internal motivational influences. The left over functions are allocated to the computers." (p. 190).

2.3 Failure to Integrate an Organization's Sociotechnical Characteristics into its Work System Design

The primary structural and process characteristics of socio-technical systems first were empirically identified in the classic long-wall coal mining studies by the Tavistock Institute in the UK over four decades ago. From this literature, four major sociotechnical system elements may be identified: The personnel subsystem, technological subsystem, organizational structure, and the external environment. These four elements interact with one another. A change to any one element affects the other three; and, if not properly planned for, often in unanticipated and dysfunctional ways (DeGreene, 1973).

Following these classic sociotechnical system studies, the critical dimensions of the technology, personnel, and external environment have been identified in terms of their relation to specific characteristics of organizational and work system structure, and empirical models of these relationships have been developed. These models can be applied to diagnosing any complex system and more optimally designing its organizational and work system structure (e.g., see Hendrick, 1986b, 1987, or 1991).

Unfortunately, as first was documented in the Tavistock Institute studies, cited above, a technology centered approach to organizational and work system design does *not* adequately consider the relevant sociotechnical system variables - not only in terms of productivity, but also in terms of their effects on employee self-worth, stress, satisfaction, and related health and safety. As a result, work systems thus designed are most often *suboptimal.*

Over the past 18 years, I have been involved with both my graduate management and human factors students in the diagnosis of over two hundred organizational units. These assessments repeatedly have validated the dysfunctional effects of these three interrelated work system design practices.

3. MACROERGONOMICS: A HUMAN-CENTERED STRATEGY

Based on the above, what is needed is a work system design approach that accomplishes the following: First, it should be human-centered; second, it should use a humanized task approach to function and task allocation; and third, it should adequately consider the relevant sociotechnical system variables in terms of their implications for organizational and work system design, and related design of jobs and human-system interfaces. One strategy that can satisfy all three of these criteria is a *macroergonomic* approach.

3.1 Macroergonomics and Work System Design

Macroergonomics may be defined as a top-down sociotechnical systems approach to the design of organizations, work systems, jobs, and related human-machine, user-system, and human-environment interfaces (Hendrick, 1986a&b; 1991). It is top-down in that it begins with an analysis of the relevant sociotechnical system variables in terms of their implications for the design of the over-all structure of the work system; and then carries these design decisions down to the micro-ergonomic level of job and work station design. It is human-centered in that decisions regarding the structure of the organization and work system require consideration of the worker's professional and psycho-social characteristics, and of the relevant characteristics of the external environment to which these humans must effectively respond (in addition to consideration of the key characteristics of the technology to be employed). By the same token, consideration of these characteristics also make it a humanized task approach to function and task allocation.

Systems theorists generally agree that complex systems are *synergistic* - that the whole is more than the simple sum of its parts. When applied to organizations, this suggests that if we truly design work systems using a macroergonomic approach, and carry this through to the micro-ergonomic design of jobs and human-system interfaces, the resulting *ergonomically harmonized* work system should result in outcomes that are more than a simple sum of the parts would indicate. Instead of the typical 10% to 25% improvements in organizational effectiveness criteria that many of us have typically experienced from purely (successful) micro-ergonomic efforts, we theoretically should see improvements of 60% or more (Hendrick, 1991). Evidence from several recent macroergonomic interventions have provided tentative validation of this hypothesis. For example, Nagamachi and Imada (1992) have reported the results of a series of macroergonomic interventions in petroleum and manufacturing firms in the U.S. and Japan which achieved from 70% to over 90% reductions in accidents and injuries. To date, these reductions have been sustained. Another study used a macroergonomic approach in implementing a total quality management (TQM) program at the L. L. Bean Corporation in the U.S.. Among other positive results, reductions in lost time accidents and injuries of over 70% were achieved in both the manufacturing and distribution divisions (Rooney, Morency and Herrick, 1993). Of particular note, approximately 80% of these savings were in reductions in soft-tissue injuries (Rooney, personal communication). Given the widespread adaption of ISO 9000 on TQM, and the specific requirements concerning worker health and safety contained therein, the Rooney, et. al study results take on an even greater significance.

3.2 Macroergonomics and VDT Job Design for Preventing WMSDs

With respect to specific job design, it is interesting to note that the same job characteristics identified by Bammer as consistently related to WMSDs are similar to those which have been identified by industrial and organizational psychologists as critical to intrinsic job motivation, employee self-worth, stress reduction, and satisfaction. These are task *variety*, *identity* or sense of job wholeness, *significance* or perceived job meaningfulness, *autonomy* or control over one's work, and *feedback* or knowledge of results (Hackman and Oldham, 1975).

Task *variety* can be incorporated into VDT jobs by (a) varying the types of computer work assigned to a given operator and (b) structuring the work system such that VDT operators also perform other administrative and clerical tasks part of the time. These kinds of job redesign also can enhance the sense of wholeness or *identity* of the job. Similarly, job *significance* or meaningfulness is likely to be enhanced by these same kinds of redesign; and by ensuring that a human truly is needed for the specific VDT tasks assigned. Job *autonomy* readily can be enhanced by allowing the VDT operators to (a) pace their own work, including micro- and mini-rest breaks, (b) work out their own schedules for when they do what, consistent with meeting necessary suspenses, and (c) by ensuring that managers do *not* over-supervise or micro-manage and, instead, treat trained operators as responsible adults. Feedback mechanisms often can be built into the software used by VDT operators *for their personal use*. What appears critical here is that these mechanisms *not* be used for *individual* monitoring by management; as such micro-control only adds to operator stress by creating a "big brother is watching you" syndrome.

Finally, as Bammer's meta-analysis indicated, it is important that work system designs allow VDT operators to meet work-related social needs. Opportunities for social interaction can be enhanced by physical workplace arrangements; and by structuring at least some administrative and clerical tasks so as to facilitate, or at least enable, social interaction.

4. CONCLUSION

Macroergonomics provides us with an intervention strategy for developing or improving WWDU work systems that overcomes the dysfunctional shortcomings of historically used design practices. As a top-down sociotechnical systems approach to organizational and work system design, it meets the criteria of being human-centered, utilizing a humanized task approach to function and task allocation, and systematically considering the key sociotechical variables related to effective VDT work system design. Using a macroergonomic approach, work systems can be structured that enable specific job designs having known desirable characteristics for enhancing employee health and other quality of work life aspects of VDT positions. Not only do such work system and job designs hold promise for reducing WMSDs, but also for humanizing VDT work, enhancing productivity, and reducing related costs. As a result, harmonized work systems that potentially can result in exponential improvements in various organizational effectiveness criteria are realizable.

Results from several recent macroergonomic interventions offer tentative validation of this conclusion. Of particular note is the potential of macroergonomics as an approach to TQM and meeting ISO 9000 requirements concerning occupational health and safety.

REFERENCES

Bailey, R. W. (1989). *Human Performance Engineering* (2nd Edition). Englewood Cliffs, NJ: Prentice-Hall.

Bammer, G. (1987). VDUs and musculoskeletal problems at the Australian National University - A case study. In B. Knave, and P. G. Wideback (Eds.), *Work With Display Units 86* (pp. 279-287). Amsterdam: North-Holland.

Bammer, G. (1990). Review of current knowledge - musculoskeletal problems. In L. Berlinguet, and D. Berthelette (Eds.), *Work With display Units 89* (pp. 113-120). Amsterdam: North-Holland.

Bammer, G. (1993). Work-related neck and upper limb disorders - social, organisational, biomechanical and medical aspects. In L. A. Gontijo, and J. de Souza (Eds.), *Segundo Congresso Latino Americano e Sexto Seminario Brasileiro de Ergonomia* (pp. 23-38). Florianopolis: Ministerio do Trabalho Fundacentro/SC.

DeGreene, K. B. (1973). *Sociotechnical Systems*. Englewood Cliffs, NJ: Prentice-Hall.

Hackman, J. R., and Oldham, G. (1975). Development of the Job Diagnostic Survey. *Journal of Applied Psychology*, 159-170.

Hales, T., Sauter, S., Petersen, M., Putz-Anderson, V., Fine, L., Ochs, T., Schleifer, L., and Bernard, B. (1992). *US West Communications (USWC): Phoenix, Arizona; Minneapolis, Minnesota; Denver, Colorado: Health Hazard Evaluation Report*. Cincinnati, OH: NIOSH, Centers for Disease Control. (HETA Report, 89-299-2230).

Hendrick, H. W. (1986a). Macroergonomics: A concept whose time has come. *Human Factors Society Bulletin, 30,* 1-3.

Hendrick, H. W. (1986b). Macroergonomics: A conceptual model for integrating human factors with organizational design. In O. Brown, Jr., and H. W. Hendrick (Eds.), *Human Factors in Organizational Design and Management-II* (pp. 467-478). Amsterdam: North-Holland.

Hendrick, H. W. (1987). Organizational design. In G. Salvendy (Ed.), *Handbook of Human Factors* (pp.470-494). New York: Wiley.

Hendrick, H. W. (1991). Human factors in orgnizational design and management. *Ergonomics, 34,* 743-756.

Nagamachi, M., and Imada, A. (1992). A macroergonomic approach for improving safety and work design. In *Proceedings of the Human Factors Society 36th Annual Meeting*. Santa Monica, CA: Human Factors Society, (pp. 859-861.

Organ, D. W., and Bateman, T. S. (1991). *Organizational Behavior*. Homewood, IL: Irwin.

Rooney, E. F., Morency, R. R., and Herrick, D. R. (1993). Macroergonomics and total quality management at L. L. Bean: A case study. In R. Neilsen and K. Jorgensen (Eds.), *Advances in Industrial Ergonomics and Safety V* (pp. 493-498). London: Taylor & Francis.

Fusion of Eastern and Western civilisations in WWDU

Hiroyuki Miyamoto

Department of Computer Science, Chiba Institute of Technology,
2-17-1, Tsudanuma, Narashino 275, Japan

Word processing by computer is now widely used in many countries, but in the way of development of this new technology, Japan has pursued a different way from that of western countries because of the particularities of Japanese language, especially *kanji*, or Chinese characters. Japanese language differs from western languages in both appearance and sound, because it has been developed under the influences of Chinese, as western languages had been influenced by Latin and Greek.

1. JAPANESE: ITS PARTICULARITIES

Many people wonder how Japanese text is handled by computer systems as this language has some mysterious characteristics as follows [1]:
- The Japanese writing system is a mixture of four different writing systems.
- Unlike English, for instance, whose alphabet of 26 letters can spell every word, the Japanese uses about 3,000 *kanji* characters in reading newspapers and books, very often more than 5,000 *kanji* characters in daily life.
- There is no universally recognised input device such as QWERTY keyboard
- Japanese text can be set horizontally or vertically.

Chinese has approximately 50,000 characters, some of which Japanese began to borrow to transcribe their proper language more than 1,500 years ago, although there is little resemblance between these two languages. *Kanji* characters are ideographic in nature, and nobody can tell how many characters exist. Besides *kanji*, Japanese uses *kana* characters that were invented from *kanji* in the 8th century in Japan: there are two styles of *kana*: *hiragana* and *katakana*. *Kana* is syllabary, or a phonetic alphabet system consisting of 50 characters and representing approximately 80 sounds. *Hiragana* are used to write native Japanese, while *katakana* represent the same set of sounds as *hiragana*, and are used primarily in two ways: to write words of foreign origin, and for emphasis like as italic in English. Japanese text is typically composed of four different writing systems: *kanji, hiragana* and *katakana*, in addition to Roman alphabet as shown in Figure 1. This makes Japanese quite complex from the orthographic point of view, and causes some problems.
Kanji are usually assigned one or more pronunciations. The typical *kanji* has at least two pronunciations, and very often more. No matter what their pronunciation, they have approximately the same meaning.

WWDUはディスプレイに関する国際会議です。

— :Hiragana
-- :Katakana
= :Kanji

WWDU is an international conference on displays.

Figure 1. Example of a Japanese text

Kanji are composed of smaller, primitive units called radicals, which are the most basic meaningful units of *kanji*. Several radicals stand alone as single, meaningful *kanji*. Radicals are stretched or squeezed so that all the radicals that constitute a *kanji* may fit into a square, a general shape of *kanji*. Radicals are positioned on the left, right, top, or bottom within *kanji*. *Kanji* may be classified into four categories: pictographic, ideographic, logical compounds, and phonetic compounds. Pictographic *kanji*, the most basic, are little pictures, and usually look like the object they means as shown in Figure 2.

Ideographic characters represent abstract concepts such as directions and numbers as shown in Figure 3. Pictographic and ideographic *kanji* may be used to represent more complex pictures, and reflect the combined meaning of its individual elements. This kind of characters are called logical compounds, some examples of which are illustrated in Figure 4.

Phonetic compounds account for more than 90 percent of *kanji*. They normally have at least two components, one to indicate pronunciation, the other to represent basic meaning as illustrated in Figure 5. There thus exist homophone problems in *kanji* system, and each distinguishable sound can represent up to 30 different *kanji*.

BC1500	present	pronunciation	meaning
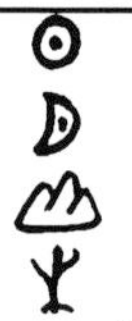 ☉	日	hi	sun
☽	月	tsuki	moon
⛰	山	yama	mountain
ᛉ	木	ki	tree

Figure 2. Examples of pictographic kanji

kanji	meaning
上	up
下	down
一	one
二	two

Figure 3. Examples of ideographic kanji

kanji	components	meaning
明	日+月	bright
林	木+木	woods
森	木+木+木	forest

Figure 4. Examples of logical compounds

kanji	meaning	meaning part	pronunciation part
板	board	木	反
販	sale	貝	反
飯	food	食	反

Figure 5. Examples of phonetic compounds

2. JAPANESE TEXT INPUT

A typewriter for western languages has some 40 to 50 keys. How one does type Japanese text? It is, indeed, no more realistic to assign *kanji* to the keys of a regular typewriter keyboard, although some mechanical typewriters existed for Japanese text; for example, lead types were arranged in a 35 by 70 matrix in phonetic order, and a skilled operator picked up leads one by one to print each character on a paper. Furthermore, traditional Japanese literature is written in vertically, and should be read from right to left column, which are totally different from western languages. The Japanese text has no space between words, but has only some punctuation marks.

3. COMPUTER SYSTEMS FOR JAPANESE TEXT INPUT

To be able to input *kanji* on a computer system, radicals and strokes are assigned to the keys of specially designed keyboard. This shape-based input method is suited to professional typists, who type from manuscripts to make a fair copy rather than compose sentences, because the typists do not have to know the pronunciation of *kanji* or even their meanings.

As the microcomputer became available, Japanese text input method of the first generation was developed, which converted a single two-byte *kanji* code into the corresponding *kanji* character as the conversion key was pushed, such as 3441 to get 漢, and 3B7A字, according to JIS encoding (JIS stands for Japanese Industrial Standard). This was, however, far from practical use. This has led to software solutions: front-end-processors (FEP) and conversion dictionaries, because sound-based input method is more natural than shape-based one, and suited to non professional users who compose sentences phonetically without thinking how each word is written in *kanji*.

Ease of input, accuracy, and speed have been the main concerns in developing a Japanese word processor. Japanese text is typically input in two stages: the user types raw keyboard input, which the computer interprets using the FEP and the conversion dictionary to display a list of candidate characters (candidate here refers to the character or characters that are mapped to the input string in the conversion dictionary). The user selects one choice from the list of candidate characters, or requests more choices. How well each stage is handled on the computer depends greatly on the quality of the input software of that machine.

A front-end-processor, Japanese text input software, handles both of these input stages. It is so named because it grabs the user's keyboard input before any other software can use it. Keyboard input can take one of two usual forms: transcribed Japanese using Roman characters such as "k" and "a" to get か, or *hiragana* input as all the *hiragana* characters can be assigned over Roman keyboard uppercases and lowercases. The FEP usually converts transcribed Japanese into *hiragana* on-the-fly, so it doesn't really matter which keyboard is used.

Once the input string is complete, it is then parsed in one of two ways: either by the user during input, or by a parser built into the FEP. Finally, each segment is run through a conversion process that consists of a lookup into a conversion dictionary. Typical conversion dictionaries have tens of thousands of entries. The more entries, the better the conversion quality. However, if the conversion dictionary is too large, users are shown a far too lengthy list of candidates. This reduces input efficiency.

Can *kanji* characters be input one at a time? While single *kanji* input is possible, there are three basic units that can be used. These units allow the user to limit the number of candidates from which the user must choose. Typically, the larger the input unit, the fewer candidates. The units are as follows:
- Single *kanji*
- *Kanji* compound
- *Kanji* phrase.

Early input programs required that each *kanji* should be input individually (single *kanji*), Nowadays it is much more efficient to input *kanji* as they appear in compounds or even phases. This means that the user may input two or more *kanji* at once by virtue of inputting their combined pronunciation. For example, the *kanji* 漢字 rather than *kan* 漢 and *ji* 字, separately.

It can be understood that there are many other *kanji* with those pronunciations, so it would take much time before finding the correct one in a long list of candidate *kanji* proposed by a *kana-kanji* conversion dictionary. This eliminated the need of learning the code. A more efficient way is to input them as one unit, namely with the input string *kanji*, which is called a *kanji* compound. This produces a much shorter list of candidates from which to choose. Along with the progress of software program based on grammatical analysis, the input strings may be phrases rather than words, and the accuracy of conversion has increased. To select between *kana-to-kanji*, conversion and raw input of *kana*, special function keys called Xfer (conversion) and Nfer (non conversion) are used. These two function keys may be often replaced by space bar for conversion and return key for non-conversion in the case of Roman keyboard. Figure 6 shows the input strings and conversion and non conversion key functions.

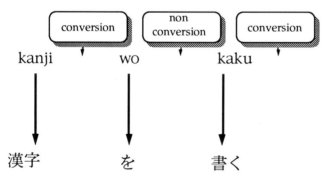

Figure 6. Conversion and non conversion keys

Result of conversion has been displayed in a special window at the bottom of display, and another key input was needed to send this result into text area to be edited as shown in Figure 7. The user's eyes thus often moved between at the end of text to be input and the bottom of display, and then a direct input replaced it.

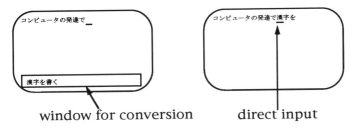

Figure 7. Input of converted string through window and direct input

A FEP provides the following operations:
- Switch between Japanese and Roman writing modes
- Convert the input string into a mixture of *hiragana, katakana, kanji*, and Roman characters
- Select from a list of candidate characters
- Validate the selected or converted string

To improve the input speed and accuracy of conversion, several features have been added, wherein automatic conversion, spelling help, self-learning function, main and personal dictionaries are included: a homophone list is ordered according to the occurrence of use of each *kanji* for example. The user may register commonly used Japanese phrases so that correct strings of characters may be retrieved by a few key strokes.

4. COMPUTER SYSTEMS FOR JAPANESE TEXT OUTPUT

Once Japanese text is input and edited by a proper software, it must be displayed on a computer monitor, or printed out on a paper. A dot-matrix printer of 8 by 5 pins have not been sufficient, nor 16 by 16 pins, because some complex *kanji* cannot be correctly presented with these resolutions. *Kanji* fonts of 24 by 24 dots may be adopted to use on display such as 72 dpi (dots per inch) although this resolution is not yet sufficient for some *kanji*. To get a clear and pleasing high quality Japanese text hard copy, it is necessary to use different sizes of bit mapped fonts of 180 dpi or more, and now outline fonts. It takes sometimes several megabytes to store a whole set of *kanji, kana* and other accompanying characters of one typeface.

5. JAPANESE TEXT AND COMPUTER TECHNOLOGY

The Japanese text processing software with above functions has not been realised until a large capacity of memory, high performance CPU, and sufficient resolution of display and printer became available. Furthermore, input software such as FEP had to be developed to convert input string into *kana* and *kanji* correctly and without special efforts.

That makes a contrast with the progress of Roman word-processing software that was initially a simple replacement of mechanical typewriter, and needed no dictionary. Spell correction and thesaurus have been added later when a larger memory capacity became common.

Other countries in Asia such as China and Korea have their character sets, and need some appropriate input software. Most Western language input software assume that one character corresponds to one byte, but some Eastern languages such as Japanese, Chinese and Korea use multiple-byte characters, and special input software had to be developed to handle their languages properly. Not only input but also output of text of these languages need studies on how the text should be handled with an appropriate software and displayed on computer monitor. That deeply depends on the civilisation and for each of which the technology should be developed.

6. ICON: IDEOGRAPHIC KANJI

It is remarked that many people now use emoticons, or smileys in exchanging e-mail. Figure 8 shows some typical smileys, wherein some facial expression may be read when looked at sideways. With an emoticon, a combination of a few characters, they can add some nuance to the context, which would be difficult to tell with text.

:-)	happy
%:-)	happy confused
:-(	sad
%:-(	sad confused
:-||	angry
:-D	laughing
;-)	winking
:-}	grinning
:'-(	crying

Figure 8. Examples of emoticon

Along with the progress of computer technology, it becomes much easier to handle not only characters but also images. GUI (Graphical User Interface) has been introduced for more intuitive operations, where the icon, a kind of ideograph, plays an important role. In this sense, *kanji* has been a kind of icon. Eastern civilisation has developed practical input methods suited for its large number of characters by using a standard Roman typewriter keyboard, while Western civilisation has begun adopting ideographs. Though the exchange of experiences, Eastern and Western civilisations will move closer to make Work With Display Units more productive and creative in the near future. ;-)

REFERENCE
1. Ken Lunde, Understanding Japanese Information Processing, O'Reilly & Associates, Inc., Sebastopol, 1993.

ICHAC Statement on the European Directive on work with display screen equipment

The General Assembly of the International Commission on Human Aspects in Computing (ICHAC) has adopted this Statement in Milan on the 2nd of October, 1994. The Statement has been prepared by an ICHAC Scientific Committee:

T. Stewart*, chair, U. Bergqvist¤, B. Piccoli#, P.G. Widebäck¤

*System Concepts, 2 Savoy Court, Strand, London WC2R OEZ, UK
¤National Institute of Occupational Health, S-171 84 Solna, Sweden
#Institute of Occupational Health, University of Milan, Via San Barnaba 8 I-201 22 Milan, Italy

Table of contents
1. Background and purpose of this Statement
2. General description of the Directive
2.1. Aim of the VDU Directive
2.2. The structure of the VDU Directive
2.3. Transposition into national regulation
3. Critique of the Directive
3.1. What´s missing from the Directive?
4. Conclusions
A 1. Comments on the preamble
A 2. Comments on Section I, General Provisions
A 3. Comments on Section II, Employers Obligations (Articles 3-8)
A 4. Comments on Section II, Employers Obligations (Article 9)
A 5. Comments on Section III, Miscellaneous Provisions
A 6. Comments on the Annex, Minimum Requirements

1. BACKGROUND AND PURPOSE OF THIS STATEMENT

Work with Visual Display Units (VDUs) has been implicated as a cause of adverse reactions among those using display screen equipment, or using such equipment in certain work situations. A comprehensive review was published by the World

Health Organization in 1987 (updated in 1990). This review discussed the specific occurrence in VDU work situations of primarily eye discomforts, musculoskeletal disorders and stress-related problems. Other adverse reactions to VDU work have also been suggested: eye injuries, adverse reproductive outcomes or skin problems, but at present, the specific occurrences of these in VDU work situations have not been verified. Nor have, as yet, health impacts of electric or magnetic fields as they exist in work situations around VDUs been shown to exist.

Nevertheless, a number of health problems are related to work with Visual Display Units. By and large, such health problems should be amendable by utilizing prudent ergonomic and work organization principles. The adaptation of these principles to the specific conditions found in VDU work is an ongoing process around the world.

The Council of the European Communities has issued a Council Directive of 29 May 1990 on the "minimum safety and health requirements for work with display screen equipment" (90/270/EEC). See the Official Journal of the European Communities, L 156 p 14-18 (21 June 1990) with a corrigendum in OJ L 170 p 30 (4 July 1990). This is referred to below as the "VDU Directive" or the "Directive".

The International Commision on Human Aspect of Computing (ICHAC) has issued this Statement in order to describe, clarify and offer critique on the VDU Directive. We feel that the Directive and this Statement will be of importance not only to those within the European Community, but also as a guidance to many individuals and organizations outside the Community.

2. GENERAL DESCRIPTION OF THE DIRECTIVE

2.1. Aim of the VDU Directive

The Directive on the minimal safety and requirements for work with display screen equipment (henceforth the "VDU Directive") was adopted by the Council of the European Communities because of its obligation to "adopt, by means of Directives, minimum requirements designed to encourage improvements, especially in the working environment, to ensure a better level of protection of workers´ safety and health" (Preamble).

In the preamble, the general purpose is given as to improve "safety and health of workers at work", while the specific aim of this Directive is directed towards ergonomic aspects since they "are of particular importance for a workstation with display screen equipment". This implies to us that the aim of the VDU Directive includes also protection against discomforts and effects that could be transient. In this context a positive attempt has been made on the part of the Directive to formulate some initial pointers for health surveillance as well as for the application of ergonomic principles in the work environments.

Unfortunately, the VDU Directive is not fully clear on 'what they are protecting the worker against'. Article 3 does include the phrase "possible risks to eyesight, physical problems and problems of mental stress". Use of the term "eyesight" in the Directive would indicate that the functional aspect of the problem takes precedence over other problems involving e.g. ocular surfaces and accessories - however, we do not consider that to be an adequate description. Disturbances affecting the visual apparatus that manifest themselves as eye discomforts are undoubtedly frequent among VDU operators, and have since the beginning of VDU usage been a central concern. While such discomforts are not specifically mentioned, they are clearly included in the aim of the Directive, as indicated both by the preamble, and by several specific obligations in the Annex. The ethical aspect of monitoring - translatable into terms such as personal integrity, dignity and unnecessary surveillance - is not mentioned, although it can be reasonably argued that the wording on monitoring is motivated by such concerns.

We think that the VDU Directive could have been more clear on "what are we protecting the worker against?". We would suggest the wording "eye discomforts, musculoskeletal problems, stress and lack of integrity" in that order. Furthermore, the term "visual apparatus" should be used in appropriate passages in lieu of terms that allude only to "vision". There are also other suggested health issues that seem to have influenced some wording. These include eye injury (see article 9 on "protection of workers´ eyes and eyesight"), and probably pregnancy issues (see Annex §2 (f) on radiation). The reader is left with his/her own interpretation as to whether these latter health issues are included or not in the specific aim of this Directive. To us, the inclusion of pregnancy and radiation issues is, at least at present, questionable.

2.2. The structure of the VDU Directive
The VDU Directive is divided into several parts. It begins with a preamble which basically refers to the obligation, justification and legal background for the Council´s decision to issue the VDU Directive. In Section I, the VDU Directive defines and describes the situations to which the VDU Directives applies. Section II specifies employers´ obligations. Section III includes some miscellaneous provisions: on adaptations to the Annex, and instructions to the Member States on the

VDU Directive. Finally, the Annex sets out a number of minimum requirements to be applied to VDU workstations as regards the equipment, the environment and the operator/computer interface.

The Annex is tied to the Directive by Article 10 in Section III: "The strictly technical adaptations to the Annex to take account of technical progress, developments in international regulations and specifications and knowledge in the field of display screen equipment shall be adopted...". The time span as to when the minimum requirements from the Annex are to be met by workstations is given in Article 4 and 5 of Section II.

The strict wording of the Annex, e.g. the use of the word "shall" is, however, partly neutralized by the statement that "the obligations laid down in this Annex shall apply in order to achieve the objectives of this Directive and to the extent that, firstly, the components concerned are present at the workstation, and secondly, the inherent requirements or characteristics of the task do not preclude it." Thus, it appears to us that the "minimum requirements" are not requirements, if it can be argued that the work task makes it impossible to fulfil certain obligations.

2.3. Transposition into national regulation

This VDU Directive is not (directly) directed towards employers etc, but to national governments: "Member States shall bring into force the laws, regulations and administrative provisions necessary to comply with this Directive by 31 December 1992" (Article 11, §1). Such activities have been ongoing in countries within the European Communities and the European Free Trade Association.

As indicated below, a number of items within this VDU Directive are very general, vague and open to different interpretation. Thus, it remains a possibility that this may result in fundamentally different requirements in different countries. In principle, reference to international standards within the VDU Directive would have decreased this potential for diversity. Unfortunately, relevant European standards did not (at the time of writing of the Directive) exist in final form, which presumably prevented the VDU Directive to give such references. This, again, makes the reference and use of forthcoming standards something that may vary between Member States.

3. CRITIQUE OF THE VDU DIRECTIVE

The details of our comments on specific articles and sections as well as the Annex are given in Appendices 1-6. The reader is thus referred to the appropriate Appendix for both a description and critique of the various sections. Items that - in our opinion - are missing from the Directive are discussed here in general, as it may implicate several Sections

3.1. What´s missing from the Directive?
The preamble, Articles 3-5 of Section II and the Annex are primarily directed towards workstation design, and its physical surroundings. Other considerations are referred to in Articles 6-9, namely information and training (Article 6), daily work routine (Article 7), worker consultation/participation (Article 8) and eye and eyesight tests (Article 9). Thus, there is a tendency towards a differentiation between ergonomic and organizational issues inherent in the structure of the Directive, and a higher degree of emphasis on at least the details of the ergonomic/physical situation. There are, as we see it, some problems with this distinction between the ergonomic/physical and the organizational situation.

The paucity of details on work content and work organization issues is problematic, since these are clearly of central interest in the prevention of discomforts and disorders among VDU operators. Although work organization considerations have been examined since the late 1970'ies, the attention given to such factors in various studies has - in general - been minor compared to the attention given the physical safety and ergonomic aspects of VDU work. However, increasing recognition has more recently been given to the fact that computerization of workplaces is intimately linked to the design of work and work organization. It is arguable that the caveat in the Annex makes the general clauses on e.g. work organization in article 8 more binding than the detailed ergonomic requirements in the Annex. Nevertheless, we think that the relative scarcity of work organisation details in the Annex should be rectified.

At present, some job design and work organization items are included in Section II: information on safety and health, training in the use of the workstation, employers planning breaks and/or changes in activity , and worker consultation and participation in actions taken according to the Directive. Thus, certain items relating to possible job stress factors are included, although it can be argued that this list of items is far from complete, missing e.g. such factors as workload, task complexity etc. In addition - and perhaps even more important, is the absence of any factor or factors that may modify, remedy or "balance" the presence of job stress factors, such as personal control over the task, participation in decsion making, and peer support. For example, it is arguable that the employers control ("plan") over rest breaks (article 7) may run contrary to both the efficient use of rest breaks to prevent the development of discomforts, and the users control over the work tasks.

The conceptual separation of ergonomic and organizational factors is also dubious in the causation of many health problem such as muscle problems. For example, it can be succesfully argued that organizational matters such as working hours or break opportunities influence the impact of ergonomic factors on muscle discomforts. Thus, an analysis of workstations (Article 3) should include also an analysis of the work task and its organizational context.

In this context, a point of interpretation could be mentioned: Suppose that a workstation is already in existence and fulfils those parts of the Annex not precluded by the work task, and that an analysis of the workstation has been performed according to Article 3. With a change in work task, but unchanged workstation, to what degree should both adherence to the Annex and to Article 3 be reconsidered? The VDU Directive does not - as we see it - give sufficient guidance on this.

As already mentioned above, there is a contrast between the degree of details given certain items such as image quality requirements on the one hand, and the broad and general directions given areas such as work organization or software ergonomics on the other. We think that some general statements of intention on all matters including ergonomics would have been valuable, followed by specific requirements where such can be made. For example, relevant parts of §§1b, 1c, 1d, 2b and 2c in the Annex could have been preceeded with a requirement of "good visual ergonomic conditions as regards to eye task objects". A parallell declaration could then be made as to work organizational items that should - in our opinion - also be included in the Annex. (It is noteworthy that the section on operator/computer interface already include such a general statement, see clause 3.e in the Annex.)

Despite the number of items concerning visual ergonomics in the Annex, individualization of risk factors from which the worker should be protected are often insufficiently specific. An analysis of the present literature results in the suggestion of several such factors, that can be grouped as:

a/ factors related to the type of visual tasks. Many authors underline the importance of the prolonged near point observation presumably causing fatigue to structures controlling accommodation and fusional convergence. Overloading of these structures appear clearly indicated by the symptomatology of VDU users, as well as confirmation from experimental investigations.

b/ It is probable that certain chemical and physical pollutants or factors such as formaldehyde or dry air may also affect the ocular surface. The impact of such factors may be reinforced by an increased gaze angle due to the position of the VDT leading to an increased ocular surface being exposed to ambient conditions. Indications of at least some such problems are also given by the symptomatology of users.

These types of factors may furthermore have different effects on the workers according to their ophthalmological characteristics. Thus, subjects suffering from hypermetropia, binocular vison impairments or alterations of the lacrimal film composition appear to be more susceptible (compared to other subjects) in developing eye discomforts. Attention should also be given to the type of correction devices (monofocal, bifocal, progressive spectacles or lenses) offered to the user.

Experience clearly tells us that situations may develop quite differently when an adverse situation is initially handled correctly or incorrectly. There is a lack of guidance on what to do in situations where a worker develops an adverse health reaction - this is left to the individual Member State. Without criticizing the Directive for the lack of instructions on this, we still would like to emphasize the importance of guidance or further comments in this respect.

4. CONCLUSIONS

In our opinion, the VDU Directive can be seen as an important and valuable tool for "improvements in the safety and health of workers". We feel, however, that the background for the issuing of the Directive, namely the specific health situation of VDU workers, have not been sufficiently taken into consideration in the recommended actions. This could be remedied by a clear statement as to what the Directive is protecting against (and what it is not), further considerations of both organizational and visual ergonomic factors, additional details on conditions and positive actions for prevention, and a better integration of such factors. Such development would - in our opinion - increase the importance of this Directive as as a guidance to both member state legislators as well as to other parties concerned with the underlying issues.

It is intended that comments on the implementation of this Directive, as well as the effect on work practice in various European nations will be forth-coming.

A 1. COMMENTS ON THE PREAMBLE

The preamble gives, as already described, a motivational and legal background for the VDU Directive.

An important statement is the obligation of the employers to "keep themselves informed of the latest advances in technology and scientific findings concerning workstation design so that they can make any changes necessary so as to be able to guarantee a better level of protection of workers´ safety and health". The mention, apart from workstation design, also of work task and organizational findings would have been valuable here - if the goal of a "guarantee" is to be met. This obligation is further dealt with in Articles 3, 6 and 8.

A 2. COMMENTS ON SECTION I, GENERAL PROVISIONS

Articles 1 and 2 form together a definition of who or what is subject to this Directive.

Certain special situations are excluded, such as computer systems on board a means of transport, control cabs, public use system, portable systems if used for short times and calculators or typewriters. The definition "display screen equipment" does not, however, highlight the most characteristic element of this equipment - that it is computer-based or -linked. A more suitable description could be "screen computer-based equipment". Furthermore, no distinction or description is made between different technologies by which this equipment is based, such as CRT, liquid crystal etc. Such distinctions are of fundamental importance in the Annex. A mention could be made here, so that it is clear that equipment based on such different technologies are all included.

Of importance is an exclusion found under definitions (Article 2), namely that workers who do not "habitually use display screen equipment as a significant part of his normal work" are excluded. The words "habitually", "significant" and "normal" can obviously be given different meanings. Either a more specified statement, or an example, would have been better. For example, the word "significant" could have been replaced by "at least 1 hour per day".

The definition of workstation (article 2) should include, together with the alphanumeric or graphic display screen equipment, any other monitor connected to the computer.

A clearer distinction should also be made between the concepts of "hardware" and "software". The categorization of equipment and their use is often done by the type of hardware. This appear unsatisfactory both from an ergophthalmological and work organizational point of view. Indeed, sophisticated "hardware" is sometimes used with relatively simple "software" (requiring e.g. low visual effort), while in other cases common computers are used with complex and mentally or visually taxing software. These and other distinctions need to be addressed, and should be identified in the definitions.

It should also be pointed out, that although some situations are excluded from the mandatory requirements based on this Directive, some such situations could benefit from the basic principles for good work conditions on which the Directive is based. Thus, beyond the formal application of the Directive, its information content should be useful as guidance. This use would be further extended by a number of suggestions made in this text - including extended definitions as suggested here.

A 3. COMMENTS ON SECTION II, EMPLOYERS OBLIGATIONS (ARTICLES 3-8)

Article 3 requires that the employer "...perform an analysis of workstations in order to evaluate the safety and health conditions to which they give rise for their workers, particularly as regards possible risks to eyesight, physical problems and problems of mental stress". Secondly, the "employers shall take appropriate measures to remedy the risks found...". This is a central obligation, in that it places the responsibility on the employer. It is not sufficient to 'wait for problems to develop'. As already stated, this article should have been reformulated to include also work tasks etc. It would be suitable to include in this analysis the average time of use within a specified period of time (e.g. one year) and the type of work performed. For the latter, the classification proposed by the WHO could be used (see WHO Offset Publication No 99, "Visual Display Terminals and Workers' Health", Geneva 1987).

Articles 4 and 5 tie the minimum requirements of the Annex to the Directive by giving a time limit for their implementation: 31 December 1992 for new workstations and 31 December 1996 for existing workstations. Within the Annex are requirements for software ergonomics, but little guidance as to what should be done in explicit terms. It is thus not very clear how existing workstations shall be made to comply by December 31st, 1992. Hopefully, this will be translated into a demand for such guidance.

In Article 6, the workers and/or their representatives are assured of information of safety and health relevant to the workstations, and training in the use of these. Practice has shown this information and training to be essential for good working conditions. Specification of the term "training in use of the workstation" should have been valuable, we consider for example both training in the ergonomics of use, and training in the use of software to be valuable. A practical point could also have been made on the follow-up training after a period of time. Consultation and participation of workers and/or their representatives are also covered in Article 8.

Article 7 states the requirement that "the employer must plan the worker's activity in such a way that daily work on a display screen is periodically interrupted by breaks or changes of activity reducing the workload at the display screen".

This very general statement contains, as we see it, both a powerful tool for improvement and a number of problems. With emphasis on the word "plan" and "periodically", its implementation could lead to a carefully planned, and thus highly regimented, work schedule with precise breaks. There is strong research evidence that short, informal rest breaks taken at the employee's discretion are helpful in reducing at least musculoskeletal health complaints. Rigid, fixed restbreaks may conceivably do more harm than good, because of the lack for variability in task structure that they engender. A different emphasis would be to increase the variability and especially the flexibility of the work task planning by the worker.

Furthermore, the phrasing carries the implication that "reducing the workload at the display screen" leads to a reduction of the workload of the worker". In general, this is not correct. Numerous examples of a lower workload with non-VDU work do indeed exist, but there are also many opposite situations, where the VDU work situation represents a reduced workload compared to the same individual's non-VDU work situation. From an ergophthalmologic point of view, however, work during "alternative activities" should not use similar near visual efforts. For musculoskeletal aspects, alternative work should involve a variation in position, thus employing different muscles and joint postures.

Finally, Article 7 could have been supplemented with a statement as to some action alternatives when a worker develops discomforts or other health problems despite a carefully designed ergonomic situation - further changes in activity and/or rest break opportunities offer additional ways to deal with these problems and help individuals with such problems.

A 4. COMMENTS ON SECTION II, EMPLOYERS OBLIGATIONS (ARTICLE 9)

This Article is probably the one with the most immediate impact on the VDU work conditions, since it requires that every VDU worker (except those excluded in Articles 1 and 2) shall be entitled to appropriate eye and eyesight tests. This shall be performed "before commencing VDU work, at regular intervals thereafter, and if the worker experience visual difficulties which may be due to display screen work". Further requirements on ophthalmological examinations ("if necessary") and special corrective appliances are also made.

These requirements are in many ways very similar to those that have been in existence in Sweden for a number of years. Experience suggests that this is a way of reducing certain discomfort problems, but that its implementation is also beset with a number of difficulties. What should be made clear is:

- what it is protecting against. The phrasing implies "eye and eyesight" problems. Current knowledge is more specific, this is essential for the elimination of eye and neck discomfort problems, probably with emphasis on the latter, caused by visual problems that may or may not be explicitly experienced. Thus, the phrasing in the text of "experience <u>visual</u> difficulties" is unfortunate, it would have been better to eliminate the word "visual". Alternatively, the phrasing could have been "experience difficulties or problems such as visual or musculoskeletal discomforts". Secondly, there are clearly other changes in the individual´s visual system which - regardless of VDU work or not - require health care attention. The distinction between these "normal" processes and those specific for VDU work situations should be made more clear - as a guidance to each nation´s balance between actions based on this VDU Directive and the nation´s normal health care system. Since eye discomforts are frequently not too specific, and there are - generally - a large number of possible contributing factors, it may not be possible to establish clear and reliable cause-effect relationships. This must be kept in mind when considering the phrasing "which may be due to display screen work".

- who should do the eye and eyesight test. This is obviously a decision where different countries may well take different approaches. Nevertheless, the sheer number of tests made necessary with this provision, makes this an extremely important question. Screening may be cost effective for identifying and eliminating from further consideration users who need no further action. Critera needs to be explicitly stated and should be both general and specific in order to take into account the characteristics of both the work situation and the operator.

- what are "regular" intervals. This may, on the other hand, be difficult to generalize across countries with rather different approaches to both occupational and national health care services. It should however be clear that such tests should preferably be incorporated into existing health care services. Since presbyope individuals with incorrect refraction constitute the major problem situation which these requirements are intended to eliminate, considerations for shorter intervals above the age of 40 may be relevant.

- what is the relevant work situation. This clearly calls for specific information for that worker´s situation, especially visual distances, to be available for the person evaluating the results of the test. Furthermore, problems caused by visual problems (manifested as visual, muscle and/or headache complaints) may be caused by changes in refraction - which motivates these tests - but the cause of the problem may also be elsewhere, e.g. glare. Thus, a reappraisal of e.g. the obligations in the Annex - under Article 3 - should also be called for.

- what is "special corrective appliances". We consider those to be such with a refraction different from that which the worker would use in his or her "normal" (non-work or non-VDU work) situation. What is not involved here are special "protective" glasses against "dangerous emissions" such as ultraviolet radiation etc.

Careful adherence to precise and correct formulation is essential for an adequate handling of these requirements. As indicated above, the formulation in the VDU Directive is not sufficiently precise for this - adding to the likelihood that different approaches to this will be taken by different Member States.

A 5. COMMENTS ON SECTION III, MISCELLANEOUS PROVISIONS

Articles 10 to 12 concern adaptations to the annex and instructions to the Member States (as already described above).

"Member States shall report to the Commission every fourth year on the practical implementation of the provisions of this Directive...". Depending on the system of evaluation, its comparability between countries etc, this may provide an excellent tool for further development of health protection of VDU workers.

A 6. COMMENTS ON THE ANNEX, MINIMUM REQUIREMENTS

The Annex is setting out obligations concerning the equipment (display screen, keyboard, work table or work surface, and work chair), the environment (space requirements, lighting, reflections and glare, noise, heat, radiation, and humidity) and the operator/computer interface. The phrasing of certain obligations are specific, while others are more general. Most specific requirements within the Annex do appear well motivated. Thus, our comments are mostly of a general nature.

There is an obvious need to link the requirements within this Annex to relevant standards. This would provide additional guidance for Member States when implementing the VDU Directive. Guidance is also needed for employers who are - in accordance with the preamble and Article 3 - responsible for keeping up with requirements and changes in them. The obligation of the employer under Article 3 is not limited to the evaluation of conditions specified in the Annex, but all conditions likely to result in increased risks. Managers therefore need to consult standards for more detailed guidance.

A problem already mentioned is the variation in details. The parts directed towards ergonomic situations are detailed and could thus give the impression that they are complete, something that is not the case. For example, the importance of the vertical position of the keyboard is not explicitly mentioned. Thus, there is a need for some general statements on the intentions within the ergonomic parts - such as emphasizing functional rather than product oriented specifications. This would bring it in parallell to the general statements on operator/computer interface, as has already been suggested. We would also stress the importance of flexibility. Work stations should also be designed in a way that permits the operator the maximum possibility of alternative display placement. Another example is that of "satisfactory lighting conditions and an appropriate contrast." These statements are insufficiently precise. A reference to an appropriate standard by e.g. the ISO/CEN would alleviate such imprecisions.

Likewise, the requirement that "adequate level of humidity shall be established and maintained" is problematic. This includes both the decision what is meant by "adequate", and the implementation, if "adequate" means, say, more than 20 or 30 per cent relative humidity. Again, a problematic omission is that no mention is made of temperature - which is linked to relative humidity, and which probably is at least as important for certain health concerns. No mention has been made of eye irritating airborne substances - such substances may also in VDU work situations be responsible for eye irritation. A clause as to the control of such substances could be made - with a phrasing similar to that of radiation (point "f").

The general statement on radiation is very unclear and is an obvious candidate for different interpretations. The phrasing "...shall be reduced to negligible levels from the point of view of the protection of workers' safety and health" - does it mean that levels shall be negligible, or that risks shall be negligible? By current international recommendations e.g. by the International Radiation Protection Association (IRPA), the levels of electric and magnetic fields due to VDUs are negligible - but is this the intended comparison?

Finally, the section on operator/computer interface is, as already stated, difficult to implement without further guidance. Here, the European Standard EN 29241 is under development. It has a number of parts which could be used. We do emphasize the importance of this part of the Annex. Software ergonomics is very important and has to be taken seriously by all concerned, especially software developers.

We would emphasize that monitoring is an issue relating to aspects of ethics, of stress and of work quality. The statement given in the Directive - "no quantitative or qualitative checking facility may be used without the knowledge of the workers (§3 b)" - implies that the ethical part has been considered. We would also like to point out that monitoring is also a health issue in that its impact on stress conditions are important. Furthermore, monitoring often emphasizes quantity of work and may thus overlook quality aspects - e.g. when the worker is dealing with customers. To summarize, we would emphasize that monitoring should be controlled by the employee, and be arranged in such a way that it gives a better feedback of the function of the system, thus enabling the creation of an improved mental model for the employee.

In §3 (c) of the Annex, the wording is that "systems must provide feedback to workers on their performance". This appear to be a requirement on monitoring of the operator, conflicting with the general intention of the §3 (b), where a reluctance to monitoring is implied. The original (French) version should have been translated as "systems must provide feedback to workers on its performance", i.e. the performance of the system, not the worker. As such, this is indeed an important factor in reducing potential stress situations, especially during customer contact.

COUNCIL DIRECTIVE

of 29 May 1990

on the minimum safety and health requirements for work with display screen equipment (fifth individual Directive within the meaning of Article 16 (1) of Directive 87/391/EEC)

(90/270/EEC)

THE COUNCIL OF THE EUROPEAN COMMUNITIES,

Having regard to the Treaty establishing the European Economic Community, and in particular Article 118a thereof,

Having regard to the Commission proposal (¹) drawn up after consultation with the Advisory Committee on Safety, Hygiene and Health Protection at Work,

In cooperation with the European Parliament (²)

Having regard to the opinion of the Economic and Social Committee (³),

Whereas Article 118a of the Treaty provides that the Council shall adopt, by means of Directives, minimum requirements designed to encourage improvements, especially in the working environment, to ensure a better level of protection of workers' safety and health;

Whereas, under the terms of that Article, those Directives shall avoid imposing administrative, financial and legal constraints, in a way which would hold back the creation and development of small and medium-sized undertakings;

Whereas the communication from the Commission on its programme concerning safety, hygiene and health at work (⁴) provides for the adoption of measures in respect of new technologies; whereas the Council has taken note thereof in its resolution of 21 December 1987 on safety, hygiene and health at work (⁵);

Whereas compliance with the minimum requirements for ensuring a better level of safety at workstations with display screens is essential for ensuring the safety and health of workers;

Whereas this Directive is an individual Directive within the meaning of Article 16 (1) of Council Directive 89/391/EEC of 12 June 1989 on the introduction of measures to encourage improvements in the safety and health of workers at work (⁶); whereas the provisions of the latter are therefore fully applicable to the use by workers of display screen equipment, without prejudice to more stringent and/or specific provisions contained in the present Directive;

Whereas employers are obliged to keep themselves informed of the latest advances in technology and scientific findings concerning workstation design so that they can make any changes necessary so as to be able to guarantee a better level of protection of workers' safety and health;

Whereas the ergonomic aspects are of particular importance for a workstation with display screen equipment;

Whereas this Directive is a practical contribution towards creating the social dimension of the internal market;

Whereas, pursuant to Decision 74/325/EEC (⁷), the Advisory Committee on Safety, Hygiene and Health Protection at Work shall be consulted by the Commission on the drawing-up of proposals in this field,

HAS ADOPTED THIS DIRECTIVE:

SECTION I

GENERAL PROVISIONS

Article 1

Subject

1. This Directive, which is the fifth individual Directive within the meaning of Article 16 (1) of Directive 89/391/EEC, lays down minimum safety and health requirements for work with display screen equipment as defined in Article 2.

2. The provisions of Directive 89/391/EEC are fully applicable to the whole field referred to in paragraph 1, without prejudice to more stringent and/or specific provisions contained in the present Directive.

(¹) OJ No C 113, 29. 4. 1988, p. 7 and OJ No C 130, 26. 5. 1989, p. 5.
(²) OJ No C 12, 16. 1. 1989, p. 92 and OJ No C 113, 7. 5. 1990.
(³) OJ No C 318, 12. 12. 1988, p. 32.
(⁴) OJ No C 28, 3. 2. 1988, p. 3.
(⁵) OJ No C 28, 3. 2. 1988, p. 1.

(⁶) OJ No L 183, 29. 6. 1989, p. 1.
(⁷) OJ No L 185, 9. 7. 1974, p. 15.

3. This Directive shall not apply to:

(a) drivers' cabs or control cabs for vehicles or machinery;

(b) computer systems on board a means of transport;

(c) computer systems mainly intended for public use;

(d) 'portable' systems not in prolonged use at a workstation;

(e) calculators, cash registers and any equipment having a small data or measurement display required for direct use of the equipment;

(f) typewriters of traditional design, of the type known as 'typewriter with window'.

Article 2

Definitions

For the purpose of this Directive, the following terms shall have the following meanings:

(a) *display screen equipment:* an alphanumeric or graphic display screen, regardless of the display process employed;

(b) *workstation:* an assembly comprising display screen equipment, which may be provided with a keyboard or input device and/or software determining the operator/machine interface, optional accessories, peripherals including the diskette drive, telephone, modem, printer, document holder, work chair and work desk or work surface, and the immediate work environment;

(c) *worker:* any worker as defined in Article 3 (a) of Directive 89/391/EEC who habitually uses display screen equipment as a significant part of his normal work.

SECTION II

EMPLOYERS' OBLIGATIONS

Article 3

Analysis of workstations

1. Employers shall be obliged to perform an analysis of workstations in order to evaluate the safety and health conditions to which they give rise for their workers, particularly as regards possible risks to eyesight, physical problems and problems of mental stress.

2. Emyployers shall take appropriate measures to remedy the risks found, on the basis of the evaluation referred to in paragraph 1, taking account of the additional and/or combined effects of the risks so found.

Article 4

Workstations put into service for the first time

Employers must take the appropriate steps to ensure that workstations first put into service after 31 December 1992 meet the minimum requirements laid down in the Annex.

Article 5

Workstations already put into service

Employers must take the appropriate steps to ensure that workstations already put into service on or before 31 December 1992 are adapted to comply with the minimum requirements laid down in the Annex not later than four years after that date.

Article 6

Information for, and training of, workers

1. Without prejudice to Article 10 of Directive 89/391/EEC, workers shall receive information on all aspects of safety and health relating to their workstation, in particular information on such measures applicable to workstations as are implemented under Articles 3, 7 and 9.

In all cases, workers or their representatives shall be informed of any health and safety measure taken in compliance with this Directive.

2. Without prejudice to Article 12 of Directive 89/391/EEC, every worker shall also receive training in use of the workstation before commencing this type of work and whenever the organization of the workstation is substantially modified.

Article 7

Daily work routine

The employer must plan the worker's activities in such a way that daily work on a display screen is periodically interrupted by breaks or changes of activity reducing the workload at the display screen.

Article 8

Worker consultation and participation

Consultation and participation of workers and/or their representatives shall take place in accordance with Article 11 of Directive 89/391/EEC on the matters covered by this Directive, including its Annex.

Article 9

Protection of workers' eyes and eyesight

1. Workers shall be entitled to an appropriate eye and eyesight test carried out by a person with the necessary capabilities:

— before commencing display screen work,

— at regular intervals thereafter, and

— if they experience visual difficulties which may be due to display screen work.

2. Workers shall be entitled to an ophthalmological examination if the results of the test referred to in paragraph 1 show that this is necessary.

3. If the results of the test referred to in paragraph 1 or of the examination referred to in paragraph 2 show that it is necessary and if normal corrective appliances cannot be used, workers must be provided with special corrective appliances appropriate for the work concerned.

4. Measures taken pursuant to this Article may in no circumstances involve workes in additional financial cost.

5. Protection of workers' eyes and eyesight may be provided as part of a national health system.

SECTION III

MISCELLANEOUS PROVISIONS

Article 10

Adaptations to the Annex

The strictly technical adaptations to the Annex to take account of technical progress, developments in international regulations and specifications and knowledge in the field of display screen equipment shall be adopted in accordance with the procedure laid down in Article 17 of Directive 89/391/EEC.

Article 11

Final provisions

1. Member States shall bring into force the laws, regulations and administrative provisions necessary to comply with this Directive by 31 December 1992.

They shall forthwith inform the Commission thereof.

2. Member States shall communicate to the Commission the texts of the provisions of national law which they adopt, or have already adopted, in the field covered by this Directive.

3. Member States shall report to the Commission every four years on the practical implementation of the provisions of this Directive, indicating the points of view of employers and workers.

The Commission shall inform the European Parliament, the Council, the Economic and Social Committee and the Advisory Committee on Safety, Hygiene and Health Protection at Work.

4. The Commission shall submit a report on the implementation of this Directive at regular intervals to the European Parliament, the Council and the Economic and Social Committee, taking into account paragraphs 1, 2 and 3.

Article 12

This Directive is addressed to the Member States.

Done at Brussels, 29 May 1990.

For the Council
The President
B. AHERN

Annex

MINIMUM REQUIREMENTS

(Articles 4 and 5)

Preliminary remark

The obligations laid down in this Annex shall apply in order to achieve the objectives of this Directive and to the extent that, firstly, the components concerned are present at the workstation, and secondly, the inherent requirements or characteristics of the task do not preclude it.

1. EQUIPMENT

   (a) General comment

   The use as such of the equipment must not be a source of risk for workers.

   (b) Display screen

   The characters on the screen shall be well-defined and clearly formed, of adequate size and with adequate spacing between the characters and lines.

   The image on the screen should be stable, with no flickering or other forms of instability.

   The brightness and/or the contrast between the characters and the background shall be easily adjustable by the operator, and also be easily adjustable to ambient conditions.

   The screen must swivel and tilt easily and freely to suit the needs of the operator.

   It shall be possible to use a separate base for the screen or an adjustable table.

   The screen shall be free of reflective glare and reflections liable to cause discomfort to the user.

   (c) Keyboard

   The keyboard shall be tiltable and separate from the screen so as to allow the worker to find a comfortable working position avoiding fatigue in the arms or hands.

   The space in front of the keyboard shall be sufficient to provide support for the hands and arms of the operator.

   The keyboard shall have a matt surface to avoid reflective glare.

   The arrangement of the keyboard and the characteristics of the keys shall be such as to facilitate the use of the keyboard.

   The symbols on the keys shall be adequately contrasted and legible from the design working position.

   (d) Work desk or work surface

   The work desk or work surface shall have a sufficiently large, low-reflectance surface and allow a flexible arrangement of the screen, keyboard, documents and related equipment.

   The document holder shall be stable and adjustable and shall be positioned so as to minimize the need for uncomfortable head and eye movements.

   There shall be adequate space for workers to find a comfortable position.

   (e) Work chair

   The work chair shall be stable and allow the operator easy freedom of movement and a comfortable position.

   The seat shall be adjustable in height.

   The seat back shall be adjustable in both height and tilt.

   A footrest shall be made available to any one who wishes for one.

2. ENVIRONMENT

   (a) Space requirements

   The workstation shall be dimensioned and designed so as to provide sufficient space for the user to change position and vary movements.

   (b) Lighting

   Room lighting and/or spot lighting (work lamps) shall ensure satisfactory lighting conditions and an appropriate contrast between the screen and the background environment, taking into account the type of work and the user's vision requirements.

   Possible disturbing glare and reflections on the screen or other equipment shall be prevented by coordinating workplace and workstation layout with the positioning and technical characteristics of the artificial light sources.

   (c) Reflections and glare

   Workstations shall be so designed that sources of light, such as windows and other openings, transparent or translucid walls, and brightly coloured fixtures or walls cause no direct glare and **no distracting** * reflections on the screen.

   Windows shall be fitted with a suitable system of adjustable covering to attenuate the daylight that falls on the workstation.

   (d) Noise

   Noise emitted by equipment belonging to workstation(s) shall be taken into account when a workstation is being equipped, in particular so as not to distract attention or disturb speech.

   (e) Heat

   Equipment belonging to workstation(s) shall not produce excess heat which could cause discomfort to workers.

   (f) Radiation

   All radiation with the exception of the visible part of the electromagnetic spectrum shall be reduced to negligible levels from the point of view of the protection of workers' safety and health.

   (g) Humidity

   An adequate level of humidity shall be established and maintained.

3. OPERATOR/COMPUTER INTERFACE

   In designing, selecting, commissioning and modifying software, and in designing tasks using display screen equipment, the employer shall take into account the following principles:

   (a) software must be suitable for the task;

   (b) software must be easy to use and, where appropriate, adaptable to the operator's level of knowledge or experience; no quantitative or qualitative checking facility may be used without the knowledge of the workers;

   (c) systems must provide feedback to workers on their performance;

   (d) systems must display information in a format and at a pace which are adapted to operators;

   (e) the principles of software ergonomics must be applied, in particular to human data processing.

---

* Correction indicated here taken from Official Journal, L 171/30.

AUTHOR INDEX

Abe, S. 95
Åborg, C. 63
Akiya, S. 119
Alessio, L. 89
Alfano, G. 323
Almgren, S. 351
Andersson, B. 335
Ankrum, D.R. 131
Apostoli, P. 89
Armstrong, T.J. 375
Arnetz, B. 335
Assini, R. 369
Asterland, P. 167

Bachinger, S. 459
Bagolini, B. 161
Bailey, I.L. 77, 107
Balogh, I. 167
Baumgartner, A. 259
Bellucci, R. 161
Berg, M. 335
Bergqvist, U. 83, 345, 363, 491
Bernazzani, G. 299
Berny, P. 265
Besuijen, J. 311
Bettendorf, R.F. 439
Biemans, P. 455
Blomkvist, A.C. 351
Bocchi, G. 299
Boles Carenini, B. 161
Borra, S. 161
Boucsein, W. 233
Bracci, C. 203
Braun, D.B. 143
Breysse, P. 173
Bruno, N. 187
Byström, J. 167

Çakir, A.E. 283
Camerino, D. 67
Capobianco, A. 113
Carayon, P. 39, 57
Ceccarelli, C. 161
Chereisky, M. 427

Coccia, G. 161
Colombini, D. . . . 73, 149, 155, 299
Compagno, L. 387
Crosignani, P.G. 33

d'Ambrosio, F.R. 323
Danckwardt, C. 143
de Lange, M. 259
De Angeli, A. 187
De Marco, F. . . . 73, 149, 155, 299
Den Buurman, R. 271
Di Bari, A. 161
Donagi, A. 427
Durndell, A. 51
Dürr, J. 143

Ericson, M.O. 63
Eriksson, N. 357

Faßbender, K. 143
Fasolino, G. 113
Fernström, E. 63
Ferrario, M. 67
Ferretti, G. 67, 73
Focosi, F. 113
Fostervold, K.I. 137
Franzblau, A. 375
Fraschini, F. 369
Fregoso, M. 73, 393
Frontali, C. 89

Gale, A.G. 101
Galletta, G. 73, 393
Garetti, R. 209
Georgi, M. 143
Gerbino, W. 187
Göbel, M. 409
Graf, M. 293
Granda, R.E. 465
Grieco, A. 1
Grießer, K. 253
Grignolo, F.M. 161

Hackl-Gruber, W. 459

Hagberg, M. 381
Hagen, R.H. 455
Hansen, E.E. 131
Hansson, G.-A. 167
Hendrick, H.W. 479
Hirose, N. 119
Hjelmquist, E. 403
Höög, J. 357
Horberry, T.J. 101

Ibi, K. 119
Iwasaki, T. 119

Jansson, B. 403
Jaschins Kruza, W. 125
Jenny, A. 259
Johansson, A. 21
Johnson, P.W. 375

Karwowski, W. 473
Kellermann, M. 167
Knave, B. 9, 83, 363
Kohlisch, O. 241
Koizumi, N. 449
Kraus-Mackiw, E. 143
Kroemer, K.H.E. 277
Krueger, H. 293

Langlet, I. 335
Lavano, P. 67
Le Leu, L.A. 191
Leino, T. 45
Lepore, D. 161
Lidén, S. 335
Lie, I. 137
Lightbody, P. 51
Lim, S.Y. 57
Linder, G. 363
Lindström, K. 45
Locarno, C.M. 113
Lordong, G. 265
Lucchini, R. 89
Luchini, L. 33
Luczak, H. 409

Maina, G. 161

Malcangi, A. 73
Manganelli, C. 113
Martin, B.J. 375
Masseroni, L. 393
Masuyama, E. 329
Mayer, H. 143
Medhage, Ö. 363
Melin, L. 335
Meroni, M. 149, 155
Miglior, M. 161
Milanesi, L. 183
Miyamoto, H. 289, 485
Molle, F. 161
Molnar, M. 459
Molteni, G. 67
Monaco, E. 161
Morbio, R. 161

Nemeth, K.J. 131
Newsham, G.R. 305
Noro, K. 289
Novara, F. 215

O'Neill, M.J. 433
Occhipinti, E. . . . 73, 149, 155, 299
Ohlsson, K. 167
Okubo, T. 227
Orsini, S. 183

Parazzini, F. 33
Pasini, I.C. 305
Pearce, B. 15
Pedotti, A. 397
Petri, A. 149, 155, 299
Piccoli, B. 179, 369, 491
Pribil, A. 459
Puhakainen, M. 45

Rauterberg, M. 221, 259, 265
Rechichi, C. 161
Reiterer, H. 247
Rempel, D.M. 375
Ricci, B. 161
Robertson, M.M. 433
Rubino, G.F. 161

Saito, Shin 95
Saito, Sujumo. 95, 119
Sandström, M. 357
Sang Park K. 227
Sawdon, D. 339
Schaefer, F. 241
Schäfer, S. 247
Schmidt, A. 265
Schmidt, H. 421
Scullica, L. 161
Shahnavaz, H. 21
Sheedy, J.E. 77, 107
Sibour, G. 161
Smith, M.J. 197
Soccio, A. 149, 155, 299
Sotoyama, M. 95
Spenkelink, G.P.J. 311
Springer, J. 409
Stanners, S.L. 465
Stenberg, B. 27, 357
Stewart, T.F.M. 415, 445, 491
Styger, E. 259
Suzuki, T. 119
Sweitzer, G. 317

Taptagaporn, S. 95
Taylor, M. 203
Taylor, S.P. 101
Thum, M. 233
Tiller, D.K. 305
Torstila, I. 45
Tosatto, E. 149, 155, 299
Troiano, P. 161
Turbati, M. 161

Villanueva, M.B.G. 95
Vimercati, C. 149, 155
Voskamp, P. 455

Wadman, C. 363
Wahl, J. 143
Wibom, R. 83
Wideback, P.G. 491
Widebäck, G. 9
Winkel, J. 167
Wu, C.-S. 289

Zemp, M. 265
Zülch, G. 253
Zürcher, T 265